UNDERSERVED AND SOCIALLY DISADVANTAGED GROUPS AND LINKAGES WITH HEALTH AND HEALTH CARE DIFFERENTIALS

RESEARCH IN THE SOCIOLOGY OF HEALTH CARE

Series Editor: Jennie Jacobs Kronenfeld

Recently Volumes:

Volume 24: Access, Quality and Satisfaction with Care: Concerns Of Patients, Providers and Insurers, 2007

Volume 25: Inequalities and Disparities in Health Care and Health: Concerns Of Patients, Providers and Insurers, 2007

Volume 26: Care for Major Health Problems and Population Health Concerns: Impacts on Patients, Providers, and Policy, 2008

Volume 27: Social Sources of Disparities in Health and Health Care and Linkages to Policy, Population Concerns and Providers of Care, 2009

Volume 28: The Impact of Demographics on Health and Healthcare: Race, Ethnicity, and Other Social Factors, 2010

Volume 29: Access to Care and Factors that Impact Access, Patients as Partners in Care and Changing Roles of Health Providers, 2011

Volume 30: Issues in Health and Health Care Related to Race/Ethnicity, Immigration, SES and Gender, 2012

Volume 31: Social Determinants, Health Disparities and Linkages to Health and Health Care, 2013

Volume 32: Technology, Communication, Disparities and Government Options in Health and Health Care Services, 2014

Volume 33: Education, Social Factors, and Health Beliefs in Health and Health Care Services, 2015

Volume 34: Special Social Groups, Social Factors and Disparities in Health and Health Care, 2016

Volume 35: Health and Health Care Concerns among Women and Racial and Ethnic Minorities, 2017

Volume 36: Gender, Women's Health Care Concerns and Other Social Factors in Health and Health Care, 2018

RESEARCH IN THE SOCIOLOGY OF HEALTH CARE
VOLUME 37

UNDERSERVED AND SOCIALLY DISADVANTAGED GROUPS AND LINKAGES WITH HEALTH AND HEALTH CARE DIFFERENTIALS

EDITED BY

JENNIE JACOBS KRONENFELD
Arizona State University, USA

United Kingdom – North America – Japan
India – Malaysia – China

Emerald Publishing Limited
Howard House, Wagon Lane, Bingley BD16 1WA, UK

First edition 2019

British Library Cataloguing in Publication Data
A catalogue record for this book is available from the British Library

ISBN: 978-1-83867-055-9 (Print)
ISBN: 978-1-83867-054-2 (Online)
ISBN: 978-1-83867-056-6 (Epub)

ISSN: 0275-4959 (Series)

Printed and bound by CPI Group (UK) Ltd, Croydon, CR0 4YY

ISOQAR
REGISTERED
ISOQAR certified Management System, awarded to Emerald for adherence to Environmental standard ISO 14001:2004.

Certificate Number 1985
ISO 14001

INVESTOR IN PEOPLE

CONTENTS

LIST OF FIGURES

LIST OF TABLES

Chapter 4

Chapter 5

Chapter 6

Chapter 8

Chapter 10

Chapter 11

Chapter 12

ABOUT THE CONTRIBUTORS

Zinobia C. Bennefield is an Assistant Professor of Sociology at the University of North Carolina, Charlotte. Her research interests include childhood and adolescent mental health, structural inequality and health, and the application of intersectionality theory in health research.

Jennifer M. Brailsford is an Instructor in the Care, Health, and Society program at The University of Arizona. As a medical sociologist, her research focuses on the impacts of social and physical environments on human health. Her research interests include neighborhood contexts, environmental hazards, and the stress process.

Amy M. Burdette is Professor of Sociology and an associate in the Pepper Institute on Aging and Public Policy at Florida State University. Amy M. Burdette is Professor of Sociology and an associate in the Pepper Institute on Aging and Public Policy at Florida State University. Amy M. Burdette's research investigates connections between religious involvement, neighborhood context, and health. Her research has examined social variations in health and health behaviors at virtually every stage of the life course from birth (e.g., low-birth weight), to adolescence (e.g., HPV vaccination, substance use), to young adulthood (e.g., BMI, sexual activity), to adulthood (e.g., breastfeeding, obesity, psychological distress, prescription drug misuse), and old age (e.g., cognitive functioning, mobility). Much of her research has paid special attention to disadvantaged populations, including low-income urban mothers.

Claudia Chaufan is Associate Professor of Health Policy and Global Health at York University in Toronto. She practiced medicine in her native Argentina, before shifting to an academic career. Her background spans medicine, sociology, comparative political economy, and philosophy. Her research and intellectual interests include the politics of health and global health in the context of capitalist globalization, medicalization and social control, language/power/discourse, and the scholarship of teaching and learning. She teaches about, and has published on, these topics in *Social Science & Medicine*, the *International Journal of Health Services*, and *Critical Public Health*. She is Editorial Board Member and Reviewer of academic journals, and a long-time supporter of organizations opposing Western intervention in the Global South.

Jessica Eckhardt is Assistant Professor of Sociology and Social Justice at Northland College, an environmental liberal arts school on the south shore of Lake Superior. As an environmental health sociologist, she uses frameworks and methodologies from medical sociology, environmental justice, social epidemiology, and public health to explore differential exposures to environmental hazards and how those hazards impact human health.

Terrence D. Hill is Associate Professor in the School of Sociology and a Scientific Member of the Arizona Center on Aging at the University of Arizona. His research examines the social distribution of health and health-relevant behaviors. To date, he has published over 100 peer-reviewed journal articles and book chapters. According to Google Scholar, his published work has been cited across a range of disciplines nearly 4,000 times.

Charley Henderson received MA in Sociology from Texas State University in 2018. She has been working on several research projects with Atsuko Kawakami, PhD, at Tarleton State University since 2015. While conducting research with Dr Kawakami, Ms Henderson completed her MA and published an article, "Hepatitis C and the Social Hierarchy: How Stigma Is Built in Rural Communities," as her research interests include medical sociology, rural sociology, stigma, and viral infections.

Andrew K. Jorgenson is Professor and Chair in the Department of Sociology and Professor of Environmental Studies at Boston College. The primary area of his research is the human dimensions of global environmental change, with a focus on the drivers of greenhouse gas emissions, energy consumption, industrial pollution, and land cover change. He also conducts research on the political-economic and environmental conditions that shape population health outcomes, uneven development, income inequality, and environmental concern.

Karen E. Joseph-Kent is an Assistant Professor at DeSales University and is Director of the MBA program. She has taught health services administration for over 20 years at Xavier University and Penn State and has an extensive background in health administration leadership as an Administrator for Johns Hopkins Medicine. She received her PhD from Miami University of Ohio in Social Gerontology. She dedicates this study to Ian Kent and the myriad of caring professionals who improve the lives of people with ASD.

Atsuko Kawakami is Associate Professor of Sociology at Tarleton State University. She received PhD in sociology from Arizona State University and MA in sociology from Doshisha University, Kyoto, Japan. Her research interests include, but are not limited to, the following areas: support systems among various groups, living arrangement and health service utilization among the elderly population, and transnational identity of immigrants.

Jennie Jacobs Kronenfeld is Professor Emerita in the Sociology Program, Sanford School of Social/Family Dynamics, Arizona State University. Her research areas are medical sociology and aging with special focus on health policy, health care utilization, and health behavior. She is Coeditor of *Health* and Associate Editor-In-Chief for *American Journal of Health Promotion*. She is a past Chair of Medical Sociology Section, American Sociological Association and past President of Sociologists for Women in Society.

Jennifer McDonald's research interests include women's health and international health policy. She has presented research at the American Sociological Association Conference, has spoken at the Canadian Coalition for Global Health Research University Conference, and has been a delegate at the World Health Assembly. Jennifer enjoys traveling and plans to attend medical school in the next two years.

Kristine M. Molina, PhD, is Associate Professor of Psychology at the University of California-Irvine. She earned a joint PhD in Psychology (Personality & Social Contexts) and Women's Studies from the University of Michigan. Her research focuses on how different dimensions of inequality, often resulting from racism, become embodied at multiple levels to affect health across the life course among racialized groups.

Ethel Nicdao, PhD, is Professor and Chair of Sociology at California State University, San Bernardino. Trained as a medical sociologist, her work centers on health disparities among minority populations. Her current research applies a community-based participatory research and intersectionality approach to examine the mental health and well-being of adults in San Joaquin and San Bernardino counties. She completed her doctoral training at the University of New Mexico and postdoctoral fellowship at the University of Washington.

Ignatius Uche Nwankwo, PhD, is Associate Professor of Medical Sociology at the Department of Sociology/Anthropology, Nnamdi Azikiwe University, Awka, Anambra State, Nigeria. He has taught sociology for more than a decade and served as Head of Department from 2012 to 2014. Currently, he is the Sub-Dean for Postgraduate Studies in the Faculty of Social Sciences. His research interests cut across health policy and finance, gender and health, sociocultural determinants of health services access, evaluation of health programs and the administration of public health law, etc.

Kim Price-Glynn, PhD, is Associate Professor of Sociology at the University of Connecticut. She was the inaugural recipient of the University of Connecticut College of Liberal Arts and Sciences Faculty Achievement Award for Excellence in Teaching. Her research examines gender, labor, health and caregiving in diverse organizational settings, from nursing homes to strip clubs. She is the author of *Strip Club: Gender, Power and Sex Work*, New York University Press (2010). She has also published in *Gender & Society; Sociology of Health & Illness; Research in the Sociology of Health Care;* and *Work, Employment & Society*, as well as other journals and the edited volume, *Caring on the Clock*.

Valentina Raffa, PhD, is a Researcher of Sociology in the Department of Cognitive Science, Educational and Cultural Studies (CSECS), University of Messina. Her research focuses on social exclusion, social marginality, social movements, new political identities, postcolonial studies, urban art, sociology of development, and sociology of health. She worked on several national and international projects.

Carter Rakovski, PhD, is Professor of Sociology at California State University Fullerton. She studies gender and work. She also applies statistical methods in her interdisciplinary work. Her research has been published in a range of journals including the *Sociology of Health and Illness*, *Work, Employment and Society*, *Disability and Rehabilitation*, and the *Journal of Accounting Research*.

Fernando I. Rivera is Professor of Sociology and Director of the Puerto Rico Research Hub at the University of Central Florida. His research interests and activities are in the sociology of health/medical sociology, disasters, and race and ethnicity. He earned his MA and PhD in Sociology from the University of Nebraska-Lincoln. He also completed a postdoctoral fellowship at Rutgers University.

Anne Scheer is Assistant Professor at the Department of Population Science and Policy at Southern Illinois University School of Medicine. She holds a master's degree in Anthropology and a PhD in Sociology – both from Freie Universität Berlin, Germany. Her research interests include obesity and nutritional health in rural communities, school discipline in US public education, and the ways in which childhood trauma/toxic stress relate to children's health and their experiences with school discipline. As a qualitative childhood sociologist, she has conducted extensive research with elementary school-aged children, using participant observation and interviews, including research about punitive disciplinary policies in a large Midwestern school district, and her current study about rural children's perspectives on health, well-being, and nutrition.

Juyeon Son is Associate Professor in Sociology at University of Wisconsin Oshkosh. She received her MA in Women's Studies from Rutgers University in 1998 and her PhD in Sociology from the University of Oregon in 2007. Dr Son is a medical sociologist and has published articles that examine issues such as health service utilization and immigrant incorporation, postpartum care, health disparities, transnationalism, and technology. Her current research is on end-of-life and palliative care.

Jessica Valles is a Doctoral Student in the Department of Sociology, and a Research Fellow for the Office of Diversity, Equity and Inclusion at the University of Alabama at Birmingham. She received her MA in Sociology from the University of North Florida in 2014. Her research focuses on mental health for immigrant and aging populations, as well as racial and ethnic disparities in caregiving and familial support.

Francesca Alice Vianello, PhD, is Lecturer in Sociology of Work at the University of Padua (Italy). Her main areas of research are migration, gender, and labor. She leads the research project "Migration and Occupational Health: Understanding the Risks for Eastern European Migrant Women" funded by the University of Padua under the STARS Grants program. She is one of the regional representatives for Europe of the RC 32 "Women in Society" of the International Sociological Association.

PART I
INTRODUCTION TO VOLUME

UNDERSERVED AND SOCIALLY DISADVANTAGED GROUPS AND LINKAGES WITH HEALTH AND HEALTH CARE DIFFERENTIALS

Jennie Jacobs Kronenfeld

ABSTRACT

Purpose – *This chapter provides an introduction to the volume along with a very brief review of literature on underserved and socially disadvantaged groups and health and health care differentials.*

Methodology/Approach – *This chapter uses the approach of a literature review.*

Findings – *The chapter argues for the importance of greater examination of underserved and socially disadvantaged groups in consideration of health and health care differentials.*

Originality/Value of Paper – *The author reviews the issues of underserved and socially disadvantaged groups in consideration of health and health care differentials and previews this book.*

Keywords: Income; education; underserved; socially disadvantaged; health care differentials; health differentials

This chapter provides an introduction to Volume 37 in the *Research in the Sociology of Health Care* series, "Underserved and Socially Disadvantaged Groups and Linkages with Health and Health Care Differentials." The beginning of this chapter will briefly review some of the more important material

Underserved and Socially Disadvantaged Groups and Linkages with Health and Health Care Differentials
Research in the Sociology of Health Care, Volume 37, 3–11

ISSN: 0275-4959/doi:10.1108/S0275-495920190000037002

about underserved and socially disadvantaged groups in consideration of health and health care differentials. The second part of this chapter will review the overall contents of the volume and the structure of the volume.

UNDERSERVED AND SOCIALLY DISADVANTAGED GROUPS AND OTHER SOCIAL FACTORS AS LINKED TO HEALTH DISPARITIES AND HEALTH CARE DISPARITIES

When one uses the terms underserved and socially disadvantaged groups, it could mean many different things. In this volume, it mostly means people of color including Asian Americans and Latinx Americans, as well as rural Americans, and aging populations. In addition, it means issues related to women and gender both as recipients of care and providers of care. Also, a few chapters look at issues of underserved groups outside of the American context. In addition, many of the chapters relate to a variety of other social factors, including but not limited to components of socioeconomic status (SES) such as income, education and occupation, demographic social factors such as age and gender and factors linked to the family such as marriage or divorce and factors linked to employment such as job stress or unemployment. The literatures covering these different groups and factors are huge, and the literature on health inequalities and health care inequalities is also quite large. This chapter will not cover any of this in a comprehensive manner but will focus in a brief section on what we mean by health and health care inequalities. There is also a brief section on the linkage of a few major social factors such as income, education and race and ethnicity with health and health care inequalities.

HEALTH INEQUALITIES, HEALTH CARE INEQUALITIES, AND HEALTH DISPARITIES

One area of growing interest within medical sociology in the past 20 years has been research in health disparities and this is also true within public health and medicine as well as medical sociology more specifically. The interest in health care disparities has expanded beyond researchers to also become an area of high interest to providers of care and policymakers, especially within the United States. The definition of health disparities or differences in health care is important to review. The Institute of Medicine (IOM) defines health care disparities as differences in treatment or access between population groups that cannot be justified by different preferences for services or differences in health (McGuire, Alegria, Cook, Wells, & Zaslavsky, 2006). Within the United States, much of the focus on health care disparities has turned to differences in access and quality across racial and ethnic groups, although these are not the only social characteristics that are of interest either sociologically or from a policy perspective. Differences based on SES and its components including education and income are of both research and policy interest. Beyond research and thinking about policy implications, health care disparities matter even more if they result in health disparities, defined as differences in health outcomes across population groups (Schnittker & McLeod, 2005).

One interesting study that demonstrates the growth in research about social differences in health and health disparities was summarized well by the Adler and Rehkopf (2008) review of US disparities in health by examining literature for the term "health disparities" and finding that while this was a key word in only one article in 1980, and fewer than 30 in the 1990s, it went up to over 400 articles from 2000 to 2004. If the term "health inequalities" was used instead, the pattern of increase was similar.

The United States is not the only country with growing interest in this topic. Great Britain and more recently some European countries also have interest in the topic. Interest in the topic in Great Britain goes back to 1980, when the Black Report was one of the first in that country to apply the term inequality to an examination of health differences. In the United States in this same time period, studies did link together death and health information with information on SES from sources such as the Current Population Study, the US Census, and Social Security Administration records (Kitagawa & Hauser, 1978; Kliss & Scheuren, 1978).Within the US, some of these earlier studies and traditions in various fields including sociology of research into variation in health, health care utilization and health services issues by SES and race/ethnicity led to the now well-known efforts in the United States to examine and try to eliminate health disparities due to race/ethnicity and SES in the *Healthy People* series. From the federal government level, one of the pushes for more research on health care inequalities came from the passage of Public Law 106–129, the Health Care Research and Quality Act of 1999. A first National Health Care Disparities Report came out in 2005 and built on previous efforts in the federal government, especially Healthy People 2010 (U.S. Department of Health & Human Services, 2000) and the IOM Report, Unequal Treatment: Confronting Racial and Economic Disparities in Health Care (Smedley, Stith, & Nelson, 2003). Elimination of disparities in health was a goal of Healthy People, 2010. Unequal Treatment extensively documented health care disparities in the United States and focused on those related to race and ethnicity, but not on SES, a weakness of the report. The IOM report on Unequal Treatment also looked at factors related to providers of care and argued that providers' perceptions and, from that, their attitudes toward patients can be influenced by patient race or ethnicity (Smedley et al., 2003).

Federal government focus on these efforts has continued, and much of it is discussed in the Healthy People 2020 publications, much of which is now easily obtainable through United States government websites including access to data from the 2020 objectives (U.S. Department of Health & Human Services, 2019). For the 2020 effort, the report points out that in Healthy People 2000, the goal was to reduce health disparities among Americans, and in Healthy People 2010 the goal was to eliminate, not just reduce, health disparities. By Healthy People 2020, that goal was expanded even further: to achieve health equity, eliminate disparities, and improve the health of all groups. Healthy People 2020 defines health equity as attaining the highest level of health for all people. In addition, the Centers for Disease Control and Prevention (CDC) is another US federal agency that works on issues of health differences and health disparities in addition to many other concerns about diseases. In a special report they issued in 2011, the agency consolidated the most recent national data available on disparities in mortality, morbidity, behavioral risk factors, health care access, preventive health services, and social determinants of critical health problems in the United States by using selected indicators (Truman et al., 2011).

One of the newest federal government-related efforts to focus on health equity is an effort by the Centers for Medicare & Medicaid Services (CMS). They have collaborated with a wide variety of stakeholders to support work in all three areas of their path to equity: increasing the understanding and awareness of disparities and their causes, developing and disseminating solutions, and implementing sustainable actions. To increase understanding and awareness of disparities, CMS sponsored a special issue of Health Services Research (James, 2019) with a goal of contributing to the conversation on health disparities and emphasizing the value of continuing research in this area (Caro, 2019). This is an important new publication to consult related to these concerns.

Beyond the role of the federal government, private foundations such as the Commonwealth Foundation have programs that focus on health differences and health disparities (Commonwealth Fund, 2015). The goals of the Commonwealth Fund's Program on Health Care Disparities are to improve the overall quality of health care delivered to low-income and minority Americans, and to eliminate racial and ethnic health disparities. In addition to issues of health differences and health disparities as many of these reports have examined, another issue related to health disparities has to do with dissatisfaction with the health care system. Recent research that compares the United States with other countries reports that Americans often report low levels of satisfaction and it does not appear to be correlated with per capita health expenditures as it is in many other countries (Hero, Blendon, Zaslavzk, & Campbell, 2016). There is also variation in satisfaction by factors such as income, with greater income associated with greater satisfaction.

UNDERSERVED AND SOCIALLY DISADVANTAGED GROUPS

Many social factors are important in health and health care inequalities. Among the most important factors are aspects of SES such as education, income, and occupation, because these factors often create and shape patterns of disease, patterns of health care utilization, and patterns of inequalities. People who have greater advantages in SES live longer than those without such advantages (Kunst, Feikhe, Mackenbach, & the EU Working Group on Socioeconomic Inequalities in Health, 1998). This is true at the beginning of life in terms of differences in infant mortality as well as across the lifespan (Gortmaker & Wise, 1997). It has also been true across time and is true in many different countries, not just the United States.

More recent research in medical sociology has especially focused on some broader approaches to SES and other social factors, an approach now known as the fundamental cause approach (Link & Phelan, 1995; Link & Phelan, 1996). This is a sociologically based explanation for persistent associations between SES and disease. The argument is that the reason SES is so consistently associated with disease is that resources such as knowledge, money, power, and prestige, all factors embodied in the SES concept, can be used in many different ways and in many different situations to avoid risks for diseases and even death. More socioeconomically advantaged people can better avoid risks and also take up protective strategies to improve health and well-being and can modify these over time to take advantage of new knowledge and approaches in the medical arena. This makes the relationship a dynamic one. If new risk factors emerge, for example, such as lack of exercise or changes in nutritional information, those with the most resources are better able to avoid risks and take advantage of protective factors. The same is true for knowledge about new treatments; the most advantaged people not only often have better health insurance that allows people to use the treatments, but are more likely to learn about the treatments, seek out health providers who familiar with such treatments and be able to pay for the treatment with their own resources if the new treatments are not yet covered by standard health insurance.

Turning away from more theoretical discussions to actual data, the United States government reports have recently been working on ways to create some simpler indicators of such factors as health-related quality of life. They have developed the HALex score which provides one individual-level measure of health-related quality of life (HRQL) that can be used to monitor health status as well as examine inequalities in morbidity across time and groups (Truman et al., 2011). This measure provides a numerical based measure that combines information on self-rated health and activity limitation as reported in nationally representative surveys. The scores on HALex can theoretically range from 1.00 for persons who have no activity limitation and are in excellent health to 0.10 for persons who are limited in activities of daily living (ADL) and are in poor health. For example, a person in excellent health with ADL disabilities is considered as healthy, with an assigned HALex score of 0.47, as is a person in poor health with no disabilities. The average HALex and inequality for HALex among US adults for 1997–2007 is estimated to show a declining trend from 0.8766 in 1997 to 0.8662 in 2007. During the same period, health inequality among individual persons, as measured by the Gini index for HALex, fluctuated, varying from 0.084 to 0.093, and experienced an overall declining trend from 0.093 in 1997 to 0.087 in 2007.

As part of the same research efforts, agencies within the government have been examining the socioeconomic circumstances of persons and the places where they live and work because studies have indicated that these strongly influence their health. The risk for mortality, morbidity, unhealthy behaviors, limited access to health care, and poor quality of care increases with decreasing socioeconomic circumstances. The two most common indicators used are educational attainment and family or household income. To assess disparities in the prevalence of non-completion of high school and poverty, the CDC analyzed data from the 2005 to 2009 Integrated Public Use Microdata Series – Current Population Survey (IPUMS-CPS). This provides a cross-sectional monthly household survey of a representative sample of the civilian, non-institutionalized US household population and is conducted jointly by the US Census Bureau and the Bureau of Labor Statistics. Group disparities in age-standardized prevalence of non-completion of high school and poverty (poverty income ration (PIR) <100% of federal poverty level (FPL)) were assessed according to sex, race/ethnicity, age, education, PIR, and disability (Beckles & Truman, 2011). In the 2009 population, statistically significant disparities were identified in non-completion of high school for all characteristics studied. Except for non-Hispanic Asian/Pacific Islander males, the absolute differences between the age-standardized percentages of each non-white racial/ethnic group and non-Hispanic whites who had not completed high school were statistically significant. The degree of racial/ethnic relative disparity varied markedly among the non-white racial/ethnic groups, ranging from three to nine times greater for Hispanics than for other groups. During 2009, the group disparities in poverty observed were similar to those for non-completion of high school No statistically significant differences were identified between relative disparities in poverty observed for 2005 and 2009.

This section has presented only a small bit of the data linked to social factors and health and health care that is available from US government sources. Because this introduction to this material is in no way comprehensive, these paragraphs are illustrative of the types of information available on CDC and other US government websites such as the Healthy People reports. They are excellent sources for researchers interested in pursuing these topics in greater depth.

Also, previous volumes in this series have presented brief reviews of issues linked to gender and health and health care as well as to race and ethnicity (Kronenfeld, 2012; Kronenfeld, 2015; Kronenfeld, 2016). Consultation of the introductory essays to these volumes will also provide additional information as do the literature review sections of a number of the chapters in this volume.

REVIEW OF CONTENTS OF THE VOLUME

This volume is divided into five parts. The first part is the introduction to this volume and contains only this chapter. The second part is on mental health related issues and contains three chapters, all of which look partially at mental health issues as related to issues of race and ethnicity. The chapter by Bennefield explores mental health pathways for girls of color. The purpose of this study was to examine whether girls of color had more or less social support than their peers and whether that affected their likelihood of experiencing the symptoms of anxiety and depression. Using data from the National Comorbidity Survey, Adolescent Supplement, path analysis found that among adolescents with both low and high SES, girls of color had significantly less family support. Despite this fact, they were not more likely to experience symptoms of anxiety and depression. The second chapter by Valles looks at familial support and mental health services use and especially examines differences among first and second generation Asian American and Latinx Older Adults. She finds that familial support partially attenuates the relationship between immigrant generation and mental health service use, but only for Latinx groups. Furthermore, the effect of familial support did not vary by age, suggesting that familial support is not significantly different for older adults than that of those younger in age. The last chapter in this part by Rivera, Molina, and Nicdao examines psychological distress differentials as a function of subjective social status among Latino subgroups in the United States. Data used were from the Latino sample (N = 2,554) of the National Latino and Asian American Study (NLAAS). A series of weighted multivariable linear regressions were the main analytical approach. Results showed that subjective social status was associated with reduced psychological distress. The chapter also demonstrates how the associations analyzed varied by Latino sub-ethnicity, an important step to fully understand the different social processes associated with the mental health of different Latina/o groups.

The third part covers four chapters related to other types of health problems, including environmental inequality and health, autism spectrum disorders (ASDs), Hepatitis C and overall perspectives on health, well-being and nutrition. The first chapter by Brailsford and colleagues points out that although theoretical models suggest that race differences in physical health are partially explained by exposures to environmental toxins, there is little empirical evidence to support this. This chapter formally tests whether black–white differences in self-rated physical health are mediated by the embodiment of environmental toxins. It uses cross-sectional data from the National Health and Nutrition Examination Surveys (2007–2008) and conducts ordinary least squares regression to model environmental toxins (from urine specimens) and overall self-rated health as a function of race and ethnicity. The authors find that non-Hispanic black respondents tend to exhibit *higher* levels of total toxins, lead, and cadmium in their urine and *poorer* physical health than non-Hispanic whites, even with adjustments for age, gender, and SES. Mediation analyses suggest that blacks may exhibit *poorer* physical health than whites because they tend to embody *higher* levels of cadmium.

The other three chapters in this part each look at different types of health problems, but all employ qualitative research approaches to better understand these issues. The second chapter in this part examines ASDs. Joseph-Kent illuminates the experiences of adults diagnosed with ASDs and intellectual disabilities (ID) and their challenges and successes in receiving quality health care services. Individuals with developmental disabilities often experience health issues associated with aging at earlier ages and at higher rates than the general population. This population has a higher incidence of chronic health conditions that require regular medical attention. This chapter is a qualitative study conducted with semi-structured interviews with 12 adults diagnosed with ASD and/or their guardians/caregivers. Some of the adults interviewed experienced negative health outcomes and suboptimal relationships with health care providers;

others seemed to have positive relationships. Barriers to accessing health care services existed in many forms.

The chapter on Hepatitis C by Kawakami, Son and Henderson focuses on better understanding the key factors that affect the quality of care that Hepatitis C patients are likely to receive in rural communities. It also discusses how to build a more effective health support system for the rural residents. Using a grounded theory approach, the researchers draw a conceptual map of the occurrence while informants had the opportunity to contemplate and share their thoughts on the issues. Local leaders held a romanticized view toward rural life while the disadvantaged reported a sense of powerlessness to bring about the needed changes to help them battle Hepatitis C. The last chapter in this part by Scheer has a broader focus than some of the other chapters in this part, with the purpose of this study being an exploration of rural children's own perspectives on health, well-being, and nutrition. Using a qualitative ethnographic research design theoretically informed by the "new" Sociology of Childhood and methodologically informed by constructivist grounded theory, the study uses as subjects fifth-grade students in an elementary school in a small rural school district in central Illinois.

Preliminary findings of this pilot study suggest that many aspects often discussed in the context of pediatric obesity, especially in rural settings, including knowledge or education about healthy eating, increasing physical activity levels, or access to healthy foods, are complex and multifaceted and do not easily lend themselves to standard interventions. Findings also indicate that children's ideas about healthy eating deviate from their own eating practices. Families' rules surrounding food selection and consumption as well as rules regarding the use of children's free time emerge as central categories for analysis.

Part IV has two chapters, both linked to gender concerns in underserved and socially disadvantaged groups.

Part V is the last section and includes three chapters discussing issues linked to health care workers. While the first chapter has a focus gender politics as an important factor for health care workers, the other two chapters examine issues of socially disadvantaged groups who are health care workers, one as vulnerable caregivers in long-term care settings and in the final chapter of the volume, migrant women who work as home care assistants.

REFERENCES

Adler, N. E., & Rehkopf. (2008). U.S. disparities in health: Descriptions, causes and mechanisms. *Annual Review of Public Health*, *29*, 235–252.

Beckles, G. L., & Truman, B. L. (2011, January 14). Education and income – United States, 2005 and 2009. *Morbidity and Mortality Weekly Report. Supplements*, *60*(01), 13–17.

Caro, J. (2019). Putting patients first: Today's disparities research leading to health equity tomorrow. *Health Services Research*, *54*(S1), 203–295. doi:10.1111/1475–6773.13107

Commonwealth Fund. (2015). *Heath care disparities*. Retrieved from http://www.commonwealthfund.org/Program-Areas/Archived-Programs/Health-Care-Disparities.aspx

Gortmaker, S. L., & Wise, P. H. (1997). The first injustice: Socioeconomic disparities, health services technology and infant mortality. *Annual Review of Sociology*, *23*, 147–170.

James, C. V. (2019). Health Services Research. Putting patients first: Today's disparities lead to health equity tomorrow. *Health Services Research*, 54(S1), 199–319. Retrieved from https://doi.org/10.1111/1475–6773.13107. Accessed on January 21, 2019.

Hero, J. O., Blendon, R. J., Zaslavzk, A. M., & Campbell, A. L. (2016). Understanding what makes americans dissatisfied with their health care system: An international comparison. *Health Affairs*, *35*(3), 502–509.

Kitigawa, E., & Hauser, P. (1978). *Differential mortality in the United States*. Cambridge, MA: Harvard University Press.

Kliss, B., & Scheuren, F. J. (1978). The 1973 CPS-IRS-SSA exact match study. *Social Security Bulletin*, *42*, 14–22.

Kronenfeld, J. J. (2012). Health care system issues and race/ethnicity, immigration, SES and gender as sociological issues linking to health and health care. In J. J. Kronenfeld (Ed.), *Issues in health and health care related to race/ethnicity, immigration, SES and gender* (Vol. 30). Bingley: Emerald Publishing.

Kronenfeld, J. J. (2015). Education, other social factors and health beliefs and health care services. In J. J. Kronenfeld (Ed.), *Education, social factors, and health beliefs in health and health care services* (Vol. 33). Bingley: Emerald Publishing.

Kronenfeld, J. J. (2016). Gender, women and other social factors in health and health care. In J. J. Kronenfeld (Ed.), *Gender, women's health care concerns and other social factors in health and health care* (Vol. 36). Bingley: Emerald Publishing.

Kunst, A. E., Feikhe, G., Mackenbach, J. P.; the EU Working Group on Socioeconomic Inequalities in Health. (1998). Occupational class and cause specific mortality in 11 European countries: Comparison of population based studies. *British Medical Journal*, *316*, 1636–1642.

Link, B. G., & Phelan, J. C. (1995). Social conditions as fundamental causes of disease. *Journal of Health and Social Behavior*, Special issue, 80–94.

Link, B. G., & Phelan, J. C. (1996). Understanding socioeconomic differences in health – The role of fundamental social causes. *American Journal of Public Health*, *86*, 471–473.

McGuire, T., Alegria, M., Cook, B. L., Wells, K. B., & Zaslavsky, A. M.(2006). Implementing the institute of medicine definition of disparities: An application to mental health care. *Health Services Research*, *41*, 1979–2005.

Schnittker, J., & McLeod, J. D. (2005). The social psychology of health disparities. *Annual Review of Sociology*, *31*, 75–103.

Smedley, B. D., Stith, A. Y., & Nelson, A. R. (Eds.). (2003). *Unequal treatment: Confronting racial and ethnic disparities in health care. Institute of Medicine*. Washington, DC: National Academies Press.

Truman, B. I., Smith, C. K.., Roy, K., Chen, Z., Moonesinghe, R., Zhu, J., … Zaza, S. (2011, January 14). Rationale for regular reporting on health disparities and inequalities – United States. *Morbidity and Mortality Weekly Report*, *60*(01), 3–10.

U.S. Department of Health and Human Services. Healthy People. (2010). (2000, November). *With understanding and improving health and objectives for improving health* (2nd ed.). Washington, DC: US Government Printing Office.

U.S. Department of Health and Human Services. (2019). *DATA 2020*. Retrieved from http://www.healthypeople.gov/2020/data-search/. Accessed on January 22, 2019.

PART II
MENTAL HEALTH RELATED ISSUES

DISADVANTAGE BEGETS DISADVANTAGE? EXPLORING MENTAL HEALTH PATHWAYS FOR GIRLS OF COLOR

Zinobia C. Bennefield

ABSTRACT

Purpose – *The purpose of this study was to examine whether girls of color (GOC) had more or less social support than their peers and whether that affected their likelihood of experiencing the symptoms of anxiety and depression.*

Methodology/Approach – *The National Comorbidity Survey – Adolescent Supplement (*n = *10,123) is a nationally representative study of mental disorder in US adolescents. GOC made up roughly 10% of the sample (*n = *1,016). Structural equation models were used to analyze the relationship between family support and psychological distress for the entire sample and then analyzed for GOC, boys of color, White girls and boys, and Latino girls and boys to compare across groups. Because of the inextricable relationship between socioeconomic status and race, three-way interactions between class, race, and gender were used to examine class differences within groups.*

Findings – *Path analysis revealed the following: (1) among adolescents with both low and high socioeconomic status, GOC had significantly less family support than their peers; (2) surprisingly, despite the fact that GOC had significantly less family support than their peers, they were not more likely to experience symptoms of anxiety and depression.*

Underserved and Socially Disadvantaged Groups and Linkages with Health and Health Care Differentials
Research in the Sociology of Health Care, Volume 37, 15–32

ISSN: 0275-4959/doi:10.1108/S0275-495920190000037005

Research Limitations/Implications – *Research limitations include cross-sectional data and limited measures. However, this study adds to the understanding of adolescent mental health and mental health of vulnerable adolescent populations. This is important because mental disorders, particularly anxiety and depression, are increasing in prevalence among American youth, and youth with multiple social disadvantages may be more likely to experience them.*

Originality/Value of Paper – *GOC, regardless of their socioeconomic backgrounds, were at a marked disadvantage regarding their perceptions of social support, a known buffer of anxiety and depression. Yet despite this disadvantage, GOC were no more likely to experience a mood disorder than their peers. These findings suggest the following: (1) family support may have less of a protective effect on the mental health of GOC than their peers; (2) GOC may be using other resources to protect their mental health; and (3) as mental health patients, GOC require unique interventions.*

Keywords: Adolescent mental health; psychological distress; intersectionality; family support; girls of color; social disadvantage

INTRODUCTION

Young Black women, here on out referred to as girls of color (GOC), are a unique socially disadvantaged group because they are disproportionately born into low socioeconomic strata within a White patriarchal system of power exposing them to institutionalized racism and sexism, and their age limits their ability to cope, change, or improve their circumstances. Research has not yet examined how these social disadvantages affect their mental health. Notably, no empirical study has examined whether GOC lack the vital forms of social support that buffer against some of the most prevalent mental disorders. This study addressed this gap in the literature and was guided by the following research question: Do GOC have more or less family support than their peers and how does that affect their likelihood of experiencing psychological distress, a predictor of serious mental disorder?

To the best knowledge of the author and at the time of the study, there were no estimates on the rates of mental illness among GOC. There were, however, estimates of mental illness in the general adolescent population and comparisons of mental illness between girls and boys and Blacks, Latinos, and Whites. Current estimates suggest that one out of every three to four adolescents meet the criteria for some form of disorder, the most common being anxiety (about 32%) and mood disorders, that is, depression (about 12%) (Costello, Erkanli, & Angold, 2006; Merikangas et al., 2010). Rates of anxiety and depression tend to be greater among girls than among boys (Kessler, Andrews, Mroczek, Ustun, & Wittchen, 1998; McGee et al., 1990). Some studies have found Black adolescents experience increased rates of anxiety disorders when compared to White adolescents (e.g., Merikangas et al., 2010), while other studies have found White and Latino adolescents have higher rates of depression than Blacks (Angold, Erkanli, & Farmer, 2002). One predictor of whether or not a child meets the diagnostic criteria for anxiety or depression is whether they experience psychological distress.

Psychological distress is defined as a state of emotional suffering characterized by symptoms of anxiety and depression (Wheaton, 2007) that may impact the social functioning and day-to-day living of individuals (Horwitz, 2007; Ridner, 2004). Untreated, psychological distress could lead to serious mental disorders like depression and generalized anxiety disorder (Horwitz, 2007; Payton, 2009). Research suggests low socioeconomic status, racial discrimination, and gender differences may be related to increased vulnerability which can limit coping abilities and exasperate distress (Aneshensel, 2009). Thus GOC may be especially susceptible.

One of the key factors that determines whether or not a person experiences mental illness is social support (Demaray, Malecki, Davidson, Hodgson, & Rebus, 2005; Helsen, Vollebergh, & Meeus, 2000). For all youth, the family is the main source of social support (Merikangas et al., 2010) and is essential to the development of positive psychological well-being (Grusec, 2011). Higher levels of parental support are consistently found to be associated with lower depression (Newman et al., 2007). Cheng and colleagues (2014) found that among adolescents, perceptions of having a caring adult in the home was positively associated with hope and negatively associated with depressive and post-traumatic stress symptoms.

Communication and closeness are two dimensions of family support that have been demonstrated to affect mental health. Open communication refers to members of the family feeling heard and able to openly share their own thoughts and opinion. Being able to express one's opinions, having input in decision-making, and a space to talk about personal issues may be important to combating psychological distress. Closeness refers to the amount of physical and emotional closeness created within the family. A supportive family setting in which youth feel close, connected, and supported by family and parents is central to development of self-esteem and other skills necessary for positive mental health outcomes (Bean, Bush, McKenry, & Wilson, 2003). Family closeness, created by positive family interactions, helps youth feel a part of a unit, safe, and stable. Such feelings are related to positive decision-making and reduced negative behavior (Ackard et al., 2006).

Similar to studies on mental illness, there are no current estimates on perceptions of family support among GOC, but studies on family support were compared between girls and boys and Blacks, Latinos, and Whites. Overall, research has indicated that racial/ethnic minorities and females tend to report higher levels of family support than their counterparts. Research has found family support is integral to young Black Americans' academic achievement and self-esteem (Brooks-Gunn & Markman, 2005; Causey, Livingston, & High, 2015; Taylor & Roberts, 1995). Among Latinos, family support is associated with advantages in mental health (Mulvaney-Day, Alegria, & Sribney, 2007). Walen and Lachman (2000) found family support reduced the effects of stress for girls more so than boys. Consequently, lower perceptions of support have been found to have greater negative effects on girls than on boys (Operario, Tschann, Flores, & Bridges, 2006; Størksen, Røysamb, Holmen, & Tambs, 2006).

At this point, we know that GOCs, due to their young age, gender, race, and socioeconomic position that is inextricably linked to their race, are at a unique set of social disadvantages. But there is very limited understanding of how these social disadvantages affect the pathways by which mental illness is created. One such pathway, family support -> psychological distress, is worthy of study because family support is the most salient form of social support for adolescents and psychological distress if an indicator of the most prevalent mental disorders. Therefore, this study examined this common pathway for GOC and compared them to their peers.

METHOD

Sample and Procedure

This study utilized data from the National Comorbidity Survey: Adolescent Supplement (NCS-A). The NCS-A is a nationally representative, face-to-face survey of 10,148 adolescents in the United States. Data were collected between February 2001 and January 2004 (Kessler et al., 2009). The NCS-A was carried out at the request of the National Institute of Mental Health (NIMH) as a late addition to the National Comorbidity Survey Replication (NCS-R) to meet a request from Congress to provide national data on the prevalence and correlates of mental health indicators among US youth (Kessler et al., 2009). The NCS-A was designed to estimate the lifetime-to-date and current prevalence, age-of-onset distributions, course, symptoms, and comorbidity of Diagnostic and Statistical Manual-IV (DSM-IV) disorders among adolescents in the United States; to identify risk and protective factors for the onset and persistence of these disorders; to describe patterns and correlates of service use for these disorders; and to lay the groundwork for subsequent follow-up studies that can be used to identify early expressions of adult mental disorders (Kessler et al., 2009). The overall response rate was 82.9%.

To ensure the target sample of 10,000 adolescents was reached, the NCS-A relied on a dual-frame design that added a school-based sample to the household sample. In the household sample, one random adolescent was selected by a computer program when more than one adolescent resided in the household. In the school sample, the adolescent was identified by the school roster. A representative sample of all accredited eligible schools was selected with probabilities proportional to the size of the student body in the classes relevant to the target sample in each of the counties or county clusters that made up the primary sampling units (PSUs) of the nationally representative NCS-R sample. Within each school, a random sample of 40–50 eligible students was selected using a systematic selection procedure. Recruitment and consent procedures were overseen and approved by both the Human Subjects Committees of Harvard Medical School and the University of Michigan.

After data collection, cases were weighted for variation in household probability of selection in the household sample and residual discrepancies between sample and population sociodemographic and geographic distributions. The household sample weights were already developed for the NCS-R. They were added to the adolescent data and adjusted for differential probability of selection of adolescents in the household. These data were then compared with nationally representative census data on basic sociodemographic characteristics for purposes of post-stratification. Weighting for the school sample was based on weights that controlled for three sets of variables: Quality Education Data which include data on the characteristics of all schools in the United States, Public Use Microdata Sample (PUMS), and Block Group (BG) level data. More detailed information regarding weighting procedures can be found in Kessler et al. (2009). Recruitment and consent procedures were approved by the Human Subjects Committees of both Harvard Medical School and the University of Michigan.

The sample consisted of 10,148 adolescents (5,648 Whites, 1,955 Blacks, and 1,922 Latinos). Due to the small number of respondents who identified as "other" ($n = 623$) and the potential ethnic variation within that subgroup, this category was omitted from the analysis. The sample included 4,965 males and 5,183 females. The average age was 15.2 years. GOC made up 10% of the total sample ($n = 1{,}016$). GOC reported higher psychological distress than the other youth in the sample (Table 1). GOC reported lower family support than the other youth in the sample except Latina females. All the youth in the sample reported similar levels of family closeness.

Measures

Psychological distress was measured using the Kessler 6 or K6, which is a six-item scale that assesses how frequently an individual has experienced six symptoms of major depression and generalized anxiety disorder in the month prior to the interview. It was based on item response theory models to ensure consistent precision and sensitivity to the distress spectrum across age groups (Kessler et al., 2002), and it is also predictive of serious mental illness in adolescents

Table 1. Mean Value of Psychological Distress and Family Support for Disaggregated Sample.

	White Males	White Females	Black Males	Black Females	Latino Males	Latino Females
Psychological distress	1.52	1.6	1.63	1.73	1.56	1.69
Family communication	2.64	2.63	2.63	2.57	2.59	2.48
Family closeness	2.78	2.75	2.8	2.76	2.8	2.7

(Kessler et al., 2010). The six questions are as follows: during the last 30 days, (1) about how often did you feel nervous? (2) about how often did you feel hopeless? (3) about how often did you feel restless or fidgety? (4) about how often did you feel that everything was an effort? (5) about how often did you feel so sad that nothing could cheer you up? and (6) about how often did you feel worthless? Response choices were measured on a 1–5 Likert scale: 1 = none of the time, 2 = a little of the time, 3 = some of the time, 4 = most of the time, and 5 = all of the time ($\alpha = 0.76$).

Family support was created by parceling together two latent scales, family communication and family closeness. Family communication was created using a five-item scale: (1) How often family members easily expressed opinions? (2) How often members each had input on major decisions? (3) How often children have a say in their discipline? (4) How often family members talk about feelings? and (5) How often family members talk when sad/worried? Family closeness included the following five items: How often family members felt close to each other? How often family members did things together? How often members willingly did what family decided? How often family shared interests and hobbies? How often family members compromise? Response choices ranged from 1 ("all of the time") to 4 ("never").

Live with biological mother/father entire life were coded 0 = no and 1 = yes. Birth order was dummy coded into three dummy variables: oldest (reference category), *middle*, and *youngest*. *Siblings* was a continuous variable. *Parent employment* was dummy coded: 1 = currently employed and 0 = not currently employed; this was collected from the primary guardian. *Parent marital status* had categories for married, separated, widowed, divorced, and never married and was recorded 1 = married 0 = not married. *Parent self-rated mental health* was measured on a 0–10 scale with 0 = poor mental health and 10 = excellent mental health.

Race/ethnicity was a categorical variable that measured self-reported racial identification: Hispanic, non-Hispanic Black, non-Hispanic White (reference category), or other. Due to the small number of respondents who identified as "other" ($n = 623$) and the potential ethnic variation within that subgroup, this category was dropped from the analysis. *Total household income* was collected from the parent data. *Parent's education* was measured by asking adolescent's the higher level of schooling completed by parents/legal guardian. If there were two parents, the higher level was recorded. Education was a continuous variable coded 1–9, representing years of education ranging from less than a high school education to college graduate or advanced degree. *Subjective Social Status* was a measure developed by the MacArthur socioeconomic status (SES) and Health Network to determine where adolescents believed they ranked in relation to others in their community. *Gender* was a binary variable coded male "0" and female "1." *Age* was a continuous variable that ranged from 13 to 18. Residence in either urban or rural areas is commonly cited as a risk factor mental disorder, though evidence of this relationship is inconclusive (Breslau, 2014). Nevertheless, *urbanicity* was included in the analysis as a categorical variable captured by three dummy variables: metropolitan area, other urban area, and rural area (reference category). Because there was a sizeable Latino population, nativity was included as a control. *US Born* was coded 1 = US born and 0 = foreign born.

Analysis

Mediated moderation approach was used to simultaneously analyze social support – psychological distress pathway varied across and within groups. Mediated moderation is used to analyze directional relationships that may be simultaneously affected by a mediator and a moderator (Morgan-Lopez & MacKinnon, 2006; Muller, Judd, & Yzerbyt, 2005). Analysis was conducted using Structural Equation Models (SEMs). SEM is useful in that it allows for testing multiple relationships, simultaneously and serves as more fully theorized model (Bauer, 2014). Models were analyzed using full information likelihood estimation for missing data (FIML). FIML retrieves as much information as possible from observations by assuming joint normality of all variables and missing values are missing at random (MAR) (Arbuckle & Marcoulides, 1996; Enders & Bandalos, 2001).

The chi-square statistic, comparative fit index (CFI), and root-mean-square of approximation (RMSEA) were used to determine whether there were any sources of misfit, in which case modification indices were used to improve the fit of the model. To assess the differential effects of SES by race/ethnicity and gender, cross product terms were created between race, SES, and gender (Szklo & Nieto, 2014). The continuous variables were centered before the interaction terms were created to reduce multicollinearity between cross product and lower-order terms (Mirowsky, 1999). When applicable, scales were reverse coded for analyses. All analyses were conducted using Stata 14.1.

Results

A baseline model represented in Table 2 (CFI 0.958 and RMSEA 0.025) was fit to examine the relationship between family support and psychological distress for the entire adolescent population. Many of the findings have been established within the literature and set a foundation for more complex models. The first panel examines the relationship between the covariates and the family support. Higher perceptions of status were associated with higher perceptions of family support ($\beta = 0.062$, $p < 0.000$). Living with biological parents, both father ($\beta = 0.133$, $p < 0.000$) and mother ($\beta = 0.084$, $p < 0.000$) were associated with higher perceptions of family support. Birth order was also associated with family support. Middle children (ref: oldest) was associated with lower perceptions of family support ($\beta = -0.077$, $p < 0.007$). Higher parental self-rated mental health was associated with higher perceptions of family support ($\beta = 0.021$, $p < 0.001$). Living in a metropolitan area was associated with decreases in perceptions of family support ($\beta = -0.053$, $p < 0.009$). Girls, contrary to the literature, had lower perceptions of family support than boys ($\beta = -0.058$, $p < 0.000$).

Table 2. Structural Equation Model Estimates of the Association between Family Support and Psychological Distress.

	Family Support	Psychological Distress
Family support		−0.174***
		(0.030)
Live with biological father	−0.054	0.133***
	(0.030)	(0.025)
Live with biological mother	−0.052*	0.084*
	(0.023)	(0.032)
Middle (ref: oldest)	−0.015	−0.077**
	(0.021)	(0.027)
Youngest (ref: oldest)	−0.004	−0.040
	(0.020)	(0.021)
Siblings	0.010	−0.0174
	(0.010)	(0.010)
Parent employment	−0.010	−0.040
	(0.024)	(0.023)
Parent marital status	0.023	0.032
	(0.030)	(0.027)
Parent self-rated mental health	−0.045***	0.021**
	(0.006)	(0.010)
Black (ref: White)	0.056	0.050
	(0.031)	(0.025)
Latino (ref: White)	0.004	0.021
	(0.020)	(0.023)
Subjective social status	−0.021***	0.062***
	(0.010)	(0.005)
Total family income	−0.005	−0.003
	(0.004)	(0.005)
Parent education	−0.017	−010
	(0.012)	(0.012)
Gender	0.100***	−0.058***
	(0.020)	(0.012)
Age	0.021	−0.020
	(0.012)	(0.013)
Metropolitan (ref: rural)	0.059*	−0.053**
	(0.025)	(0.019)
Suburban (ref:rural)	0.024	−0.022
	(0.028)	(0.025)
US born	0.049*	−0.0196
	(0.024)	(0.036)
R^2		0.20

Notes: $*p < 0.05$; $**p < 0.01$; $***p < 0.001$.

The second panel examines the relationship between the covariates, family support, and psychological distress. Higher perceptions of family support were associated with lower psychological distress ($\beta = -0.174$, $p < 0.000$). Higher parental mental health was associated with lower symptoms of anxiety and depression ($\beta = -0.045$, $p < 0.000$). US-born children had lower anxiety and depression than foreign-born children ($\beta = 0.049$, $p < 0.047$). Living in a metropolitan area was associated with higher symptoms of psychological distress ($\beta = 0.059$, $p < 0.022$). Girls had higher symptoms of anxiety and depression than boys ($\beta = 0.099$, $p < 0.000$). Living with biological mother was associated with lower anxiety and depression ($\beta = -0.051$, $p < 0.027$).

Because the focus of the study was on the experience of GOC, interaction effects were added to the model (CFI 0.957 RMSEA 0.023) represented in Table3. Two-way interactions were first added to examine socioeconomic differences within racial/ethnic (White, Black, and Latino) and gender (girls and boys) groups. Research has demonstrated that subjective measures of status are

Table 3. Structural Equation Model Estimates of the Association between Family Support and Psychological Distress with Two-way Interactions.

	Family Support	Psychological Distress
Family support		0.173***
		(0.030)
Live with biological father	−0.055	0.134***
	(0.030)	(0.025)
Live with biological mother	−0.051*	0.083*
	(0.023)	(0.032)
Middle (ref: oldest)	−0.014	−0.075**
	(0.021)	(0.026)
Youngest (ref: oldest)	0.003	−0.039
	(0.020)	(0.021)
Siblings	0.006	−0.018*
	(0.009)	(0.009)
Parent employment	−0.012	−0.039
	(0.024)	(0.023)
Parent marital status	−0.024	0.029
	(0.029)	(0.027)
Parent self-rated mental health	−0.045***	0.021**
	(0.007)	(0.006)
Black (ref: White)	0.089*	−0.061**
	(0.037)	(0.021)
Latino (ref: White)	0.009	0.039
	(0.023)	(0.030)
Gender	0.111***	−0.052**
	(0.021)	(0.016)

Table 3. *(Continued)*

	Family Support	Psychological Distress
Subjective social status	−0.013*	0.060***
	(0.005)	(0.006)
Black*SSS	−0.014	−0.030*
	(0.016)	0.015
Latino*SSS	−0.009	0.005
	(0.016)	(0.013)
Gender*SSS	−0.011	0.018*
	(0.011)	(0.008)
Black*Gender	−0.060	−0.016
	(0.050)	(0.038)
Latino*Gender	−0.014	−0.035
	(0.044)	(0.036)
Total family income	−0.005	−0.003
	(0.004)	(0.005)
Parent education	−0.016	−0.009
	(0.012)	(0.012)
Age	0.020	−0.018
	(0.012)	(0.013)
Metropolitan (ref: rural)	0.059*	−0.053**
	(0.025)	(0.019)
Suburban (ref: rural)	0.024	−0.021
	(0.028)	(0.025)
US born	−0.047*	−0.022
	(0.023)	(0.037)
R^2		0.203

Notes: $^{*}p < 0.05$; $^{**}p < 0.01$; $^{***}p < 0.001$.

better predictors of health than objective measures (Bennefield, 2018; McLaughlin, Costello, Leblanc, Sampson, & Kessler, 2012); therefore, interaction effects were only created using the subjective social status. Exploratory analysis (results not shown here) for interaction effects between objective measures and the race variables were insignificant. The first panel shows the relationship between the covariates, interaction effects, and family support. The significant interaction effect between Blacks and status ($\beta = -0.030$, $p < 0.05$) indicates that the relationship between status and family support is stronger for Whites than Blacks. The significant interaction effect between gender and status indicates that the relationship between status and family support is stronger for girls than boys ($\beta = 0.018$, $p < 0.018$). In line with the baseline model, higher perceptions of status were associated with higher perceptions of family support

($\beta = 0.059$, $p < 0.000$). Adolescents with parents with high self-rated mental health had higher perceptions of family support than adolescents with parents with low self-rated mental health ($\beta = 0.021$, $p < 0.001$).

The second panel shows the relationship between the covariates, family support, the interaction effects, and psychological distress. None of the interaction effects were significant. However, in line with the baseline model, higher perceptions of social status were associated with decreases in symptoms of anxiety and depression ($\beta = -0.012$, $p < 0.026$). Black adolescents had higher symptoms of anxiety and depression than Whites ($\beta = 0.089$, $p < 0.022$). Higher parental self-rated mental health was associated with lower symptoms of anxiety and depression ($\beta = -0.045$, $p < 0.000$). Girls had higher symptoms of anxiety and depression than boys ($\beta = 0.111$, $p < 0.000$).

Finally, three-way interactions (CFI 0.957 RMSEA 0.022) represented in Table4 were added to the model to examine the relationship for GOC specifically as well as to be able to examine the relationship between family support and psychological distress within and across race/gender/class groups. The first

Table 4. Structural Equation Model Estimates of the Association between Family Support and Psychological Distress with Three-way Interactions.

	Family Support	Psychological Distress
Family support		−0.172
		(0.030)
Live with biological father	−0.054	0.134***
	(0.030)	(0.026)
Live with biological mother	−0.053*	0.085*
	(0.023)	(0.032)
Middle (ref: oldest)	−0.014	−0.075**
	(0.021)	(0.027)
Youngest (ref: oldest)	−0.003	−0.039
	(0.020)	(0.021)
Siblings	0.007	−0.018*
	(0.009)	(0.009)
Parent employment	−0.011	−0.038
	(0.024)	(0.023)
Parent marital status	0.023	0.029
	(0.029)	(0.027)
Parent self-rated mental health	−0.046***	0.021**
	(0.007)	(0.006)
Black	0.091*	0.058***
	(0.038)	(0.021)
Latino	0.006	0.039
	(0.022)	(0.028)

Table 4. (*Continued*)

	Family Support	Psychological Distress
Gender	0.112***	−0.053**
	(0.021)	(0.016)
Subjective social status	−0.007	0.052***
	(0.007)	(0.006)
Black*SSS	−0.033	−0.001
	(0.027)	(0.011)
Latino*SSS	−0.027	0.013
	(0.018)	(0.017)
Gender*SSS	−0.024*	0.031**
	(0.011)	(0.009)
Black*Gender	−0.067	−0.007
	(0.051)	(0.039)
Latino*Gender	−0.009	−0.035
	(0.044)	(0.036)
Black*Gender*SSS	0.039	−0.060*
	(0.030)	(0.027)
Latino*Gender*SSS	0.041	−0.018
	(0.022)	(0.021)
Total family income	−0.005	−0.003
	(0.004)	(0.005)
Parent education	−0.015	−0.010
	(0.012)	(0.012)
Age	0.019	−0.017
	(0.012)	(0.013)
Metropolitan (ref: rural)	0.060*	−0.054**
	(0.024)	(0.020)
Suburban (ref: rural)	0.024	−0.021
	(0.027)	(0.026)
US born	0.046*	−0.022
	(0.022)	(0.037)
R^2 0.205		0.205

Notes: $*p < 0.05$; $**p < 0.01$; $***p < 0.001$.

panel examines the relationship between the covariates and interaction effects and family support. The focal point in this model is the significant cross product between the three-way interaction between race, gender, and status ($\beta = -0.060$, $p < 0.028$). This indicates that Black girls, with both high and low status, reported significantly less family support than their peers. As in the previous models, having parents with high self-rated mental health and living with biological parents were associated with increases in perceptions of family support.

The second panel examines the relationship between the covariates, family support, interaction effects, and psychological distress. None of the interaction effects were significant. As in the previous models, higher perceptions of family, higher parental self-rated mental health, and living with the biological mother were associated with lower symptoms of anxiety and depression. And being born in the United States and living in a metropolitan area was associated with higher symptoms of anxiety and depression.

DISCUSSION

The central focus of this study was on the mental illness experience of GOC, defined here as Black American girls. Because GOC have multiple disadvantaged social identities, the study examined whether they lacked the most influential form of social support available to youth, family support. Further, I examined whether diminished social support affected their likelihood of experiencing psychological distress. Such inquiries become of increasing importance, because as youth become a greater proportion of the mental health patient population, the most vulnerable youth may be at increased risk.

The results from the study found that GOC with both low and high perceptions of status had significantly less family support than their peers (White boys, White girls, Black boys, Latino boys, and Latino girls). The fact that increased socioeconomic status had little effect on family support for GOC was unsurprising because earlier studies on socioeconomic status and race have consistently shown that the benefits of class are diminished for Blacks (Farmer & Ferraro, 2005). Although such studies on socioeconomic status and race were conducted on adult populations, this study demonstrated similar findings among adolescents. This is important because it highlights the fact that children are just as negatively affected by the interconnected nature of racism and class. Yet because GOC have significantly less ability to change their socioeconomic circumstances, as compared to their adult counterparts, this disadvantage could have a more severe impact on their lives and health. Though it was unsurprising that increased socioeconomic status had little effect on family support, it was surprising that, overall, GOC had significantly less family support than their peers.

Studies on family support and gender has demonstrated that girls almost consistently report more family support than boys (Cheng & Chan, 2004). Further, studies on family support and race have demonstrated that racial/ethnic minorities, particularly Black Americans, report having more family support than Whites (Brooks-Gunn & Markman, 2005; Causey et al., 2015). An educated guess would assert that GOC would then have high levels of family support. But studies that utilize an intersectional approach, either theoretically or methodologically, show why such additive, educated guesses are flawed (Brown & Hargrove, 2013). Identities cannot be summed up (Bowleg, 2008). Instead, it is much more appropriate to think of identities as interacting multiplicatively, and the findings from this study support such arguments. This is important because there are many populations, both adult and adolescent, that sit at the center of complex interactions (Rosenfield, 2012) and research has yet to examine their health experiences specifically. This study found that the relationship between race, gender, and family is quite complex. The question remains, why would GOC have significantly less family support than their peers?

Gendered and racialized understandings of the family unit can help contextualize these findings. Gender roles within the family dictate that girls are more likely than boys to be socialized to take on responsibilities within the home such as caring for younger siblings, cooking, and cleaning. Further, Black American families are often characterized by large extended kin networks and multigenerational homes (Franklin, 2007). It is plausible then that GOC cook, clean, and care for a greater number of relatives causing the family to be a source of stress and altering their perception of the supportive nature of their family network. This makes sense when one considers that Black women across their *lifecourse o*ften lack familial support. For example, Black women are more likely than their peers to be the head of their household or single mothers, and elderly Black women are more likely than their peers to be raising grandchildren with less than adequate support. Black women, across the lifecourse, bear an undue burden within their families, and it makes sense that this would begin in childhood and adolescence.

Despite low levels of family support when compared to their peers, this study found no increase in the symptoms of anxiety and depression for GOC. Studies on different populations have found that lower social support is associated with higher anxiety and depression (Newman et al., 2007). Yet this study did not find evidence of this, and again highlights the complexity of studying multiple intersecting identities. While there were no variables in the analysis that could account for these findings, the literature holds some clues.

First, it is possible that other components of family support are associated with anxiety and depression for GOC. This study examined family communication and closeness because previous studies have identified them as important parts of family support (Bean et al., 2003; Erickson, 1968). But other components such as family integration, discipline within family, and relationships with family members are just as important. It is plausible that communication and closeness are not the most important factors of family support and that decreases in other components of family support could be associated with increases in symptoms of anxiety and depression for GOC. This should be investigated further in other quantitative studies that have measures of family support and a large sample of GOC.

Another explanation for why GOC did not have increased anxiety and depression despite their decreased familial support is that they may be given tools to handle the undue burden their families place on them. Studies on Black home culture (Feagin, 2013) have found that Black Americans have constructed coping mechanisms to enable them to deal with chronic stressors. Those coping mechanisms could be extended to GOC in that they are empowered to be the bearers of burdens. One example of this is the "Black Girl Magic" movement which praises Black girls for, among many things, their resilience and ability to handle enormous amounts of stress with grace and beauty. While there are no variables like this in the current dataset, it is worth exploring through ethnographic and other qualitative means in order to better understand these findings.

In conclusion, this study highlights the complexities of social disadvantage and mental health. Many mental health patients would be considered members of vulnerable populations with multiple intersecting marginalized identities. This studies show that the path from social identity to mental health and illness is not a straight one. Disadvantaged identities do not necessarily mean disadvantages in mental health. Even when disadvantage in the pathways that effect health are documented, that does not mean that those disadvantages will be seen in mental health. This is particularly evident for GOC.

Despite the findings that GOC are not at an increased risk of anxiety and depression, when compared to their peers, it is important to emphasize that they are still at risk. The findings suggest that family may be a good place to focus interventions as it is a nexus for stress and support. Health professionals assessing GOC should be aware of the complexities surrounding the family for GOC and utilize interventions tailored to this population. Further, although this study found that low familial support had no effect on psychological distress that does not mean that the relationship between GOC and their families should not be improved. The literature is clear that family support is vital to the mental health of adolescents. Because this study only looked at one mental health outcome, it is very plausible that low family support could negatively impact GOC's self-esteem, self-identities, or likelihood to engage in risky behavior.

These findings are not interpreted without caution. The NCS-A is a cross-sectional data set which limited the ability to examine the relationship between family support and psychological distress across time. As adolescents age, the relationship between support systems and psychological distress may change as they rely on newly developing friendship groups and become independent of their families. Future studies should utilize longitudinal data in order to understand the nature of these relationships across time.

Another issue of concern was reverse causality as the subjective measure or status (*X*) could be confounded with psychological distress (*Y*). This study does not address the issues of causality because it can only be tested in longitudinal data and "specifications about directionality concern observed variables only" (Kline, 2011). Because of the potential for confounding issues, a few precautions were taken: (1) the hypothesized relationship (status->mental health) was based on theoretical reasons. Studies suggest the causal relationship from SES to mental health is more common than the reverse (Hudson, 2005; Miech, Caspi, Moffitt, Wright, & Silva, 2000); (2) the study utilized SEMs which are well suited for estimating the correlations between latent variables in cross-sectional data;and (3) other presumed causes of distress (other measures of SES, parent mental health) were included in the analysis as covariates. Thus while, the data are not best suited for causal analysis, the research engages foundational issues around correlation and the nature of the relationship between SES, social support and mental health in the adolescent population in order to ask questions about causality in the future.

Finally, the coefficients had notably small magnitudes. Family closeness and communication were used as measures of family support; however, family support networks are complex multidimensional networks that are not fully represented here. Other dimensions of family support should be evaluated in its relation to psychological well-being in order to gain more information about the correlates of mental health. Further, there was no measure of stress, an important correlate of anxiety and depression. The omission of such variables was made to focus the study, but may partially explain the small magnitudes of the coefficients as well as the low amount of explained variance.

Notwithstanding the limitations, this study is, to the best knowledge of the author, the first study to use a nationally representative data set to examine the mental health of GOC. And the findings add to the empirical literature on adolescent mental health in general and the mental health of GOC specifically. Further, this study speaks to the conversation on social disadvantage. As evidence is continually brought forth that many mental disorders are the function of social location, this study shows that the pathways by which social identity affects mental health is multi-faceted. Finally, this study highlights an amazingly complex population, whose experiences could tell us something about mental health across the lifecourse.

REFERENCES

Ackard, D. M., Neumark-Sztainer, D., Story, M., & Perry, C. (2006). Parent–child connectedness and behavioral and emotional health among adolescents. *American Journal of Preventive Medicine*, *30*(1), 59–66.

Aneshensel, C. S. (2009). Toward explaining mental health disparities. *Journal of Health and Social Behavior*, *50*, 377–394.

Angold, A., Erkanli, A., & Farmer, E. (2002). Psychiatric disorder, impairment, and service use in rural African American and White youth. *Archives of General Psychology*, *59*, 893–901.

Arbuckle, J. L., & Marcoulides, G. A. (1996). Full information estimation in the presence of incomplete data. *Advanced Structural Equation Modeling: Issues and Techniques*, *243*, 277.

Bauer, G. R. (2014). Incorporating intersectionality theory into population health research methodology: Challenges and the potential to advance health equity. *Social Science and Medicine*, *110*, 10–17.

Bean, R. A., Bush, K. R., McKenry, P. C., & Wilson, S. M. (2003). The impact of parental support, behavioral control, and psychological control on the academic achievement and self-esteem of African American and European American adolescents. *Journal of Adolescent Research*, *18*(5), 523–541.

Bennefield, Z. (2018). School and family correlates of positive affect in a nationally representative sample of US adolescents. *Child and Adolescent Social Work Journal*, *35*(5), 541–548.

Bowleg, L. (2008). When Black + lesbian + woman ≠ Black lesbian woman: The methodological challenges of qualitative and quantitative intersectionality research. *Sex Roles*, *59*(5–6), 312–325.

Brooks-Gunn, J., & Markman, L. (2005). The contribution of parenting to ethnic and racial gaps in school readiness. *The Future of Children*, *15*(1), 139–168.

Brown, T. H., & Hargrove, T. W. (2013). Multidimensional approaches to examining gender and racial/ethnic stratification in health. *Women, Gender, and Families of Color*, *1*(2), 180–206.

Causey, S. T., Livingston, J., & High, B. (2015). Family structure, racial socialization, perceived parental involvement, and social support as predictors of self-esteem in African American college students. *Journal of Black Studies*, *45*(7), 655–677.

Cheng, S., & Chan, A. (2004). The multidimensional scale of perceived social support: Dimensionality and age and gender differences in adolescents. *Personality and Individual Differences*, *37*(7), 1359–1369.

Cheng, Y., Li, X.-C., Lou, C., Sonenstein, F. L., Kalamar, A., Jejeebhoy, S., ... Ojengbede, O. (2014). The association between social support and mental health among vulnerable adolescents in five cities: Findings from the study of the well-being of adolescents in vulnerable environments. *Journal of Adolescent Health*, *55*(6), S31–S38.

Costello, J. E., Erkanli, A., & Angold, A. (2006). Is there an epidemic of child or adolescent depression?*Journal of Child Psychology and Psychiatry*, *47*(12), 1263–1271.

Demaray, M. K., Malecki, C. K., Davidson, L. M., Hodgson, K. K., & Rebus, P. J. (2005). The relationship between social support and student adjustment: A longitudinal analysis. *Psychology in the Schools*, *42*(7), 691–706.

Enders, C. K., & Bandalos, D. L. (2001). The relative performance of full information maximum likelihood estimation for missing data in structural equation models. *Structural Equation Modeling*, *8*(3), 430–457.

Farmer, M. M., & Ferraro, K. F. (2005). Are racial disparities in health conditional on socioeconomic status?*Social Science and Medicine*, *60*(1), 191–204.

Feagin, J. R. (2013). *The white racial frame: Centuries of racial framing and counter-framing*. New York, NY: Routledge.

Franklin, J. H. (2007). African American families. In H. P. McAdoo (Ed.), *Black families* (pp. 3–6). Thousand Oaks, CA: Sage.

Grusec, J. E. (2011). Socialization processes in the family: Social and emotional development. *Annual Review of Psychology*, *62*, 243–269.

Helsen, M., Vollebergh, W., & Meeus, W. (2000). Social support from parents and friends and emotional problems in adolescence. *Journal of Youth and Adolescence*, *29*(3), 319–335.

Horwitz, A.V. (2007). Distinguishing distress from disorder as psychological outcomes of stressful social arrangements. *Health*, *11*(3), 273–289.

Hudson, C. G. (2005). Socioeconomic status and mental illness: Tests of the social causation and selection hypotheses. *American Journal of Orthopsychiatry*, *75*(1), 1–18.

Kessler, R. C., Andrews, G., Mroczek, D., Ustun, B., & Wittchen, H. (1998). The World Health Organization composite international diagnostic interview short-form (CIDI-SF). *International Journal of Methods in Psychiatric Research*, *7*(4), 171–185.

Kessler, R. C., Andrews, G., Colpe, L. J., Hiripi, E., Mroczek, D. K., Normand, S. L., ... Zaslavsky, A. M. (2002). Short screening scales to monitor population prevalences and trends in non-specific psychological distress. *Psychological Medicine*, *32*(6), 959–976.

Kessler, R. C., Avenevoli, S., Costello, J., Green, J. G., Gruber, M. J., Heeringa, S., ... Zaslavsky, A. M. (2009). National comorbidity survey replication adolescent supplement (NCS-A): II. Overview and design. *Journal of American Academy Child Adolescent Psychiatry*, *48*(4), 380–385.

Kessler, R. C., Green, J. C., Gruber, M. J., Sampson, N. A., Bromet, E., Cuitan, M., & Zaslavsky, A. M. (2010). Screening for serious mental illness in the general population with the k6 screening scale: Results from the WHO World Mental Health (WMH) survey initiative. *International Journal of Methods in Psychiatric Research*, *19*(S1), 4–22.

Kline, R. B. (2011). *Principles and practice of structural equation modeling* (3rd edn.). New York, NY: The Guilford Press.

McGee, R., Feehan, M., Williams, S., Partridge, F., Silva, P. A., & Kelly, J. (1990). DSM-III disorders in a large sample of adolescents. *Journal of the American Academy of Child and Adolescent Psychiatry*, *29*(4), 611–619.

McLaughlin, K. A., Costello, J., Leblanc, W., Sampson, N. A., & Kessler, R. C. (2012). Socioeconomic status and adolescent mental disorders. *American Journal of Public Health*, *102*(9), 1742–1750.

Merikangas, K. R., He, J., Brody, D., Fisher, P. W., Bourdon, K., & Koretz, D. S. (2010). Prevalence and treatment of mental disorders among US children in the 2001–2004 NHANES. *Pediatrics*, *125*(1), 75–81.

Miech, R. A., Caspi, A., Moffitt, T. E., Wright, B. R., & Silva, P. A. (2000). Low socioeconomic status and mental disorders: A longitudinal study of selection and causation during young adulthood. *American Journal of Sociology*, *104*(4), 1096–1131.

Mirowsky, J. (1999). Subjective life expectancy in the US: Correspondence to actuarial estimates by age, sex and race. *Social Science & Medicine*, *49*(7), 967–979.

Morgan-Lopez, A. A., & MacKinnon, D. P. (2006). Demonstration and evaluation of a method for assessing mediated moderation. *Behavior Research Methods*, *38*(1), 77–87.

Muller, D., Judd, C. M., & Yzerbyt, V. Y. (2005). When moderation is mediated and mediation is moderated. *Journal of Personality and Social Psychology*, *89*(6), 852–863.

Mulvaney-Day, N. E., Alegria, M., & Sribney, W. (2007). Social cohesion, social support, and health among Latinos in the United States. *Social Science and Medicine*, *64*(2), 477–495.

Newman, B. M., Newman, P. R., Griffen, S., O'Connor, K., & Spas, J. (2007). The relationship of social support to depressive symptoms during the transition to high school. *Adolescence*, *42*(167), 441–459.

Operario, D., Tschann, J., Flores, E., & Bridges, M. (2006). Brief report: Associations of parental warmth, peer support, and gender with adolescent emotional distress. *Journal of Adolescence*, *29*(2), 299–305.

Payton, A.R. (2009). Mental health, mental illness, and psychological distress: Same continuum or distinct phenomena? *Journal of Health and Social Behavior*, *50*(2), 213–227.

Ridner, S. H. (2004). Psychological distress: Concept analysis. *Journal of Advanced Nursing*, *45*(5), 536–545.

Rosenfield, S. (2012). Triple jeopardy? Mental health at the intersection of gender, race, and class. *Social Science and Medicine*, *74*(11), 1791–1801.

Størksen, I., Røysamb, E., Holmen, T. L., & Tambs, K. (2006). Adolescent adjustment and well-being: Effects of parental divorce and distress. *Scandinavian Journal of Psychology*, *47*(1), 75–84.

Szklo, M., & Nieto, F. J. (2014). *Epidemiology: Beyond the basics*. Burlington, MA: Jones & Bartlett Publishers.

Taylor, R. D., & Roberts, D. (1995). Kinship support and maternal and adolescent well-being in economically disadvantaged African-American families. *Child Development*, *66*(6), 1585–1597.

Walen, H. R., & Lachman, M. E. (2000). Social support and strain from partner, family, and friends: Costs and benefits for men and women in adulthood. *Journal of Social and Personal Relationships*, *17*(1), 5–30.

Wheaton, B. (2007). The twain meet: Distress, disorder and the continuing conundrum of categories (comment on Horwitz). *Health*, *11*(3), 303–319.

FAMILIAL SUPPORT AND MENTAL HEALTH SERVICE USE: DIFFERENCES AMONG FIRST- AND SECOND-GENERATION ASIAN AMERICAN AND LATINX OLDER ADULTS

Jessica Valles

ABSTRACT

Purpose – *Drawing from theories of modernization and socioemotional selectivity, this study investigates the effect of familial support on the relationship between immigrant generation and mental health service use for Asian American and Latinx older adults.*

Methodology/Approach – *Using the data from the National Latino and Asian American Study (NLAAS) 2002–2003, nested logistic regressions (*N *= 810) were used to test the effects of familial support (parent–child relationship quality) on the relationship between immigrant generation and the use of mental health services. Differences in familial support between older adults and their younger counterparts were also accounted for.*

Findings – *The results indicate that familial support partially attenuates the relationship between immigrant generation and mental health service use, but only for Latinx groups. Familial support was not significantly different for older adults than that of those younger in age.*

Underserved and Socially Disadvantaged Groups and Linkages with Health and Health Care Differentials
Research in the Sociology of Health Care, Volume 37, 33–52

ISSN: 0275-4959/doi:10.1108/S0275-495920190000037006

Research Limitations/Implications – *Findings suggest the need for a better understanding of familial support as it relates to mental health service use for these groups. Approaches to improving the access to, and the overall use of, mental health services should be sensitive to ethnic variation. Immigrant groups may also endure stressors associated with legal and citizenship status. Future research should consider the effect of these political identities on mental health. Studies on parent–child relationship quality should also be longitudinal in order to better understand the dynamic nature of familial support across the life course.*

Originality/Value of Paper – *This chapter addresses gaps in the literature as Asian Americans are relatively understudied group with regard to mental health. Previous studies showed that US-born Asian American and Latinx populations are more likely to use mental health services than their foreign-born counterparts, but the effects of generation status and familial support for older adults are unclear.*

Keywords: Familial support; parent–child relationships; mental health; service use; Asian American; Latinx; ethnicity; immigrant health

INTRODUCTION

Immigration and aging are two dynamic social processes. Given the nondiscriminatory nature of the aging process, virtually everyone will find themselves subject to inevitable changes in their cognitive and physical abilities. Immigration is an issue that continues to gain attention, particularly in the United States. According to the Office of Immigration Statistics Annual Flow Report, 1,051,031 persons became new lawful permanent residents (LPRs) of the United States, with Asia as a leading country of origin, accounting for 40% of total LPRs (U.S. Department of Homeland Security, 2017). Latinx are the largest minority group, accounting for approximately 17% of the total US population – a ninefold increase since 1960 (Pew Research Center, 2016). This population accounted for about 35% of foreign-born immigrants in 2014 (Pew Research Center, 2016). With Asian American and Latinx families both bearing a strong sense of family cohesion and familial support, it would seem intuitive that the duties of caregiving and emotional support for aging family members would occur in the home. This thesis seeks to measure the relationship between familial support and the use of mental health services. This relationship will compare first- and second-generation older adults of Asian and Latinx ancestry.

The population of those aged 65 and older is projected to increase, accounting for 20% of the total population by 2050 – a 105% increase from 2014 (US Census Bureau, 2014). The immigration of working age groups is projected to slow the aging of the population (US Census Bureau, 2014). Immigration will create a far more racially and ethnically diverse population of older adults.

This growing population is expected to demand more care resources and may present challenges in various sectors of the health care system such as policy, social security, and insurance programs. At the microlevel, these demographic changes will also affect families and the nature of caregiving within them (Ortman, Velkoff, & Hogan, 2014).

According to Fuligni, Tseng, and Lam (1999), American families of Asian descent have often been characterized as placing a strong emphasis on familial responsibility and obligation. Filial piety refers to the traditional Confucian view that children – particularly sons – are responsible for the obligatory physical and emotional care of their aging parents (Ng, Phillips, & Lee, 2002). Existing literature suggests that although behaviors believed to satisfy obligations of filial piety are undergoing modification as a result of modernization, the notions of obligation and obedience still bear strong sentimental value and influence in Eastern regions of the world (Cheng & Chan, 2006).

Familism, a core component of Hispanic culture, is the collective focus of well-being; it refers to the prioritized sentiment of family well-being over that of the individual (Landale & Oropesa, 2007). It emphasizes the importance of family closeness, the trust between family members, loyalty, and the overall family orientation (Lorenzo-Blacno & Cortina, 2013; Rivera, 2007). Similar to that of filial piety, existing literature suggests that while its observable practice has changed over time, the attitudes of familism still remain (Lara, Gamboa, Kahramanian, Morales, & Hayes, 2005; Sabogal, Marin, Otero-Sabogal, Marin, & Perez-Stable, 1987).

Family Support

Foreign-born populations and subsequent generations advance through the life course in a Western context. As such, questions of consistency in the obligation and active engagement toward familial support arise. Acculturation and assimilation are the immediate *and* latent mechanisms by which immigrants come to adapt to their new country of residence (Gans, 2007). These mechanisms may also affect the ways in which different immigrant generations provide care and support to their parents emotionally. In the Asian context, family support comes through filial piety. In the Latinx context, the concept of familism is important. Further, these mechanisms may also affect whether aging parents will use mental health services. According to the data compiled from the National Survey on Drug Use and Health, Asian Americans are found to be the *least* likely to utilize mental health services compared to all other racial groups, and Latinx follow closely with the second lowest service use rate (Substance Abuse & Mental Health Services Administration, 2015). Although overall formal health service use is likely to be lower among foreign-born Asian American and Latinx immigrants (Abe-Kim et al., 2007; Alegria et al., 2007), a little is known about the effect familial support on generational differences in mental health service use, particularly for older adults.

THEORETICAL BACKGROUND

As their children mature, aging parents begin to experience a transitory period of role and status change, characterized by Merton's (1957) "status sequence." Rosow (1977) extends this process to the socialization of older adults, where these transitional experiences are more of a discontinuation in their major roles. As parents age, they exit various roles and statuses: as a parent with the absence of their adult children's dependence, as a worker with retirement, and as a spouse with the passing of their partners (Kim, Hurh, & Kim, 1993). As adult children lose their dependency on their parents, parents may become dependent on their adult children.

Socioemotional Selectivity Theory

Socioemotional selectivity theory (Carstensen, 1992) further elaborates on this notion of parental dependence on their adult children. As adults age, social exchanges and interactions are no longer motivated by instrumental desires, such as acquiring information. Instead, older adults increase their emotional investments in relationships with significant others – often their children or aging siblings – which translates into increasingly selective interactions with others in advancing age. While several studies have tested this theory empirically, there is a lack of its application in studying the immigrant populations and the generational differences in mental health service use.

Modernization

The economic characteristics of where someone and/or their parents are born may also affect the strength of familial traditions. According to Cowgill (Su & Ferraro, 1997), societies with a more advanced economic standing tend to lower the status of older adults. Goode (1963) emphasizes changes in the economic demands of full-time employment in industrialized societies and how that may affect the value of the extended family in an effort to focus on the nuclear family. While the aging process is one of inevitability, taking into account context – namely time and place – may offer an explanation of the variability in help-seeking behaviors, medicalization, and the care of the aging process given the emphasized nature of filial support and familism or "familismo" in Asian American families and Latinx families, respectively. That is, where someone and/or their parents are born may affect the strength of such familial traditions. With that said, it is important to acknowledge the role of age–period–cohort effects. Age effects speak specifically to the aforementioned inevitability of aging and are those that arise from the biological and social processes specific to aging (Yang, 2008). Period effects refer to those that arise from larger and external factors that may affect all age groups within a particular calendar time. Cohort effects are those that result from unique exposures to a certain group of people as they move through time (Yang, 2008). Therefore, in focusing on older adults by immigrant generation, the data and models in this analysis would speak more so to cohort and aging effects than to period effects.

How do industrialized Western economies affect the strength and consistency of family cohesion and familial obligation across generations of immigrants? Modernization theory would suggest that second-generation Asian American and Latinx older adults would have lower levels of familial support and be more likely to use mental health services. Socioemotional selectivity theory would predict that the effect of familial support on mental health services would be greater at older ages.

LITERATURE REVIEW

Existing literature analyzes immigrant populations, health, and family cohesion. However, there is little research on generational differences among immigrants in the care of older Asian American and Latinx adults and the effects that these differences may have on the utilization of mental health services.

Beliefs and Behaviors in Mental Health Services

There are cultural and structural reasons that Asian Americans and Latinx may not utilize mental health services; however, the literature on these reasons is relatively inconsistent. As previously mentioned, the rates of mental health service use are low for Asian American and Latinx populations, compared to all other racial groups. Alternatively, the rates of complementary and alternative medicine (CAM) are relatively high for both populations (Gallant, Spitze, & Grove, 2010). Asian Americans may frame their mental health in the context of somatic complaints. According to Lin and Cheung (1999), Asian Americans tend to hold traditions that view the body and mind as one unit, resulting in a patient's focus on more physically symptomatic ailments. Further, the existence of mental illness is often only acknowledged if it presents itself with disruptive behavior (Leong & Lau, 2001). A lack of service use may also be attributed to the behaviors and beliefs about accepting health services. Stigma and shame have been shown to act as barriers in seeking and utilizing mental health services (Leong & Lau, 2001). In a study by Tabora and Flaskeurd (1997), the fear of shame and the avoidance of damaging the family's reputation acted as a barrier to care for Chinese immigrant women. However, it has also been suggested that Asian Americans of Chinese descent rely heavily on friends and neighborhood networks for health-related help (Pang, Jordan-Marsh, Silverstein, & Cody, 2003). In a study of Korean Americans, Jang, Kim, Hansen, and Chiriboga (2007) also found that cultural beliefs played a significant role in shaping attitudes toward mental health services. Although Asian culture places an emphasis on the secrecy of personal problems or stress, Lee, Heo, Lu, and Portman (2013) found that elderly Asian Americans still found counseling to be important. This is particularly important, as "first-generation immigrants experience less depression and greater positive well-being than their native born [persons] of similar demographic and family background" (Harker, 2001, p. 969).

Latinx also experience cultural differences that may act as a barrier to mental health service use. When coping with mental health issues, Latinx tend to exercise greater levels of self-reliance, which may reduce formal service use (Chapman & Mullis, 2000). In tandem with personal beliefs, self-rated health has also been found to be a mediator on the relationship between mood disorders and mental health services for Latinx immigrant elders.

Informal caregiving can be an indicator of structural inadequacies, such as lack of health insurance coverage and low income. Immigrants tend to lack health literacy for accessing information in the health care system. In addition to language barriers, Chinese elders have suggested that "the American health care system [is] very confusing and intimidating" with policies and treatment coverage that seemed unclear (Pang et al., 2003, p. 869). Further, Pang et al. (2003) found that language efficiency is particularly important for navigating the health care system, including pharmaceutical inquiries and medication regimens. Limited English proficiency (LEP) was has also been found to significantly decrease Latinx immigrants' odds of using mental health services (Kim et al., 2011). The lack of bilingual clinicians may lead to inaccurate diagnoses or insufficient treatment remedies for mental health disorders that would also affect specialized mental health service use (Alegria et al., 2007).

Immigrant populations often struggle with Medicare coverage through more objective barriers, such as employment and insurance policies. Immigrant populations struggle with insurance coverage largely because of the amount of time that must pass before they can obtain sufficient work credits to qualify (Siddhartan, 1991). Even after adjusting for insurance coverage, low-income Latinx have significantly lower access to specialty service care than non-Latinx whites (Alegria et al., 2002). Thus, the use of mental health services – and overall health care system engagement – may be lower among first-generation Asian Americans and Latinx than among second-generation counterparts.

However, the transition to more positive views and heightened acceptance of health services is possible. The engagement in remedial programs for older adults can help diminish harsh effects of role emptying and status change (Kim et al., 1993). That is, as older adults begin to age out of major life roles, the socioemotional impacts may be less severe via role substitution – transitioning from parents to grandparents – alongside language programs, or training programs for volunteer work and/or activities that would enable older adults to take on meaningful roles for those they are helping, and themselves. Similarly, perceptions of counseling services, although met with some hesitancy, are improving (Lee et al., 2013). Despite the support in the literature for the strong function of stigma and secrecy for illness among Asian groups, it has also been suggested that some groups, including Chinese adults, rely heavily on friend and neighborhood networks for health-related assistance (Gallant et al., 2010). The importance and/or function of these same networks for Latinx, however, is less clear (Gallant et al., 2010). Altogether, these cultural and structural factors can affect the help-seeking behaviors – including service use – of foreign-born persons.

Filial Piety

Filial support can serve as a form of social support, particularly in Asian populations where norms of filial piety traditionally emphasize obligatory obedience and respect toward aging parents, caring for parents, regardless if healthy or sick, and coresidence (Cheng & Chan, 2006). However, the power of filial norms that emphasize coresidence of aging parents and adult children may be weakening (Lai & Surood, 2009). Trends in coresidence can vary when taking into account family structure. Coresidence between parents and their children is more common in bilateral family systems, like those in Thailand, the Philippines, and Malaysia, with daughters often having more prominent roles (Ofstedal, Knodel, & Chayovan, 1999). In contrast, sons have more prominent roles in caretaking in patrilineal or patriarchal family systems, such as in China and in India. Gender patterning in coresidence tends to be more pronounced when children are married (Ofstedal et al., 1999). When caregiving extends beyond coresidence, gender and marital status can be less significant. In terms of financial and material support, the gender and marital status of adult children is "muted" (Ofstedal et al., 1999). Given the slight cultural variations of who provides older adult care, this research will use familial support as a proxy for filial piety and familism.

Familism

Although very similar to practices of filial piety in Asian cultures in terms of strong devotions toward the family, familism is exclusive to Latinx culture. Familism emphasizes ties to both the extended and the nuclear family. In an effort to maintain these familial traditions, maintaining contact with all family members is important (Beyene, Becker, & Mayen, 2002). Adult children remain close to their parents and grandparents, as they often serve as a solution to the problems that may arise through daily interactions from a lack of English proficiency (Gallant et al., 2010; Hayes-Bautista, Hsu, Perez, & Gamboa, 2002). Whereas the support in filial piety is most often unidirectional from the adult children to their parents, older Latinx have been found to offer more support than they receive; they often provide assistance with household duties and childcare assistance (Sarkisian, Gerena, & Gerstel, 2007). These older adults also hold valuable roles in their children's lives, as they are often a main source for advice and help (Markides, Boldt, & Ray, 1986).

Western Influences

Fundamental changes to the structure of the family as a result of industrialization and urbanization may alter the practice of filial piety in a Western context (Cheng & Chan, 2006). As previously mentioned, Goode (1963) illustrates that the economic demands of full-time employment in industrialized society place a strong emphasis on the ability and efficiency of the individual and an overshadowing the extended family by the nuclear family (Goode, 1963). If adult children are urged to maximize their occupational mobility and efficiency, they "must distance themselves – both geographically and socially – from their parents or face socioeconomic stagnation" (Silverstein & Bengston, 1997, p. 430). This disconnect and separation of everyday affairs may lead to an insensitivity to the needs of the parents, given the focus on the adult child's own personal and familial needs (Kim et al., 1993). Thus, aging parents may need to turn to mental health services rather than their children.

Conversely, full-time employment does not necessarily conflict with caring for an aging parent or providing support. Rather, full-time employment can affect the kind of care administered. Those who work full-time are more likely to assist with daily living activities (e.g., eating, dressing, bathing) than instrumental daily living activities (e.g., household work, meal preparation, laundry) (Wolf & Soldo, 1994). Further, other conflicting arguments in the literature suggest that despite residing in a Western society that promotes and values individuality, a child's obligations to their parents continues to resonate with subsequent generations (Lai & Surood, 2009).

Shifts in Family Expectations and Networks

In Asian countries, aging parents still reside with their adult children (Ofstedal et al., 1999). It is only under "compelling situations such as manpower insufficiency, in-house inconvenience or professional incompetence [that] descendants send senior citizens to a nursing institution" (Yen-Jen, 2007, p. 126). With the transition to Western society, foreign-born immigrants begin to experience a shift in their living arrangements, as well as in their social networks.

Much of the existing literature suggests that older foreign-born Asian Americans are experiencing more independent living. Aging parents are living independently from their children, whether in their own private residences or in senior apartments. Despite this, Pang et al. (2003) found that older adults do not report having difficulty obtaining help from their adult children when requested. Conversely, Latinx are more likely to reside in multigenerational households than their non-Latinx white counterparts (Sarkisian et al., 2007). Many of these immigrant parents understand the responsibilities of their adult children in Western economic settings and try not to inconvenience their family members (Pang et al., 2003). Filial piety emphasizes that children are the product of the labor, sacrifices, and efforts of the parents. Therefore, the achievements of their children (e.g., jobs, degrees) are directly tied to their meaning of life (Lee et al., 2013). On the same note, Latinx elders continue to hold valued positions within the family and are still willing to maintain ties with their families (Beyene et al., 2002).

However, the literature exhibits a few inconsistencies. Kim, Jang, Chiriboga, Ma, and Schonfeld (2010) suggest that immigrant parents may not clearly understand the demands of American employment or the children's Western obligations. The different life conditions of immigrant parents and those of their native-born children may create misunderstandings that of which may lead to conflicts in the expectations that the parents hold for children's reverent behavior (Kim et al., 1993). Lee et al. (2013) found that some parents condemn the lack of parental support from children regardless if children are successful. On the same note, higher achievement, namely education, correlates with less familial support and obedience to parents (Lai & Surood, 2009). Older parents in China who live independently reported receiving inadequate care and financial support from their children (Ng, Phillips, & Lee, 2002). In the United States, those living in senior housing communities rely heavily on the support of neighbors, friends, and management (Pang et al., 2003). Older adults, who live independent of their children, but not in institutional settings, also rely heavily on the support from their neighbors and church communities (Kim et al., 1993). As previously mentioned, there is not enough literature to discern whether the function of neighbors operates similarly for Latinx, but church communities do serve as a vital network of support for older adults (Gallant et al., 2010).

Recall that language barriers may complicate the care for aging parents. Language barriers also initiate cultural shifts in social networks for aging parents who lack the presence of their adult children. As foreign-born parents age, living outside of their formerly familiar ethnic communities, they are limited in opportunities to build diverse social relationships (Lee et al., 2013). They are unable to socialize efficiently with other cultural groups. Further, foreign-born persons of Asian descent tend to "define themselves through their origin of birth ethnicity," and their relationships are primarily with those from the same ethnic group (Lee et al., 2013, p. 11). Unlike the diversity among Asian groups, Latinx are united by a shared language (Landale & Oropesa, 2007) which may foster better conditions for building social relationships with those who may share origins of ethnicity, but may not necessarily be of the same ethnic group.

One must also consider the potential for network shifts and inconsistencies in filial piety given the changes in life stages of adult children. Many adulthood transitions such as education completion, marriage, and childrearing have been steadily occurring later in life (Harris, 2010). As the average age difference between parents and their children increases, the ability of children to care for their aging parents becomes less certain given possible delays in financial stability and time preoccupations. These inconsistencies and complications bring into question the availability and quality of aging immigrant parents' support networks, particularly in the face of relationship changes with adult children as a result of Western influence.

DATA AND METHODS

In order to properly assess the validity and significance of these concepts, I will begin by performing secondary data analysis with data gathered in the National Latino and Asian American Study (NLAAS), 2002–2003. As part of a broader project, the Collaborative Psychiatric Epidemiology Studies (CPES), NLAAS provides nationally representative data consisting of 2,554 Latinx respondents and 2,095 Asian American respondents. It examines both the lifetime and 12-month prevalence of mental disorders, as well as the rates of mental health service use for these populations. This study aimed to assess the social, environmental, and psychosocial factors associated with mental health and mental health service use. All samples in CPES, including NLAAS, were selected using stratified probability sampling. Survey collection was conducted in 252 geographic areas or other primary sampling units across the country, 18 of which were unique to NLAAS.

Only 25% of the sample was asked mental health service questions, and another 25% of the sample was lost due to respondent's indicating they had no children; in order to be present on the familial support variable, respondents must have at least one child. Missingness for all other variables in the study was for negligible reason and were handled using listwise deletion. The final sample size was 810. Analyses were conducted as a complete case analysis in which nested logistic regressions estimated the models for missingness, ensuring a consistent sample size.

Upon collecting data from the following measures, I will conduct a series bivariate analyses and logistic regressions to test the following hypotheses:

> *H1.* Second-generation Asian Americans and Latinx are more likely to use mental health services than their first-generation counterparts.
>
> *H2.* First-generation Asian Americans and Latinx will have greater levels of familial support than their second-generation counterparts.
>
> *H3.* The relationship between immigrant generation and mental health service use is accounted for by familial support.
>
> *H4.* The effect of familial support on mental health service use varies by age.

This study seeks to understand the role of socioemotional selectivity, which focuses on older adults. However, in order to assess SST, addressed in *H4*, the general relationships between immigrant generation, familial support, and mental health service use must be analyzed. As previously noted, differences in service use between immigrant generation may in part be due to acculturative processes. Therefore, in order to test the effect of familial support on the relationship between immigrant generation and mental health service use for older adults, *H1* and *H2* must be included in my analyses before addressing *H3* and *H4*.

Variables

Mental Health Service Use

The NLAAS asks, "Did you ever in your lifetime go to see any of the following professionals for problems with your emotions, nerves or mental health, or your use of alcohol or drugs?" (i.e., psychiatrist, general practitioner, other medical doctor or specialty professional, psychologist, social worker, counselor, mental health nurse, or any other professional). A dummy variable has been created in which (1) represents those who indicate having been seen by a health professional and (0) represents those who were not.

Ancestry and Immigrant Generation

Respondents were asked whether they were born in the United States or in another country. They were also asked to indicate their ancestral origins. Dummy variables were created to encompass all those of Asian ancestry and those of Latinx ancestry. Another dummy variable was created to account for those born in and outside of the United States. Because the aim of this study is to make immigrant-generational comparisons on service use, not ancestral or ethnic comparisons, a new variable was created representing (1) first-generation Asian Americans, (2) second-generation Asians Americans, (3) first-generation Latinx, and (4) second-generation Latinx.

Familial Support

Familial support is measured by the respondent's scaled rating of their relationship with their child. The question asks, "On a scale from 0–10 where 0 means 'the worst possible relationship' and 10 means 'the best possible relationship', how would you rate your relationship with your children these days?" Because this variable is skewed – most respondents report having a good relationship with their child/children, I will be using the natural log of this variable.

Controls

Although this study focuses on older adults, those younger than 55 years of age will still be included. Because SST suggests that older adults are more likely to have closer relationships with their children than those who are younger, including younger adults will allow for comparison. Therefore, interaction analyses will be used to test whether the effect of familial support on the relationship between immigrant generation and mental health service use varies by age. Other controls to be considered are sex, income, marital status, and insurance coverage. The variables for marital status and insurance coverage have been recoded as dummy variables (Table 1).

RESULTS

Ancestry/Immigrant-generation and Mental Health Service Use

To begin, I want to test whether my independent variable – ancestry and immigrant generation – and my dependent variable – mental health service use are related. As both are categorical variables, I conducted basic bivariate analyses using a chi-square test. The results indicate a significant association between these two variables ($p < 0.05$). Regression analyses have been recorded in the tables below. As shown in Tables 2 and 3, Model 1 indicates the significant association between ancestry *and* immigrant generation, and mental health service use.

Sex, Marital Status, and Familial Support

For each model that they were included in, sex and marital status remained significant. Compared to men, women had just over twice the odds of using mental

Table 1. Descriptive Statistics and Variables for Analysis by Ancestry and Immigrant Generation ($N = 810$).

	First-generation Asians	Second-generation Asians	First-generation Latinx	Second-generation Latinx
Sex %				
Female	55.56	57.89	56.36	53.70
Male	44.44	42.11	43.64	46.30
Age	48 (12.95)	44 (14.31)†	46 (14.53)	40 (12.65)†
Marital status %				
Married	90.42	71.93†	73.64	70.37
Not married	9.58	28.07	26.36	29.63
Income	US$73,583 (62,285.3)	US$79,762 (54,527.91)	US$40,600 (47,481.18)	US$57,913 (50,892.06)†
Insurance coverage %				
Yes	86.97	89.47	66.97	80.86†
No	13.03	10.53	33.03	19.14
Mental health service use %				
Yes	14.56	28.07†	26.36	40.74†
No	85.44	71.93	73.64	59.26
Familial support*	2.21 (0.138)	2.18 (0.144)	2.22 (0.163)	2.18 (0.275)†
N	261	57	330	162

Notes: *Unlogged mean 9.15.
†Significantly different from respective first-generation ethnic group.

health services, when all other variables are controlled for ($p < 0.05$). Compared to their non-married counterparts, those who are married had about half the odds of using mental health services, when all other variables controlled for ($p < 0.05$). When introduced as the mediating variable, familial support was significant at the $p < 0.05$ level. Bearing in mind that this is a logged variable, a 1% increase in familial support decreases the odds of using mental health services by 0.32.

Hypothesis 1

H1 stated that mental health service use would be greater among the second generation Asian Americans and Latinx than that of the first generation. As shown in Table 2, Model 1 second-generation Asian Americans had 2.29 the odds of using mental health services compared to their first-generation counterparts, net of controls ($p < 0.05$). However, once controls were added, this relationship was no longer significant (Table 2, Model 2), indicating that marital status and sex explained this difference. Before adding controls, second-generation Latinx had nearly twice (1.92) the odds of using mental health

Table 2. Logistic Regression for Mental Health Service Use with First-generation Asian Americans as Reference Group Using Data of the National Latino and Asian American Survey 2002–2003, Odds Ratios (OR) and 95% Confidence Intervals (CI).

	Model 1		Model 2		Model 3		Model 4	
	OR	95% CI	OR	95% CI	OR	95% CI	OR	95% CI
Ancestry/immigrant generation (First-gen Asian Americans)								
Second-gen Asian Americans	2.29*	(1.17, 4.49)	1.97	(0.99, 3.98)	1.95	(0.97, 3.93)	1.93	(0.96, 3.89)
First-gen Latinx	2.10**	(1.38, 3.20)	2.03**	(1.29, 3.19)	2.06**	(1.31, 3.25)	2.06**	(1.31, 3.24)
Second-gen Latinx	† 4.03***	(2.53, 6.43)	† 3.87***	(2.35, 6.36)	† 3.79***	(2.30, 6.23)	† 3.74***	(2.26, 6.18)
Sex (male)								
Female			2.17***	(1.52, 3.10)	2.29***	(1.59, 3.30)	2.29***	(1.59, 3.30)
Age			0.99	(0.98, 1.01)	0.99	(0.98, 1.01)	0.99	(0.98, 1.01)
Marital status (not married)								
Married			0.52**	(0.35, 0.76)	0.56**	(0.37, 0.83)	0.56**	(0.36, 0.83)
Income			1.00	(0.99, 1.00)	1.00	(0.99, 1.00)	1.00	(0.99, 1.00)
Insurance coverage (no)								
Yes			1.35	(0.88, 2.08)	1.34	(0.87, 2.07)	1.35	(0.87, 2.08)
Familial support					0.32*	(0.12, 0.81)	0.32*	(0.12, 0.83)
Family support × age							1.02	(0.95, 1.09)
								$N = 810$

Note: †Significantly different from first-gen Latinx, $p < 0.05$.

Table 3. Logistic Regression for Mental Health Service Use with First-generation Latinx as Reference Group Using Data of the National Latino and Asian American Survey 2002–2003, Odds Ratios (OR) and 95% Confidence Intervals (CI).

	Model 1		Model 2		Model 3		Model 4	
	OR	95% CI	OR	95% CI	OR	95% CI	OR	95% CI
Ancestry/immigrant generation (First-gen Latinx)								
Second-gen Latinx	1.92**	(1.29, 2.86)	1.91**	(1.24, 2.91)	1.84**	(1.19, 2.82)	1.82**	(1.18, 2.79)
First-gen Asian Americans	0.48**	(0.31, 0.73)	0.49**	(0.31, 0.77)	0.48**	(0.31, 0.76)	0.48**	(0.31, 0.76)
Second-gen Asian Americans	†1.09	(0.58, 2.04)	0.98	(0.50, 1.89)	0.94	(48, 1.84)	0.93	(0.48, 1.83)
Sex (Male)								
Female			2.17***	(1.52, 3.10)	2.29***	(1.59, 3.30)	2.29***	(1.59, 3.30)
Age			0.99	(0.98, 1.01)	0.99	(0.98, 1.01)	0.99	(0.98, 1.01)
Marital status (not married)								
Married			0.52**	(0.35, 0.76)	0.56**	(0.37, 0.83)	0.56**	(0.36, 0.83)
Income			1.00	(0.99, 1.00)	1.00	(0.99, 1.00)	1.00	(0.99, 1.00)
Insurance coverage (no)								
Yes			1.35	(0.88, 2.08)	1.34	(0.87, 2.07)	1.35	(0.87, 2.08)
Familial support					0.32*	(0.12, 0.81)	0.32*	(0.12, 0.83)
Family support × age							1.02	(0.95, 1.09)
								$N = 810$

Note: †Significantly different from first-gen Asian Americans, $p < 0.05$.

services compared to their first-generation counterparts ($p < 0.05$). After adding considering controls, as shown in Table 3, Model 2 second-generation Latinx remained nearly twice as likely to use mental health services, although partially attenuated by sex and marital status.

Therefore, *H1* was supported for only Latinx, albeit it weak. The association was no longer significant for second-generation Asian Americans once marital status and sex were incorporated into the model.

Hypothesis 2

H2 stated that familial support would be greater for first-generation Asian American and Latinx than that of the second-generation. After running a bivariate analysis, the ANOVA test showed that the overall relationship between ancestry/immigrant generation and familial support was not significant ($p > 0.05$). However, while checking for differences between the ancestry/immigrant-generation groups, a simple linear regression showed that first-generation Latinx had a 0.042 difference on familial support compared to their second-generation counterparts. Post-tests showed that there was no significant differences in familial support between first- and second-generation Asian Americans. Although first-generation Latinx have more familial support than their second-generation counterparts, the relationship is not the same for first- and second-generation Asian Americans. Thus, there is partial support for *H2*.

Hypothesis 3

H3 stated that the relationship between immigrant generation and mental health service use is attenuated by familial support. Familial support was significant for both Asian American and Latinx second-generation immigrants. As shown in Table 2, Model 3 familial support is related to mental health service use, although the odds ratio from second-generation Asian Americans for mental health service use remained unchanged and non-significant. Recall that the relationship between mental health service and second-generation Asian Americans was explained away controls, namely sex and marital status. Thus, *H3* was not supported for Asian Americans.

As shown in Table 3 once taking into account familial support, the odd ratios for second-generation Latinx decreased from Models 2–3 (1.91–1.84), where the association remained significant. Thus, familial support explained some of the difference of mental health service use between first- and second-generation Latinx, providing partial support for *H3*.

Hypothesis 4

H4 stated that the effect of familial support on mental health service use varies by age. As shown in Tables 2 and 3, Model 4, interactions between familial support and age (centered at the mean) show that the effect of familial support on mental health service use does not vary by age. To be sure, quintiles of age were created to check for non-linear effects of age. These results were also not significant; moderating effects of age did not occur.

DISCUSSION AND LIMITATIONS

These results show that familial support partially explains the relationship between immigrant generation and mental health service use, but only for Latinx. It is possible that although family is important for these populations, the function of family with regard to mental health service use may operate differently for these two groups. Ethnic identity is an another factor to consider. Familial support can vary by ethnicity for Asian Americans, in particular. Compared to Latinx who are united by a common language – which may foster better conditions in building meaningful relationships – foreign-born persons of Asian descent tend to "define themselves through their origin of birth ethnicity" and their relationships are primarily with those from the same ethnic group (Lee et al., 2013, p. 11). Although these populations are united by being classified as Asian American, their different ethnic identities may bear implications for variation in their conditions of familial support.

Marital status and sex were significant measures for both ethnic and immigrant-generation groups. Compared to their unmarried counterparts, married Asian Americans and Latinx had half the odds of using mental health services. Asian Americans have been found to rely less on social support as a means for coping with stress when compared to their European American counterparts (Taylor et al., 2004). Latinx are far more likely to have larger families, where more than half of Latinx women in the United States have more three or more children (Pew Research Center, 2015). Family caregiving is associated with psychological distress (Schulz, Visintainer, & Williamson, 1990; Skaff & Pearlin, 1992), which is important to consider for women in large families that may experience greater levels financial burden, role strain, and overall caregiver stress. Compared to men, Asian American and Latinx women had nearly twice the odds of using mental health services. There is a growing body of literature suggesting that males are less likely to seek professional help for their health than their female counterparts (Husaini, Moore, & Cain, 1994; McKay, Rutherford, Cacciola, & Kabasakalian-McKay, 1996; Padesky & Hammen, 1981; Thom, 1986; Weissman & Klerman, 1977). Existing literature using gender and masculinity theories has posited that men are less likely to use formal health services as the result of socialization and the belief that seeking help denotes femininity and weakness (Addis & Mahalik, 2003). However, further exploration as to how these theories apply to both different ethnic populations and immigrant generations is needed.

It should also be noted that the odds of mental health service use increased for married person and women once familial support was added to the model. Future research should consider paradoxical effects of familial support including, but not limited to, aspects that may attribute to role strain – particularly when a parent is employed (Barnett & Baruch, 1985; Erdwins et al., 2001;

Pearlin, 1983) – and the varying effects of family size (Nye, Carlson, & Garrett, 1970).

There are several limitations to this study that must be addressed. To begin, because no question in the study asked specifically about whether a child felt deep obligation to their parent, I was unable to measure filial piety. However, given that familial support served as the proxy for this study, measuring closeness between parents and their children was a better measure for socioemotional selectivity theory.

It should also be noted that this is a cross-sectional analysis and provides only a snapshot of the sample's behaviors and interactions. A longitudinal analysis of these measures would provide a more accurate depiction for these associations. That is, longitudinal analyses would check trends in changes over time regarding parent–child relationships and mental health service use, as well as for effects on pattern variation by immigration period.

Original analyses attempted to account for acculturative processes that may have an effect on the relationship between immigrant generation and mental health service use. The number of years that the respondents have resided in the United States was set at a minimum of five years for those who were born in another country. However, the number of years living in the United States in this study would only apply to part of the population – only those from the first-generation of both ethnic groups.

Immigrant populations may also face stressors related to legal or citizenship status identities. Furthermore, some immigrant groups may face differing levels of acculturative stress which can affect mental health outcomes. Future analyses should not only use better measures for acculturation but also consider the effects of legal or citizenship status.

Support for modernization theories was found, indicating that the individualization processes of being a second-generation immigrant lead to greater mental health service needs. Although there is no support for socioemotional selectivity theory, it is possible that different results could be yielded if other measures were available to test SST. Questions about particular child-to-parent interactions, such as caregiving, and physical, emotional, and/or economic support may serve as better measures for this study, and for SST, in general.

CONCLUSION

The analyses in this study showed that the odds of mental health service use are significantly different for second-generation Asian Americans, but only when other sociodemographic measures are not controlled for. The odds of mental health service use for second-generation Latinx were shown to be significantly different from their first-generation counterparts, net of controls. This relationship was partially attenuated by familial support. Support for socioemotional selectivity theory to different immigrant generations was unsuccessful; however, limitations in the data set serve as implications for future research. That is, measures that are directly related to child–parent interactions – and the kinds of interactions – may yield different results for this study and also serve as more accurate measures for testing SST, in general. Doing so would also aid in applying SST to other racial and ethnic groups, as these different groups may offer different responses regarding not only their perceptions of child–parent relationships but also child-to-parent interactions such as caregiving and support.

REFERENCES

Abe-Kim, J., Takeuchi, D. T., Hong, S., Zane, N., Sue, S., Spencer, M. S., ... Alegria, M. (2007). Use of mental health–related services among immigrant and US-born Asian Americans: Results from the National Latino and Asian American study. *American Journal of Public Health*, *97*(1), 91–98.

Addis, M. E., & Mahalik, J. R. (2003). Men, masculinity, and the contexts of help seeking. *American Psychologist*, *58*(1), 5–14.

Alegria, M., Canino, G., Rios, R., Vera, M., Calderon, J., Rusch, D., & Ortega, A. N. (2002). Inequalities in use of specialty mental health services among Latinos, African Americans, and Non-Latino Whites. *Psychiatric Services*, *53*(12), 1547–1555.

Alegria, M., Mulvaney-Day, N., Torres, M., Gao, S., Oddo, V., & Woo, M. (2007). Correlates of past-year mental health service use among Latinos: Results from the National Latino and Asian American study. *American Journal of Public Health*, *97*(1), 76–83.

Barnett, R. C., & Baruch, G. K. (1985). Women's involvement in multiple roles, and psychological distress. *Journal of Personality and Social Psychology*, *49*(1), 135–145.

Beyene, Y., Becker, G., & Mayen, N. (2002). Perception of aging and sense of well-being among Latino elderly. *Journal of Cross-Cultural Gerontology*, *17*(2), 155–172.

Carstensen, L. L. (1992). Social and emotional patterns in adulthood: Support for emotional selectivity theory. *Psychology and Aging*, *7*(3), 331–338.

Chapman, P. L., & Mullis, R. (2000). Racial differences in adolescent coping and self-esteem. *Journal of Genetic Psychology*, *161*(2), 152–160.

Cheng, S.-T., & Chan, A. C. M. (2006). Filial piety and psychological well-being in well older Chinese. *Journals of Gerontology*, *61*(5), 262–269.

Erdwins, C. J., Buffardi, L. C., Casper, W. J., & O'Brien, A. S. (2001). The relationships of women's role strain to social support, role satisfaction, and self-efficacy. *Family Relations*, *50*(1), 230–238.

Fuligni, A. J., Tseng, V., & Lam, M. (1999). Attitudes toward family obligations among American adolescents with Asian, Latin American, and European backgrounds. *Child Development*, *70*(1), 1030–1044.

Husaini, B. A., Moore, S. T., & Cain, V. A. (1994). Psychiatric symptoms and help-seeking behavior among the elderly. *Journal of Gerontological Social Work*, *21*, 177–196.

Gallant, M. P., Spitze, G., & Grove, J. G. (2010). Chronic illenss self-care and the family lives of older adults: A synthetic review across four ethnic groups. *Journal of Cross-Cultural Gerontology*, *25*(1), 21–43.

Gans, H. J. (2007). Acculturation, assimilation and mobility. *Ethnic and Racial Studies*, *30*(1), 152–164.

Goode, W. J. (1963). *World revolution and family patterns*. New York, NY: Free Press.

Harker, K. (2001). Immigrant generation, assimilation, adolescent psychological well-being. *Social Forces*, *79*(3), 969–1004.

Harris, K. M. (2010). An integrative approach to health. *Demography*, *47*(1), 1–22.

Hayes-Bautista, D. E., Hsu, P., Perez, A., & Gamboa, C. (2002). The 'Browning' of the graying of America: Diversity in the elderly population and policy implications. *Generations*, *26*(3), 15–24.

Jang, Y., Kim, G., Hansen, L., & Chiriboga, D. A. (2007). Attitudes of older Korean Americans toward mental health services. *Journal of the American Geriatrics Society*, *55*(4), 616–620.

Kim, G., Aguado Loi, C. X., Chiriboga, D. A., Jang, Y., Parmelee, P., & Allen, R. S. (2011). Limited English proficiency as a barrier to mental health service use: A study of Latino and Asian immigrants with psychiatric disorders. *Journal of Psychiatric Research*, *45*(1), 104–110.

Kim, G., Jang, Y., Chiriboga, D. A., Ma, G. X., & Schonfeld, L. (2010). Factors associated with mental health service use in Latino and Asian immigrant elders. *Aging and Mental Health*, *14*(5), 535–542.

Kim, K. C., Hurh, W. M., & Kim, S. (1993). Generation differences in Korean immigrants' life conditions in the United States. *Sociological Perspectives*, *36*(3), 257–270.

Lai, D. W. L., & Surood, S. (2009). Filial piety in Chinese Canadian family caregivers. *International Journal of Sociology of the Family*, *35*(1), 89–104.

Landale, N. S., & Oropesa, R. S. (2007). Hispanic families: Stability and change. *Annual Review of Sociology*, *33*(1), 381–405.

Lara, M., Gamboa, C., Kahramanian, I. M., Morales, L. S., & Hayes, D. E. (2005). Acculturation and Latino health in the United States: A review of the literature and its sociopolitical context. *Annual Review of Public Health*, *26*(1), 367–397.

Lee, J. H., Heo, N., Lu, J., & Portman, T. A. A. (2013). Qualitative exploration of acculturation and life-span issues of elderly Asian Americans. *Adultspan Journal*, *12*(1), 4–23.

Leong, F. T. L., & Lau, A. S. L. (2001). Barriers to providing effective mental health services to Asian Americans. *Mental Health Services Research*, *3*(4), 201–214.

Lin, K.-M., & Cheung, F. (1999). Mental health issues for Asian Americans. *Psychiatric Sciences*, *50*(6), 774–780.

Lorenzo-Blanco, E. I., & Cortina, L. M. (2013). Latino/a depression and smoking: An analysis through the lenses of culture, gender, and ethnicity. *American Journal of Community Psychology*, *51*(3), 332–346.

Markides, K. S., Boldt, J. S., & Ray, L. A. (1986). Sources of helping and intergenerational solidarity: A three-generations study of Mexican Americans. *Journal of Gerontology*, *41*(4), 506–511.

McKay, J. R., Rutherford, M. J., Cacciola, J. S., & Kabasakalian-McKay, R. (1996). Gender differences in the relapse experiences of cocaine patients. *Journal of Nervous and Mental Disease*, *184*, 616–622.

Merton, R. (1957). *Social theory and social structure*. Glencoe, IL: Free Press.

Ng, A. C. Y., Phillips, D. R., & Lee, W. K. (2002). Persistence and challenges to filial piety and informal support of older persons in a modern Chinese society: A case study in Tuen Mun, Hong Kong. *Journal of Aging Studies*, *16*(2), 135–153. doi:10.1016/S0890–4065(02)00040-3

Nye, I. F., Carlson, J., & Garrett, G. (1970). Family size, interaction, affect and stress. *Journal of Marriage and Family*, *32*(2), 216–226.

Ofstedal, M. B., Knodel, J., & Chayovan, N. (1999). Intergenerational support and gender: A comparison of Four Asian countries. *Southeast Asian Journal of Social Science*, *27*(2), 21–42.

Ortman, J. M., Velkoff, V. A., Hogan, H., & U.S. Department of Commerce. (2014). *An AGINGNATIOn: The older population in the United States*. Washington, DC: U.S. Government Printing Office.

Padesky, C. A., & Hammen, C. L. (1981). Sex differences in depressive symptom expression and help-seeking among college students. *Sex Roles*, *3*(1), 309–320.

Pang, E. C., Jordan-Marsh, M., Silverstein, M., & Cody, M. (2003). Health-seeking behaviors of elderly Chinese Americans: Shifts in expectations. *The Gerontologist*, *43*(6), 864–874.

Pearlin, L. I. (1983). Role strains and personal stress. In H. B. Kaplan (Ed.), *Psychological stress: Trends in theory and research* (pp. 3–32). New York, NY: Academic Press.

Pew Research Center. (2015). *Family size among mothers*. Retrieved from http://www.pewsocialtrends.org/2015/05/07/family-size-among-mothers/. Accessed on November 12, 2017.

Pew Research Center. (2016). *Statistical portrait of the foreign-born population in the United States*. Retrieved from http://www.pewhispanic.org/2016/04/19/statistical-portrait-of-the-foreign-born-population-in-the-united-states-2014/. Accessed on April 19, 2017.

Rivera, F. I. (2007). Contextualizing the experience of young Latino Adults: Acculturation, social support and depression. *Journal of Immigrant and Minority Health*, *9*(3), 237–244.

Rosow, I. (1977). *Socialization to old age*. Berkeley, CA: University of California Press.

Sabogal, F., Marin, G., Otero-Sabogal, R., Marin, B. V., & Perez-Stable, E. J. (1987). Hispanic familism and acculturation: What changes and what doesn't? *Hispanic Journal of Behavioral Sciences*, *9*(4), 397–412.

Sarkisian, N., Gerena, M., & Gerstel, N. (2007). Extended family integration among Euro and Mexican Americans: Ethnicity, gender, and class. *Journal of Marriage and Family*, *69*(1), 40–54.

Schulz, R., Visintainer, P., & Williamson, G. M. (1990). Psychiatric and physical morbidity. *Journal of Gerontology*, *45*(5), 181–191.

Siddhartan, K. (1991). Health insurance coverage of the immigrant elderly. *Inquiry*, *28*(4), 403–412.

Silverstein, M., & Bengston, V. L. (1997). Intergenerational solidarity and the structure of adult child–parent relationships in American families. *American Journal of Sociology*, *103*(2), 429–460.

Skaff, M. M., & Pearlin, L. I. (1992). Caregiving: Role engulfment and the loss of self. *The Gerontologist*, *32*(5), 656–664.

Su, Y.-P., & Ferraro, K. F. (1997). Social relations and health assessments among older people: Do the effects of integration and social contributions vary cross-culturally? *Journal of Gerontology*, *52B*(1), S27–S36.

Substance Abuse and Mental Health Services Administration. (2015). *Racial/ethnic differences in mental health service use among adults*. HHS Publication No. SMA-15–4906. Rockville, MD.

Tabora, B. L., & Flaskerud, J. H. (1997). Mental health beliefs, practices, and knowledge of Chinese American immigrant women. *Issues in Mental Health Nursing*, *18*(3), 173–189.

Taylor, S. E., Sherman, D. K., Kim, H. S., Jarcho, J., Takagi, K., & Dunagan, M. S. (2004). Culture and social support: Who seeks it and why? *Journal of Personality and Social Psychology*, *87*(3), 354–362.

Thom, B. (1986). Sex differences in help-seeking for alcohol problems-1. The barriers to help-seeking. *Addiction*, *81*(6), 777.

U.S. Census Bureau. (2014). *An agingnation: The older population in the United States*. Washington, DC: U.S. Census Bureau.

U.S. Department of Homeland Security. Office of Immigration Statistics. (2017). U.S. lawful permanent residents: 2015. *Annual flow report*. Retrieved from https://www.dhs.gov/sites/default/files/publications/Lawful_Permanent_ResidentR_2015.pdf. Accessed on October 10, 2016.

Weissman, M. M., & Klerman, G. L. (1977). Sex differences and the epidemiology of depression. *Archives of General Psychiatry*, *34*(1), 98–111.

Wolf, D. A., & Soldo, B. J. (1994). Married women's allocation of time to employment and care of elderly parents. *Journal of Human Resources*, *29*(4), 1259–1276.

Yang, Y. (2008). Social inequalities in happiness in the United States, 1972 to 2004: Age age-period-cohort analysis. *American Sociological Review*, *73*(2), 204–226.

Yen-Jen, C. (2007). More choices for families?: Changing elderly care models in Taiwan. *International Journey of Sociology of the Family*, *33*(1), 123–143.

PSYCHOLOGICAL DISTRESS DIFFERENTIALS AS A FUNCTION OF SUBJECTIVE SOCIAL STATUS AMONG LATINO SUBGROUPS IN THE UNITED STATES

Fernando I. Rivera, Kristine M. Molina and Ethel Nicdao

ABSTRACT

Purpose – *To investigate the association between subjective dimensions of socioeconomic status and psychological distress, paying particular attention to Latino subgroup differences.*

Methodology/Approach – *We used data from the Latino sample (*N = *2,554) of the National Latino and Asian American Study (NLAAS). For our main analyses, we conducted a series of weighted multivariable linear regressions.*

Findings – *The results showed that subjective social status was associated with reduced psychological distress.*

Research Limitations/Implications – *There are several key study limitations that warrant consideration. Chiefly, data utilized were cross-sectional; thus, it is unclear whether subjective socioeconomic status (SES) precedes or follows psychological distress.*

Originality/Value of Paper – *Overall, our study makes several contributions to the sociological study of mental health differentials among Latinos. We*

Underserved and Socially Disadvantaged Groups and Linkages with Health and Health Care Differentials
Research in the Sociology of Health Care, Volume 37, 53–67

ISSN: 0275-4959/doi:10.1108/S0275-495920190000037007

show the importance of the association between subjective SES indicators and psychological distress. We also demonstrate how the associations analyzed in this study varied by Latino subethnicity, which we argue is an important step to fully understand the different social processes associated with the mental health of different Latina/o groups.

Keywords: Health differentials; subjective social status; Latino/as; psychological distress; objective social status; sociocultural; Latino subethnicity

Prior research investigating the mental health of Latinos in the United States has found that, as a group, Latinos fare better than Whites (Kessler et al., 2005) despite facing a host of unfavorable social and economic conditions (Markides & Eschbach, 2005; Riosmena, Root, Humphrey, Steiner, & Stubbs, 2015). Furthermore, when compared with other racial and ethnic groups, some Latino groups (mainly Latin American immigrants and US-born Latinos) have higher life expectancies and lower mortality rates (Riosmena et al., 2015). On the surface, it seems that some Latino groups might have a health advantage, but other health differentials are displayed when looking at the social location of Latino groups within a social structure. In the US context, Latinos have higher rates of living in poverty, unemployment, and low-wage jobs, while having lower rates of educational attainment when compared to non-Latino Whites (Motel & Patten, 2012). The individual's location or position within the social hierarchy has the potential to create considerable stress if the demands of the position are incompatible with the resources available to deal with them.

To further compound these issues, the analyses of Latino subethnic groups' mental health profiles reveal significant differences. For instance, Cubans typically display the most favorable mental health outcomes, while Puerto Ricans display the worst, with Mexicans and other Latino ethnic groups falling in between (Alegría et al., 2007; Rivera et al., 2008). Several correlates have been investigated to understand these differences, including acculturation levels (Ortega, Rosenheck, Alegria, & Desai, 2000; Rivera, 2007) and other factors such as migratory history, English language proficiency (Alegría et al., 2007), nativity (Alegría et al., 2008; Dey & Lucas, 2006), and years in the United States (Cook, Alegria, Lin, & Guo, 2009). Gender differences have also been found in terms of self-reported mental health and frequency of utilizing mental health services by Latino subgroups (Ai, Appel, Huang, & Lee, 2012; Ai, Noel, Appel, Huang, & Hefley, 2013).

In this study, we proposed an underexplored explanatory pattern of health differentials, mainly the role of subjective measure of social status such as social location and perception of one's social location/standing which have been found to be important predictors of mental health, particularly among immigrant groups (Gong, Xu, & Takeuchi, 2012). With these concerns in mind, we paid close attention to the association between subjective dimensions of socioeconomic status (SES) and psychological distress among Latino subgroups, while controlling for other well-known covariates including nativity, years in the United States, English language proficiency, gender, marital status, and age.

LATINO GROUPS MENTAL HEALTH DIFFERENTIALS

Prior evidence from the Collaborative Psychiatric Epidemiology Surveys (CPES) reveal that overall Latinos had lower rates of lifetime and 12-month disorders than Whites (Alegría et al., 2007; Kessler et al., 2005; Williams et al., 2007). Yet closer inspection shows that among all Latino subgroups, Puerto Ricans had, in fact, the highest rates of lifetime and past year disorders of all Latino groups and that these rates were even higher than Whites (Alegría et al., 2007). Several explanations have been put forward to explain such differences. Some of them include the impact of residential segregation (Alegría, Molina, & Chen, 2014), acculturation (Vega & Alegría, 2001) and social support (Falcon, Todorova, & Tucker, 2009). Still, there has yet to be consensus on the specific reasons why Puerto Ricans have the worst mental health of all Latino groups.

Researchers that investigated the mental health of Mexican Americans found considerable evidence to suggest that their mental health indicators are somewhat better due to closer family ties and stronger social support networks (Almeida, Molnar, Kawachi, & Subramanian, 2009; Escobar, Nervi, & Gara, 2000). This paradox has found some support as a feasible mechanism to explain mental health differences, particularly for Mexicans but not for Puerto Ricans (Morales, Lara, Kington, Valdez, & Escarce, 2002). Additionally, as Mexicans acculturate, their mental health tends to worsen, particularly in comparison with recently arrived migrants and those with longer lengths of stay in the United States, and thus, the relation between acculturation and mental health appears more consistent for Mexicans than with other groups (Gil, Wagner, & Vega, 2000). Finally, Cubans, unlike Mexicans and Puerto Ricans, tend to have the best mental health of all Latino groups (Alegría et al., 2007), particularly as a result of their higher socioeconomic standing and favorable context of reception. Specifically, their refugee status eases the process of legal participation in the United States and upon migrating to the United States, they often come into well-established ethnic enclaves that have strong ethnic communities and access to resources (Guarnaccia, Martinez, & Acosta, 2005). However, apart from these three main groups, less is even known about other Latino groups as they are typically undersampled or not the subject of inquiry. Even among this less represented group, several processes have been identified as potential predictors of mental health including context of exit among Nicaraguans (Gil & Vega, 1996), exposure to political violence among Salvadorans (Eisenman, Gelberg, Liu, & Shapiro, 2003), and religious coping among immigrants from El Salvador and Guatemala (Dunn & O'Brien, 2009; Menjívar, 1997). In short, although the current body of literature indicates there is ample heterogeneity in the prevalence of mental health among different Latino groups and the theoretical explanations for these differences, the association between subjective dimensions of SES, such as social standing, and its relation to mental health remains underexplored.

SUBJECTIVE SES AND MENTAL HEALTH

SES may be conceptualized as having an objective component, measured by such variables as income, education, and occupation, and a subjective component. Although less examined than objective SES, subjective SES has been defined as a person's perception of their social position in the social hierarchy based on their past and current socioeconomic conditions (Diemer, Mistry, Wadsworth, Lopez, & Reimers, 2013; Singh-Manoux, Marmot, & Adler, 2005). Similar to findings of objective SES, studies investigating the relation between subjective socioeconomic position find that perceiving oneself to occupy a higher social status is associated with better health (Molina, Alegría, & Mahalingam, 2012). For example, Leu and colleagues (2008) found consistent evidence of the association between subjective social status (SSS) and mood dysfunction, and concluded that SSS was important in predicting mental health compared to traditional SES measures. Moreover, a previous study among a sample of healthy White women (Adler, Epel, Castellazzo, & Ickovics, 2000) found a strong association between SSS indicators and psychological functioning and other health indicators. Another study of low-income Mexican-origin women in Texas showed an association between subjective SES, mental health, and self-rated health, but not with physical health (Franzini & Fernandez-Esquer, 2006). Still, the logic is that higher SES allows individuals to have better life conditions, such as greater access to social and human capital resources, which leads to better mental health. This theory, better known as the social gradient theory, indicates that those at the top of the hierarchy will experience better health, while those below and each subsequent social class gradient will experience less favorable health outcomes (Marmot, 2004).

Still, few studies have analyzed the relationship between subjective SES and psychological distress among different subethnic Latino groups. The exploration of subjective SES addressed in this study fills a gap in the research literature and provides explanations on Latino subgroup differences in psychological distress, while accounting for other known covariates.

STATISTICAL ANALYSES

For our main analyses, we conducted a series of weighted multivariable linear regressions to model the association between SSS in the United States and SSS community, respectively. Given the two SSS measures were highly correlated ($r = 0.67$), we ran separate regression analyses for each SSS indicator variable. First, step 1 of our models included the main effects of SSS and sociodemographic indicators (gender, age, and marital status). Second, objective measures of SES (income, education, employment, and education) were added in step 2. Step 3 of our models further added the sociocultural indicators (Latino ethnicity, nativity, years in United States, and English proficiency). Third, to examine the effect modification by Latino ethnicity, step 4 included the SSS × Latino ethnicity interaction term, adjusting for all other main effects. We tested formally for differences in slopes associated with the product term. To better understand significant interactions, we used coefficients from the final model to calculate predicted marginal means and graphed them at each conditional effect at 1 standard deviation (*SD*) below, at the mean, and above the mean of SSS for each Latino ethnic group (Aiken, West, & Reno, 1991). We analyzed data using Stata 14 and accounted for the complex survey design by incorporating sample weights and sample design effects due to clustering and stratification.

METHODS

Sample and Procedures

We used data from the Latino sample ($N = 2{,}554$) of the National Latino and Asian American Study (NLAAS). The NLAAS is the first nationally representative, cross-sectional epidemiologic study that examined the prevalence of mental health disorders and utilization rates of mental health services among non-institutionalized Latino and Asian adults aged 18 years and older residing in the United States. Among the Latino sample, the subgroups included 495 Puerto Ricans, 577 Cubans, 868 Mexicans, and 614 Other Latinos. The mean age of participants was 38.0 years ($SD = 15.0$).

Detailed sampling procedures have been previously documented (Heeringa et al., 2004). Briefly, the survey was administered between May 2002 and November 2003. To obtain a nationally representative sample of Latino subgroups, regardless of geographic residential patterns, the sampling design included three components: (1) core sampling of primary and secondary sampling units, (2) high-density supplemental samplings of census block groups to oversample geographic areas made up of more than 5% of the targeted ethnic group, and (3) secondary respondent sampling to recruit participants from households where a primary respondent was already interviewed (Heeringa et al., 2004). Face-to-face interviews were conducted in either English of Spanish by trained, bilingual interviewers. The final weighted response rate for the Latino sample was 77.6%. All study participants provided written informed consent, and the study procedures and protocols were approved by the Institutional Review Boards at the University of Washington, University of Michigan, Cambridge Health Alliance, and Harvard University.

Measures

Psychological Distress

Non-specific psychological distress was measured with the Kessler Psychological Distress Scale (K10; Kessler et al., 2002), a 10-item inventory that assesses the prevalence of negative feelings, including depressive and anxious symptoms, over the past 30 days. Respondents reported frequency of each item on a five-point scale (1 = *all of the time* to 5 = *none of the time*). Raw variables were reverse coded and summed, with higher values indicated higher levels of psychological distress ($\alpha = 0.92$). The Kessler Psychological Distress Scale is routinely used in population health surveys and its reliability and validity are well established (Kessler et al., 2002).

Subjective Social Status (SSS)

We used the MacArthur's SSS measure (Adler et al., 2000) to assess the perceptions of social class rank. SSS was measured by having participants rank themselves with regard to their *social position in the United States* and *social position in the community*. Participants were shown a graphic representation of a ladder with 10 rungs accompanied by the following description:

> Think of this ladder as representing where people stand in the United States. At the top of the ladder are the people who are the best off—those who have the most money, the most education, and the most respected jobs. At the bottom are the people who are the worst off—those who have the least money, least education, and the least respected jobs or no job. The higher you are on the ladder, the closer you are to the people at the very top; the lower you are, the closer you are to the people at the very bottom. (Adler et al., 2000)

Respondents were then asked: "What is the number to the right of the rung where you think you stand at this time in your life, relative to other people in the United States?" Additionally, participants also ranked their perceived social position in their community following the same prompt that included "community" instead of "in the United States." Because people define community in different ways, respondents were asked to define community based on what was most meaningful for them: "What is the number to the right of the run where you think you stand at this time in your life, relative to other people in your community?"

Sociodemographic Variables

We measured several sociodemographic variables which included *gender*, *age*, and *marital status*. *Gender* was defined as a dichotomous variable, indicating whether the participant self-identified as male (reference) or female. *Age* was categorized into four groups: 18−34 (reference), 35−49, 50−64, and 65 and older. Age was categorized because age of immigration to the United States has been shown to affect mental health among immigrants (Leu et al., 2008). *Marital status* was categorized as married (reference), never married, and widow/separated/divorced.

Sociocultural Indicators

We used several social and cultural indicators (Kimbro, Gorman, & Schachter, 2012) to understand their impact on psychological distress. *Years in United States* measured the number of years a respondent has lived in the United States: 0−3 years, 4−10 years, 11−20 years, and 20+ years/US-born (reference). *English proficiency* was measured as a respondent's language proficiency in English and was coded poor/fair (reference) and good/excellent. *Latino ethnicity* was defined as a categorical variable, indicating whether the participant was self-identified as Cuban (reference), Puerto Rican, Mexican, or Other

Latino. Cubans were used as the reference group given their socioeconomic and health advantage relative to other Latino ethnic groups (Alegría et al., 2007; Daviglus et al., 2012; Guarnaccia et al., 2007).

Objective Socioeconomic Status (SES)

Objective SES measures included *household income*, *education*, and *employment*. The *income* variable was divided into four categories: US$0–14,999, US$15,000–34,999, US$35,000–74,999, and US$75,000 and over (reference). *Education* was measured in terms of years of education: 11 years or less, 12 years, 13–16 years, and 17 years or more (reference). *Employment* included the categories employed (reference) and unemployed/out of labor force.

RESULTS

Descriptive Statistics and Preliminary Analyses

Table 1 summarizes the weighted distribution of sociodemographic characteristics for the total sample and by Latino group. Significant group differences were noted across many of the selected characteristics, with the exception of the distribution of gender, age, and employment.

Table 2 displays descriptive statistics of key study variables (i.e., psychological distress, SSS community, SSS-US). Adjusted Wald tests revealed a significant overall group difference on mean levels of psychological distress ($p < 0.001$). Bonferonni-adjusted pairwise comparisons showed that Puerto Ricans reported significantly higher levels of psychological distress ($M = 13.3$, $SD = 10.8$) than Cubans ($M = 11.6$, $SD = 15.1$), Mexicans ($M = 11.3$, $SD = 4.9$), and Other Latinos ($M = 11.9$, $SD = 6.2$). No overall group differences were noted for SSS community or SSS-US.

Bivariate correlations indicated that among the total sample, SSS community and SSS-US were significantly and highly associated ($r = 0.67$, $p < 0.001$). Psychological distress was significantly and negatively correlated with both SSS community ($r = -0.18$, $p < 0.001$) and SSS-US ($r = -0.18$, $p < 0.001$).

Multivariable Linear Regression Models

Subjective Social Status in the United States

In the first step of the model (data not shown), the results showed that higher SSS in the United States was significantly associated with reduced psychological distress ($B = -0.40$, $p < 0.001$), controlling for sociodemographic indicators (gender, age, and marital status). In step 2, higher levels of SSS in the United States remained significantly associated with lower reports of psychological distress ($B = -0.35$, $p < 0.001$), even after controlling for sociodemographic and socioeconomic (household income, education, and employment) indicators. Sociocultural indicators (Latino ethnicity, years in the United States, and English proficiency) were further added to step 3; the results remained nearly identical to those in step 2. In the final step of the model (see Table 3), the

Table 1. Distribution of Sociodemographic Characteristics for Total Sample and by Latino Ethnicity.

	Total Sample			Cuban		Puerto Rican		Mexican		Other Latino		
	$N = 2{,}554$			$(n = 577)$		$(n = 495)$		$(n = 868)$		$(n = 614)$		p
	n	%	SE	%	SE	%	SE	%	SE	%	SE	
Gender												n.s.
Male	1,127	51.5	0.01	51.5	0.02	51.5	0.02	51.5	0.02	51.5	0.02	
Female	1,427	48.5	0.01	48.5	0.02	48.5	0.02	48.5	0.02	48.5	0.02	
Age												n.s.
18–34	1,068	49.0	0.02	49.0	0.03	49.0	0.03	49.0	0.02	49.0	0.03	
35–49	801	30.1	0.01	30.1	0.03	30.1	0.02	30.1	0.02	30.1	0.02	
50–64	454	13.4	0.01	13.4	0.01	13.4	0.02	13.4	0.01	13.4	0.02	
65 and over	231	7.6	0.01	7.5	0.01	7.5	0.03	7.5	0.01	7.5	0.02	
Marital status												***
Married	1,599	64.2	0.01	60.6	0.03	54.0	0.03	69.7	0.02	57.5	0.02	
W/D/S	479	14.4	0.01	17.0	0.02	17.4	0.03	12.2	0.01	17.3	0.02	
Never married	476	21.4	0.01	22.4	0.02	28.5	0.02	18.1	0.02	25.2	0.02	
Household income												**
US$0–14,999	703	27.2	0.02	21.9	0.03	25.9	0.02	29.6	0.03	23.7	0.02	
US$15k–34,999	692	28.3	0.01	23.9	0.03	22.4	0.02	30.8	0.02	26.2	0.03	
US$35k–74,999	685	27.8	0.02	25.9	0.02	29.5	0.02	26.2	0.03	30.9	0.03	
US$75k and over	474	16.7	0.01	28.2	0.04	22.3	0.02	13.4	0.01	19.3	0.03	
Education												***
11 years or less	994	44.1	0.02	21.0	0.02	32.6	0.03	53.1	0.02	34.2	0.02	
12 years	633	24.5	0.01	27.2	0.02	30.1	0.02	23.7	0.01	23.6	0.02	
13–15 years	567	21.1	0.01	26.5	0.02	26.5	0.02	15.9	0.02	28.6	0.02	
16 years or more	567	10.3	0.01	25.3	0.03	10.9	0.02	7.3	0.01	13.6	0.02	
Employment												n.s.
Employed	1,566	63.1	0.02	66.9	0.02	60.0	0.03	61.9	0.03	66.1	0.02	
Unemployed/OLF	988	36.9	0.02	33.1	0.02	40.0	0.03	38.1	0.03	33.9	0.02	
Years in United States												***
US-born	924	42.9	0.02	23.6	0.03	58.7	0.03	43.8	0.04	38.7	0.03	
Less than five years	250	9.6	0.01	21.8	0.05	2.1	0.01	9.6	0.02	10.4	0.02	
5–10 years	245	8.9	0.01	13.7	0.02	4.1	0.01	8.9	0.01	9.9	0.02	
11–20 years	411	17.9	0.01	8.2	0.02	9.9	0.01	18.3	0.02	21.4	0.02	
20 or more years	716	20.7	0.01	32.7	0.03	25.1	0.03	19.4	0.01	19.7	0.02	
English proficiency												***
Poor/fair	1,254	48.0	0.03	44.9	0.04	27.5	0.03	54.5	0.04	42.9	0.03	
Good/excellent	1,291	52.0	0.03	55.1	0.04	72.5	0.03	45.5	0.04	57.1	0.03	

Notes: W/D/S = Widowed/divorced/separated. OLF = Out of labor force. p-values are from Rao-Scott statistics for the Pearson chi-square test for contingency tables.
$^{*}p < 0.05$; $^{**}p < 0.01$; $^{***}p < 0.001$, n.s. = non-significant.

Table 2. Descriptive Statistics of Main Variables for Total Sample and by Latino Group (Weighted).

	Total Sample		Cubans		Puerto Ricans		Mexicans		Other Latinos		
Measure	*M*	*SD*	*M*	*SD*	*M*	*SD*	*M*	*SD*	*M*	*SD*	*p*-value
Psychological distress	11.7	6.7	11.6[a]	15.1	13.3[b]	10.8	11.3[a]	4.9	11.9[a]	6.2	0.001
Subjective social status in the United States	5.5	2.0	5.7	4.3	5.6	2.6	5.4	1.5	5.7	1.8	0.247
Subjective social status in the community	6.1	2.0	6.4	4.4	6.1	2.8	6.0	1.5	6.3	1.8	0.170

Notes: Different superscripts describe significant differences after Bonferroni adjustment ($p = 0.0083$). *p*-value is from Design-based Adjusted Wald test for overall test of difference in means by Latino ethnicity.

Table 3. Regression Models for Subjective Social Status Variables Predicting Psychological Distress (Weighted).

	Model A (Final Model)		Model B (Final Model)	
	B	*SE*	*B*	*SE*
Main effects of SSS				
SSS-US	−0.79***	0.16		
SSS community			−0.76***	0.18
Two-way interactions				
SSS-US × *Latino ethnicity*				
Cuban	Ref			
Puerto Rican	0.03	0.28		
Mexican	0.44*	0.17		
Other Latino	0.62*	0.27		
SSS community × *Latino Ethnicity*				
Cuban			Ref	
Puerto Rican			0.02	0.33
Mexican			0.44*	0.20
Other Latino			0.49*	0.21
Obs	2,509		2,483	
Design-based *F*-test	(24, 30) = 11.86***		(24, 30) = 9.35***	
R^2	7.80%		7.87%	

Notes: Model A included subjective social status in the United States. Model B included subjective social status in the community. Models A and B controlled for gender, marital status, household income, education, employment, years in the United States, and English proficiency.
Ref = reference group; SSS = subjective social status.
Continuous variables included in interaction terms were centered at their means.
* $p \leq 0.05$; *** $p \leq 0.001$.

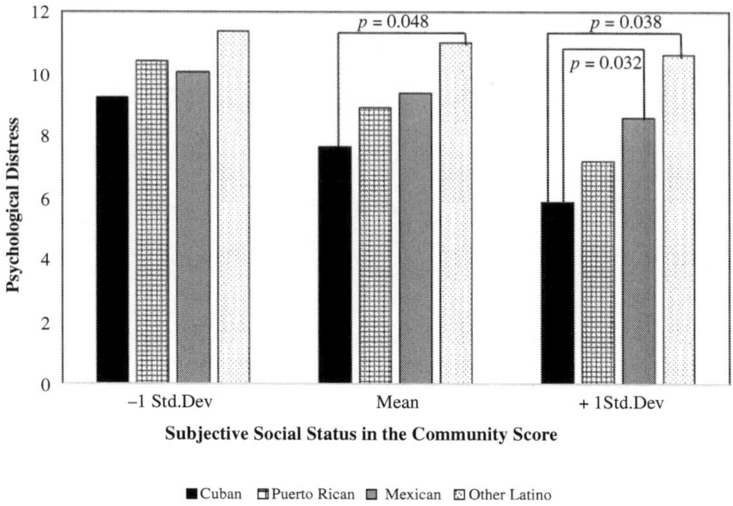

Fig. 1. Predicted Marginal Means of Psychological Distress as a Function of Subjective Social Status in the United States and Latino Group.

results showed a significant moderating effect of Latino ethnicity in the association between SSS in the United States and psychological distress.

Fig. 1 shows a bar graph with the plotted predicted marginal means of psychological distress. Cubans, compared Other Latinos, are predicted to endorse lower levels of psychological distress when at moderate levels (at the mean) of SSS in the United States. Further, Cubans, relative to Mexicans and Other Latinos, are predicted to endorse lower levels of psychological distress at high levels (1 *SD* above the mean) of SSS in the United States.

Subjective Social Status in the Community

In the first step of the model (data not shown), the results showed that higher SSS in the community was significantly associated with reduced psychological distress ($B = -0.44$, $p < 0.001$), while adjusting for sociodemographic indicators (gender, age, and marital status). In step 2, higher levels of SSS in the community remained significantly associated with lower reports of psychological distress ($B = -0.39$, $p < 0.001$), even after controlling for sociodemographic and socioeconomic (household income, education, and employment) indicators. Sociocultural indicators (Latino ethnicity, years in the United States, and English proficiency) were further added to step 3; the results remained nearly identical to those in step 2. In the final step of the model (see Table 3), the results showed a significant moderating effect of Latino ethnicity in the association between SSS in the community and psychological distress. Fig. 2 shows a bar graph for the plotted predicted

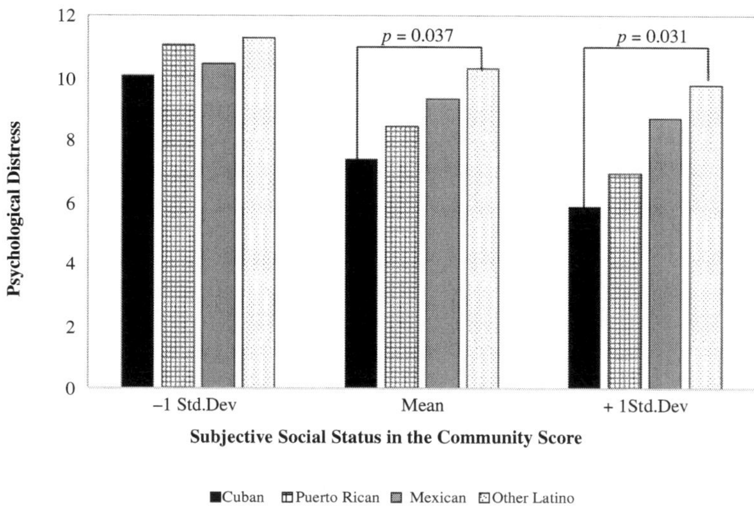

Fig. 2. Predicted Marginal Means of Psychological Distress as a Function of Subjective Social Status in the Community and Latino Group.

marginal means of psychological distress. Cubans, compared Other Latinos, are predicted to endorse lower levels of psychological distress when at moderate levels (at the mean) and at high levels (at 1 *SD* of above the mean) of SSS in the community.

DISCUSSION

Utilizing data from the NLAAS, we investigated the association between subjective dimensions of socioeconomic status and psychological distress, paying particular attention to Latino subgroup differences. In order to understand the effects of subjective dimensions of socioeconomic status, we examined SSS and its association with psychological distress, while controlling for sociocultural and sociodemographic indicators. The results showed that SSS was associated with reduced psychological distress. Furthermore, there were significant differences by Latino ethnicity, mainly that Cubans were more likely to endorse lower levels of psychological distress when endorsing higher SSS in the United States in comparison with Mexicans and Other Latino groups. The results revealed the same pattern for SSS in the community as well.

Our study reveals distinctive patterns of understanding to unpack previous explanations for the differences in psychological distress among Latino groups. First, our study revealed significant differences in psychological distress among different Latino subgroups, particularly among Puerto Ricans. This result corresponds to previous research that has found less favorable mental health outcomes among Puerto Ricans (Alegría et al., 2007; Rivera et al., 2008). This might be indicative of the effect of the overrepresentation of Puerto Ricans in unfavorable social conditions such as poverty, low education, among others (Acosta-Belén & Santiago, 2006). These results also demonstrated that even when controlling for sociocultural, sociodemographic, and socioeconomic indicators, there was no association between SSS with psychological distress among Puerto Ricans in comparison with other Latinos groups, findings that are in accordance with previous research (Morales et al., 2002; Rivera & Burgos, 2010). Second, although sociodemographic and sociocultural indicators are important, the subjective dimensions of socioeconomic status are important predictors of psychological distress. In a sense, an unfavorable perception of one's position is associated with considerable psychological distress. As suggested by Molina et al. (2012), SSS might be a better predictor for those of high status relative to those with lower objective SES. That is, the perceptions of where you stand may be more important for those who already have the objective status, whereas for those of low SES (measured objectively), any change in status may not matter much as compared to actual changes in education or income. For instance, US$100 might matter more for those without it than whether they perceive themselves higher than others.

We found significant differences for these associations between Cubans, Mexicans, and Other Latinos. At first glance, this could be the result of Cubans displaying the best social and economic indicators (see Table 1), but the association between subjective social standing remained significant even when controlling for these factors. For Mexicans, perhaps the strong role that family relations play (Molina & Alcántara, 2013) might shield them from the effects of a perceived lower social position and psychological distress. Mexicans are also more likely to be married which brings forth different sorts of privileges and status. Despite Mexicans' lower social position, the perceptions of social status may encompass seeing themselves higher than others because of their marital status, which was not captured in the measure of SSS. The significant differences in the association between SSS and psychological distress among other Latinos might be the result of merging other Latino ethnicities in another group and perhaps masking some of their unique subethnic group processes. Nonetheless, it reveals the importance of research linking sociocultural variations, described as "differential lived experiences linked to race, nativity, ethnicity, and cultural influences" (Brown, Donato, Laske, & Duncan, 2013, p. 255) to mental health.

LIMITATIONS

There are several key study limitations that warrant consideration. Chiefly, data utilized were cross-sectional; thus, it is unclear whether subjective SES precedes or follows psychological distress. For example, it may be that individuals with poor mental health are more likely to perceive themselves as being of lower social status. At the same time, it is possible that poor mental health is associated with a perceived lower socioeconomic status given the greater likelihood of ill persons being unemployed or out of the labor force. Prospective studies are necessary to capture causal directions and dynamic relations between these variables. Second, the NLAAS was conducted in 2002–2003. An individual's perceived socioeconomic status may differ if they were assessed during the current socioeconomic and political context. It will therefore be important in future studies to examine any changes in socioeconomic position across time and contexts. Qualitative studies provide a unique methodological avenue for future research in this area, as this approach can be used to assess the phenomenological experience of perceived socioeconomic position at different stages of an individual's life.

CONCLUSION

Overall, our study makes several contributions to the sociological study of mental health differentials among Latinos. We show the importance of the association between subjective and objective SES indicators and psychological distress. We also demonstrated how the associations analyzed in this study varied by Latino subethnicity, which we argue is an important step to fully understand the different social processes associated with the mental health of different Latina/o groups.

REFERENCES

Acosta-Belén, E., & Santiago, C. E. (2006). *Puerto Ricans in the United States: A contemporary portrait*. Boulder, CO: Lynne Rienner.

Adler, N. E., Epel, E. S., Castellazzo, G., & Ickovics, J. R. (2000). Relationship of subjective and objective social status with psychological and physiological functioning: Preliminary data in healthy, White women. *Health Psychology*, *19*(6), 586–592.

Ai, A. L., Appel, H. B., Huang, B., & Lee, K. (2012). Overall health and healthcare utilization among Latino American women in the United States. *Journal of Women's Health*, *21*(8), 878–885.

Ai, A. L., Noel, L. T., Appel, H. B., Huang, B., & Hefley, W. E. (2013). Overall health and health care utilization among Latino American men in the United States. *American Journal of Men's Health*, *7*(1), 6–17.

Aiken, L. S., West, S. G., & Reno, R. R. (1991). *Multiple regression: Testing and interpreting interactions*. Newbury Park, CA: Sage.

Alegría, M., Canino, G., Shrout, P., Woo, M., Duan, N., Vila, D., ... Meng, X.-L. (2008). Prevalence of mental illness in immigrant and non-immigrant US Latino groups. *American Journal of Psychiatry*, *165*(3), 359–369.

Alegría, M., Molina, K. M., & Chen, C.-N. (2014). Neighborhood characteristics and differential risk for depressive and anxiety disorders across racial/ethnic groups in the United States. *Depression and Anxiety*, *31*(1), 27–37.

Alegría, M., Mulvaney-Day, N., Torres, M., Polo, A., Cao, Z., & Canino, G. (2007). Prevalence of psychiatric disorders across Latino subgroups in the United States. *American Journal of Public Health*, *97*(1), 68–75.

Almeida, J., Molnar, B. E., Kawachi, I., & Subramanian, S. V. (2009). Ethnicity and nativity status as determinants of perceived social support: Testing the concept of familism. *Social Science & Medicine*, *68*(10), 1852–1858.

Brown, T., Donato, K., Laske, M. T., & Duncan, E. (2013). Race, nativity, ethnicity, and cultural influences in the sociology of mental health. In Aneshensel, C. S., Phelan, J. C., and Bierman, A. (Eds.), *Handbook of the sociology of mental health* (2nd ed., pp. 255–276). Dordrecht: Springer Science & Business Media.

Cook, B., Alegria, M., Lin, J. Y., & Guo, J. (2009). Pathways and correlates connecting Latinos' mental health with exposure to the United States. *American Journal of Public Health*, *99*(12), 2247–2254.

Daviglus, M. L., Gregory, A. T., Avilés-Santa, M. L., Allison, M., Cai, J., Criqui, M. H., … Stamler, J. (2012). Prevalence of major cardiovascular risk factors and cardiovascular diseases among Hispanic/Latino individuals of diverse backgrounds in the United States. *Jama*, *308*(17), 1775–1784.

Dey, A. N., & Lucas, J. W. (2006). *Physical and mental health characteristics of US-and foreign-born adults, United States, 1998–2003*. Advance data from vital and health statistics; no 369. Hyattsville, MD: National Center for Health Statistics.

Diemer, M., Mistry, R., Wadsworth, M., Lopez, I., & Reimers, F. (2013). Best practices in conceptualizing and measuring social class in psychological research. *Analyses of Social Issues & Public Policy*, *13*(1), 77–113.

Dunn, M. G., & O'Brien, K. M. (2009). Psychological health and meaning in life stress, social support, and religious coping in Latina/Latino immigrants. *Hispanic Journal of Behavioral Sciences*, *31*(2), 204–227.

Eisenman, D. P., Gelberg, L., Liu, H., & Shapiro, M. F. (2003). Mental health and health-related quality of life among adult Latino primary care patients living in the United States with previous exposure to political violence. *JAMA*, *290*(5), 627–634.

Escobar, J. I., Nervi, C. H., & Gara, M. A. (2000). Immigration and mental health: Mexican Americans in the United States. *Harvard Review of Psychiatry*, *8*(2), 64–72.

Falcon, L. M., Todorova, I., & Tucker, K. (2009). Social support, life events, and psychological distress among the Puerto Rican population in the Boston area of the United States. *Aging & Mental Health*, *13*(6), 863–873.

Franzini, L., & Fernandez-Esquer, M. E. (2006). The association of subjective social status and health in low-income Mexican-origin individuals in Texas. *Social Science & Medicine*, *63*(3), 788–804.

Gil, A. G., & Vega, W. A. (1996). Two different worlds: Acculturation stress and adaptation among Cuban and Nicaraguan families. *Journal of Social and Personal Relationships*, *13*(3), 435–456.

Gil, A. G., Wagner, E. F., & Vega, W. A. (2000). Acculturation, familism, and alcohol use among Latino adolescent males: Longitudinal relations. *Journal of Community Psychology*, *28*(4), 443–458.

Gong, F., Xu, J., & Takeuchi, D. T. (2012). Beyond conventional socioeconomic status: Examining subjective and objective social status with self-reported health among Asian immigrants. *Journal of Behavioral Medicine*, *35*(4), 407–419.

Guarnaccia, P. J., Martinez, I., & Acosta, H. (2005). Chapter 2. Mental health in the Hispanic immigrant community: An overview. *Journal of Immigrant & Refugee Services*, *3*(1–2), 21–46.

Guarnaccia, P. J., Martínez Pincay, I., Alegría, M., Shrout, P. E., Lewis-Fernández, R., & Canino, G. J. (2007). Assessing diversity among Latinos: Results from the NLAAS. *Hispanic Journal of Behavioral Sciences*, *29*(4), 510–534.

Heeringa, S. G., Wagner, J., Torres, M., Duan, N., Adams, T., & Berglund, P. (2004). Sample designs and sampling methods for the collaborative psychiatric epidemiology studies (CPES). *International Journal of Methods in Psychiatric Research*, *13*(4), 221–240.

Kessler, R. C., Andrews, G., Colpe, L. J., Hiripi, E., Mroczek, D. K., Normand, S. L., … Zaslavsky, A. M. (2002). Short screening scales to monitor population prevalences and trends in non-specific psychological distress. *Psychological Medicine*, *32*(6), 959–976.

Kessler, R. C., Berglund, P., Demler, O., Jin, R., Merikangas, K. R., & Walters, E. E. (2005). Lifetime prevalence and age-of-onset distributions of DSM-IV disorders in the national comorbidity survey replication. *Archives of General Psychiatry*, *62*(6), 593–602.

Kimbro, R. T., Gorman, B. K., & Schachter, A. (2012). Acculturation and self-rated health among Latino and Asian immigrants to the United States. *Social Problems*, *59*(3), 341–363.

Leu, J., Yen, I. H., Gansky, S. A., Walton, E., Adler, N. E., & Takeuchi, D. T. (2008). The association between subjective social status and mental health among Asian immigrants:

Investigating the influence of age at immigration. *Social Science & Medicine*, *66*(5), 1152–1164.

Markides, K. S., & Eschbach, K. (2005). Aging, migration, and mortality: Current status of research on the Hispanic paradox. *The Journals of Gerontology Series B: Psychological Sciences and Social Sciences*, *60*(Special Issue 2), S68–S75.

Marmot, M. (2004). *The status syndrome: How your social standing affects your health and life expectancy*. New York, NY: Henry Holt and Company.

Menjívar, C. (1997). Immigrant kinship networks and the impact of the receiving context: Salvadorans in San Francisco in the Early 1990s. *Social Problems*, *44*(1), 104–123.

Molina, K. M., & Alcántara, C. (2013). Household structure, family ties, and psychological distress among US-born and immigrant Latino women. *Journal of Family Psychology*, *27*(1), 147–158.

Molina, K. M., Alegría, M., & Mahalingam, R. (2012). A multiple-group path analysis of the role of everyday discrimination on self-rated physical health among Latina/os in the USA. *Annals of Behavioral Medicine*, *45*(1), 33–44.

Morales, L. S., Lara, M., Kington, R. S., Valdez, R. O., & Escarce, J. J. (2002). Socioeconomic, cultural, and behavioral factors affecting Hispanic health outcomes. *Journal of Health Care for the Poor and Underserved*, *13*(4), 477–503.

Motel, S., & Patten, E. (2012). *The 10 largest Hispanic origin groups: Characteristics, rankings, top counties*. Washington, DC: Pew Hispanic Center.

Ortega, A. N., Rosenheck, R., Alegria, M., & Desai, R. A. (2000). Acculturation and the lifetime risk of psychiatric and substance use disorders among Hispanics. *The Journal of Nervous and Mental Disease*, *188*(11), 728–735.

Riosmena, F., Root, E., Humphrey, J., Steiner, E., & Stubbs, R. (2015). The Waning Hispanic health paradox. *Pathways: A Magazine on Poverty, Inequality, and Social Policy*, *Spring*, 24–29. Retrieved from https://inequality.stanford.edu/publications/pathway/hispanics-america

Rivera, F. I. (2007). Contextualizing the experience of young Latino adults: Acculturation, social support and depression. *Journal of Immigrant and Minority Health*, *9*(3), 237–244.

Rivera, F. I., & Burgos, G. (2010). The health status of Puerto Ricans in Florida. *CENTRO: Journal of the Center for Puerto Rican Studies*, *22*(1), 199–219.

Rivera, F. I., Guarnaccia, P. J., Mulvaney-Day, N., Lin, J. Y., Torres, M., & Alegria, M. (2008). Family cohesion and its relationship to psychological distress among Latino groups. *Hispanic Journal of Behavioral Sciences*, *30*(3), 357–378.

Singh-Manoux, A., Marmot, M. G., & Adler, N. E. (2005). Does subjective social status predict health and change in health status better than objective status? *Psychosomatic Medicine*, *67*(6), 855–861.

Vega, W. A., & Alegría, M. (2001). Latino mental health and treatment in the United States. In M. Aguirre-Molina C. W. Molina, & R. E. Zambrana (Eds.), *Health issues in the Latino community* (pp. 179–207). San Francisco, CA: Jossey-Bass.

Williams, D. R., Gonzalez, H. M., Neighbors, H., Nesse, R., Abelson, J. M., Sweetman, J., & Jackson, J. S. (2007). Prevalence and distribution of major depressive disorder in African Americans, Caribbean blacks, and non-Hispanic whites: Results from the National Survey of American Life. *Archives of General Psychiatry*, *64*(3), 305–315.

PART III
OTHER HEALTH PROBLEMS

RACE, ENVIRONMENTAL INEQUALITY, AND PHYSICAL HEALTH

Jennifer M. Brailsford, Jessica Eckhardt, Terrence D. Hill, Amy M. Burdette and Andrew K. Jorgenson

ABSTRACT

Purpose – *Although established theoretical models suggest that race differences in physical health are partially explained by exposures to environmental toxins, there is little empirical evidence to support these processes. We build on previous research by formally testing whether black–white differences in self-rated physical health are mediated by the embodiment of environmental toxins.*

Methodology/Approach – *Using cross-sectional data from the National Health and Nutrition Examination Surveys (2007–2008), we employ ordinary least squares regression to model environmental toxins (from urine specimens) and overall self-rated health as a function of race and ethnicity. We employ the Sobel test of indirect effects to formally assess mediation.*

Findings – *Our results show that non-Hispanic black respondents tend to exhibit* higher *levels of total toxins, lead, and cadmium in their urine and* poorer *physical health than non-Hispanic whites, even with adjustments for age, gender, and socioeconomic status (SES). Our mediation analyses suggest that blacks may exhibit* poorer *physical health than whites because they tend to embody* higher *levels of cadmium.*

Underserved and Socially Disadvantaged Groups and Linkages with Health and Health Care Differentials
Research in the Sociology of Health Care, Volume 37, 71–86

ISSN: 0275-4959/doi:10.1108/S0275-495920190000037009

Research Limitations/Implications – *Research limitations include cross-sectional data and restricted indicators of SES.*

Originality/Value of Paper – *This study contributes to previous work by bridging the fields of social epidemiology and environmental inequality and by formally testing established theoretical models.*

Keywords: Race; health; environmental inequality; toxins; lead; cadmium

INTRODUCTION

Over the past three decades, numerous studies have shown that black adults tend to exhibit poorer physical health and shorter life expectancies than white adults (Ademuyiwa et al., 2015; Bailey et al., 2017; Dressler, Oths, & Gravlee, 2005; Farmer & Ferraro, 2005; Ferraro & Farmer, 1996; Ferraro, Kemp, & Williams, 2017; Hayward, Miles, Crimmins, & Yang, 2000; Hummer, 1996; Hummer & Chinn, 2011; Kelley-Moore & Ferraro, 2004; Krieger, Jarvis, Waterman, Rehkopf, & Subramanian, 2005; Sloan, Ayyagari, Salm, & Grossman, 2010; Williams, 2012; Williams & Collins, 1995; Williams & Sternthal, 2010; Williams, Yu, Jackson, & Anderson, 1997). Black–white differences in physical health have been documented across a range of outcomes, including obesity, diabetes, hypertension, asthma, sexually transmitted infections, disability, and subjective health. Race inequalities in life expectancy are consistent across indicators of all-cause mortality and mortality linked to specific causes like heart disease, cerebrovascular disease, malignant neoplasms, pneumonia, influenza, diabetes, injuries, homicides, and HIV.

Although this empirical literature has made significant contributions to our understanding of black–white differences in physical health, we are still working to establish the precise underlying mechanisms. Previous studies suggest that black adults tend to have poorer physical health because they tend to be disadvantaged across a range of likely pathways, including racism, individual and institutional discrimination, segregation, socioeconomic status (SES), political power, health care, living conditions, physical activity, nutrition, and physiological stress (Bailey et al., 2017; Dressler et al., 2005; Ferraro et al., 2017; Hayward et al., 2000; Hummer, 1996; Williams & Collins, 1995; Williams & Mohammed, 2013; Williams & Sternthal, 2010). Although well-known theoretical models developed by prominent scholars like Williams and Collins (1995), Robert Hummer (1996), and Ferraro, Kemp, and Williams (2017) identify "environmental exposure," "toxicity and waste," and "exposure to toxins" as important explanations for established race differences in physical health, direct empirical measurements and assessments of environmental risk are often "sorely lacking" (Brulle & Pellow, 2006). With this in mind, Brulle and Pellow (2006, p. 117) argue that the:

> next stage of research on health disparities must address the fragmented nature of existing knowledge by testing a conceptual-empirical model that includes social and environmental

factors and investigates their effects, individual and joint, on general and specific health outcomes.

In this chapter, we build on previous research by formally testing whether black–white differences in self-rated physical health are mediated by the embodiment of environmental toxins. In the pages that follow, we discuss (1) race variations in environmental risk and (2) the potential physical health consequences of embodied toxins. After describing our data, measures, and statistical procedures, we summarize the results of our analyses. We end with a discussion of our key findings and research limitations. We also describe several avenues for future research.

BACKGROUND

Race and Environmental Risk

Over the past four years, the city of Flint, Michigan has suffered from a lead water crisis that is likely to undermine community health and well-being for generations. Although President Obama called for a state of emergency in 2016, his administration did very little to address the concerns of this primarily impoverished, black community. Given that the Trump administration in general and EPA chief Scott Pruitt in particular are seemingly devoted to deregulation and the elimination of important environmental protections, the residents of Flint are unlikely to receive any serious relief for years to come.

While the media has focused on the recent water crisis in Flint, they have virtually ignored the broader structural problem of environmental inequality. In reality, Flint is not unique. Black individuals, families, and communities are disproportionately exposed to the hazards of environmental injustice (Ard, 2015, 2016; Ard, Colen, Becerra, & Velez, 2016; Brulle & Pellow, 2006; Bullard, 1993, 2000; Collins, Munoz, & JaJa, 2016; Downey & Hawkins, 2008; LaVeist, 2005; Mohai & Bryant, 1992; Mohai, Pellow, & Roberts, 2009; Morello-Frosch & Lopez, 2006; Williams & Collins, 1995). Nearly three decades ago, Bullard (1993, p. 320) noted that:

> Race is a powerful predictor of many environmental hazards, including the distribution of air pollution, the location of municipal solid waste facilities, the location of abandoned toxic waste sites, toxic fish consumption, and lead poisoning in children.

Over the years, these patterns have been replicated by numerous studies. For example, recent work confirms that blacks are especially vulnerable to airborne industrial toxins (Ard, 2015, 2016; Linder, Marko, & Sexton, 2008; Zwickl, Ash, & Boyce, 2014).

The intersection of race inequality and environmental inequality is largely explained by racism, discrimination, racial segregation, differential housing practices, and proximity to sources of environmental hazards (Ard, 2015, 2016; Ard et al., 2016; Brulle & Pellow, 2006; Bullard, 1993, 2000; Downey & Hawkins, 2008; Mohai & Bryant, 1992; Mohai et al., 2009; Morello-Frosch, 2002; Pastor, Sadd, & Hipp, 2001). Racism and discrimination restrict socioeconomic and residential opportunities for racial and ethnic minorities. Occupational and financial constraints tend to limit opportunities for safety in nutrition, housing, employment, and transportation. For example, low-income housing is often characterized by dilapidation, which exposes residents to toxins, infections, and illness (Evans & Kantrowitz, 2002; Evans & Kim, 2010). Black individuals and families are often trapped in contexts of environmental inequality because of their location within various systems of stratification, because they often lack the financial assets, legal resources, and political power to block or evade the siting of pollution-producing facilities in their communities (Brulle & Pellow, 2006; Bullard, 1993, 2000; Cushing, Morello-Frosch, Wander, & Pastor, 2015; Downey & Hawkins, 2008; Szasz & Meuser, 1997).

Environmental Risk and Physical Health

Toxins are pervasive in our environments and generally refer to a range of potential hazards like lead, arsenic, polychlorinated byphenyls, and other heavy metals and chemicals. In this study, we focus on toxic heavy metals found throughout the built environment, including arsenic, barium, cadmium, cobalt, cesium, lead, molybdenum, thallium, and tungsten. Exposure to these toxins can occur through multiple pathways, including, air pollution, water contamination, industrial fumes, and substandard housing.

The primary threats to humans from heavy metals are exposures to cadmium and lead (Järup, 2003). These toxins are worthy of investigation due to their association with numerous adverse health outcomes (Agency for Toxic Substances and Disease, 2005). Exposures to these metals occur through contaminated air, water, soil, food, and other health-related behaviors. Cadmium is consistently associated with higher rates of inflammation, diabetes, liver disease, renal failure, skeletal damage, cardiovascular disease, obstructive lung disease, breast cancer, stroke, early onset osteoporosis, developmental disabilities, all-cause mortality, and mortality from specific causes (Ciesielski et al., 2012; Gallagher, Kovach, & Meliker, 2008; Hecht, Landy, Ahn, Hlaing, & Hennekens, 2013; Järup, 2003; Larsson, Orsini, & Wolk, 2015; Lin, Rathod, Ho, & Caffrey, 2009; Mendy, Gasana, & Vieira, 2012; Peters et al., 2010; Rokadia & Agarwal, 2013; Tellez-Plaza et al., 2013; Wallia, Allen, Badon, & Muayed, 2014). Lead is also harmful to human health. Lead poisoning has been linked with higher rates of headaches, irritability, abdominal pain, nerve damage, kidney ailments, ventricular hypertrophy, hypertension, and all-cause mortality (ATSDR, 2007; Järup, 2003; Navas-Acien et al., 2005; Schober, Mirel, Graubard, Brody, & Flegal, 2006; Schwartz, 1991).

While cadmium and lead are among the most dangerous and pervasive environmental toxins, research has identified other harmful heavy metals. For example, arsenic is a heavy metal found in groundwater intended for human consumption. About 90% of all arsenic is used in preserving wood for fences, decks, and picnic tables. Arsenic is also found in pesticides and lead-acid batteries (ATSDR, 2007). Arsenic can induce vomiting, diarrhea, and fatigue in the short term. Long-term effects include skin changes, circulatory and peripheral nervous disorders, abnormal fetal development, and lung cancer (ATSDR, 2007).

The embodiment of toxins like antimony, cobalt, molybdenum, tungsten, and uranium can also occur through occupational hazards (e.g., heavy industrial work). These toxins are associated with a range of adverse health consequences, including higher rates of asthma, pulmonary fibrosis, cardiovascular disease, cerebrovascular disease, liver damage, thyroid disorders, and vision impairments (Agarwal, Zaman, Tuzcu, & Kapadia, 2011; Christensen, 2013; De Palma, Manini, Sarnico, Molinari, & Apostoli, 2010; Mendy et al., 2012; Navas-Acien et al., 2005; Shiue, 2015). There is also some evidence linking related exposures to elevations in mortality risk (Lasfargues et al., 1994; Moulin et al., 1998).

To our knowledge, only two studies have tested the connection between heavy-metal toxins and self-rated health, which is the primary outcome of this study. Shiue (2015) found that people who exhibited higher levels of urinary arsenic and heavy metals, including cadmium, cobalt, manganese, molybdenum, lead, antimony, strontium, tungsten, and uranium, were more likely to describe their general health status as poor, fair, or good than very good or excellent. Most recently, Brailsford and colleagues (2018) also showed that higher levels of urinary cadmium were associated with poorer self-rated health. Related to our conceptual model, Ard and colleagues (2016) tested whether race differences in self-rated health were mediated or explained by race differences in exposure to air toxins. The authors concluded that:

> Although African Americans had the highest estimated toxic exposure from industrial toxins, followed by Whites and Hispanics, controlling for relative exposure to air toxins was shown to have no impact on the racial gap in self-rated health. (p. 9)

In this chapter, we extend previous research by testing whether race differences in physical health are mediated by heavy-metal toxins.

Hypotheses

In accordance with previous research, we developed three hypotheses to guide subsequent analyses: (*H1*) Non-Hispanic blacks will tend to embody higher levels of environmental toxins than non-Hispanic whites. (*H2*) People who embody higher levels of environmental toxins will tend to exhibit poorer overall self-rated physical health. (*H3*) Non-Hispanic blacks will tend to exhibit poorer overall self-rated physical health than non-Hispanic whites, and this association will be at least partially mediated or explained by the embodiment of environmental toxins.

DATA

The data for this study come from the 2007–2008 cross-sectional *National Health and Nutrition Examination Surveys* (NHANES). The NHANES employs a complex, multistage, and probability sample of the non-institutionalized civilian US population (Curtin et al., 2013). Starting in 2007, a new sampling methodology was implemented. Several groups were oversampled, including adults at

Table 1. Descriptive Statistics (n = 1,792).

	Range	Mean	*SD*
Self-rated physical health	1.00–5.00	3.13	0.97
Total toxins	−0.61 to 4.27	0.00	1.00
Lead	−0.54 to 37.47	0.00	1.00
Cadmium	−0.70 to 10.10	0.00	1.00
Non-Hispanic White	0.00–1.00	0.46	
Non-Hispanic Black	0.00–1.00	0.21	
Hispanic	0.00–1.00	0.29	
Other Race/Ethnicity	0.00–1.00	0.04	
Education	1.00–5.00	3.14	1.29
Employed	0.00–1.00	0.56	
Income	0.00–2.71	1.92	0.62
Age	18.00–80.00	48.97	18.37
Female	0.00–1.00	0.50	

Note: National Health and Nutrition Examination Surveys (2007–2008).

or below 130% of federal poverty level and adults aged 80 and over. The survey consists of questionnaires administered in the home, followed by a standardized health examination in specially equipped mobile examination centers. Blood and urine samples were taken from random subgroups (about one-third) of the full sample. Our final analytic sample included 1,792 adults aged 18–80 who were tested for metal toxins in their urine. Table 1 provides descriptive statistics for all variables included in the analyses.

MEASURES

Environmental Toxins

The NHANES 2007–2008 included urine samples for arsenic, barium, cadmium, cobalt, cesium, molybdenum, lead, thallium, and tungsten. Urinary tests of heavy metals have been shown to accurately reflect the amount of heavy metals in the body (ATSDR, 2012). The amount of heavy metals present in urine shows both recent and past exposure (ATSDR, 2012). The urine collection procedure consisted of urine specimen collection and processing. Urine specimens were processed, stored, and shipped to the Division of Environmental Health Laboratory Sciences, National Center for Environmental Health, and Centers for Disease Control and Prevention for analysis.

Inductively coupled plasma-mass spectrometry (ICP-MS) was employed to quantify heavy-metal concentrations in urine (Date & Gray, 1989). This multi-element analytical technique measures the following 12 elements in urine: beryllium (Be), cobalt (Co), molybdenum (Mo), cadmium (Cd), antimony (Sb), cesium (Cs), barium (Ba), tungsten (W), platinum (Pt), thallium (TI), lead (Pb), and uranium (U) (Mulligan, Davidson, & Caruso, 1990). Most elements were measured in micrograms per liter (μg/L) (CDC 2008).

In this study, toxins are measured in two ways. We first examine a mean index of the nine toxins ($\alpha = 0.804$). To account for variations in response metrics, all toxin measures were standardized before indexing. We also examine exposures to *lead* and *cadmium* separately. Lead and cadmium are studied independently because, as noted in the discussion above, they are often found to be the most pervasive and dangerous of the metal toxins (Agency for Toxic Substances & Disease Registry, 2005; Krueger & Wade, 2016; Weidemann et al., 2015).

Self-rated Physical Health

Following recent work in environmental inequality (Ard et al., 2016; Brailsford, Hill, Burdette, & Jorgenson, 2018), we use an overall self-rated health item to measure physical health. Self-rated health is a common subjective indicator of general health status that is consistently associated with more objective health measures, including physician diagnoses and mortality risk (Idler & Benyamini, 1997). According to Idler and Benyamini (1997), self-rated health is a robust predictor of mortality risk, over and above numerous specific medical, behavioral, and psychosocial risk factors. We focus on self-rated physical health precisely because it is a subjective indicator of general health status. As a global subjective indicator, self-rated health captures symptoms and conditions that are experienced, not simply diagnosed or undiagnosed. This is important because our toxin measures may indicate embodiment in the distant past or more recently. While *recent* toxin exposures are unlikely to generate chronic conditions like liver disease, the measures of self-rated health may capture the subjective experience of subclinical symptoms (e.g., short-term pain and discomfort). Thus, overall self-rated physical health may be especially sensitive to the potential mediating influence of toxin exposures. Respondents were asked to rate their physical health on a scale ranging from (1) "poor" to (5) "excellent."

Race and Ethnicity

Race and ethnicity are assessed using a categorical measure of self-reported identification, converted into a series of dummy variables. The sample includes (1) non-Hispanic whites, (2) non-Hispanic blacks, (3) Hispanics, and (4) other races and ethnicities. In multivariate analyses, non-Hispanic whites serve as the common reference category.

Socioeconomic Status

We employ three common indicators of SES, including educational attainment, employment status, and personal income. *Education* is an ordinal measure of educational attainment. Response categories include (1) less than ninth grade, (2) 9–11 grade (including 12 grade without completion), (3) high school graduate or GED equivalent, (4) some college or AA degree, and (5) college graduate or higher. *Employed* is a dichotomous variable that asks if a respondent is (1) currently employed or (0) not. *Income* is measured in US dollars earned in the previous calendar year. The index is split into increments of $5,000, with $0 to $4,999 being the lowest increment and $100,000 or more being the largest increment. Income is logged to normalize its positively skewed distribution. All missing values on income were replaced via multiple imputations. The multiple imputation model employed all independent variables from the full model to predict income. Our final income measure reflects average estimates from 10 iterations.

SES measures were not indexed for two primary reasons. First, it is customary to examine indicators of SES separately because they are causally related to each other. According to standard life course models, these factors build upon each other (Mirowsky & Ross, 2003). Second, different indicators of SES tend to have different theoretical paths to toxin exposure. For example, education is often tied to occupational exposures because credentials shape employment opportunities while income may be more relevant for residential exposures because financial resources are necessary for housing.

Background Variables

Subsequent multivariate analyses adjust for two background variables that are known correlates of toxin exposure and self-rated health: age and gender. *Age* is measured in continuous years (18–80). *Gender* is a dichotomous variable (1 = *female*; 0 = *male*).

STATISTICAL PROCEDURES

Our primary statistical analyses proceed in two steps. In the first step, we employ ordinary least squares (OLS) regression to model the embodiment of environmental toxins (Table 2) and self-rated physical health (Table 3) by race and background variables. We acknowledge that toxin exposure is continuous while self-rated physical health is ordinal. DeMaris (2002, p. 259) notes that, in large samples, ordinal variables "with at least five levels" can be treated as "approximately interval" in OLS regression. In supplemental analyses (not shown), we replicated our regressions of self-rated physical health using ordered logistic regression. These results were substantively identical to our reported OLS models.

In the second step, we test whether race differences in health are mediated by embodied environmental toxins. There are two general approaches to testing mediation models. The first is the "coefficient change" approach, which assesses the change in the coefficient for the focal predictor across nested models (i.e., before and after the mediator variable is added to the regression equation). The second is the "indirect effect" approach, which assesses the statistical significance of an indirect effect (i.e., the product of two coefficients, the coefficient for the effect of the focal predictor on the mediator and the coefficient for the effect of the mediator on the outcome). In this study, we employ the indirect effect

Table 2. Ordinary Least Squares Regression of Toxin Exposure ($n = 1{,}792$).

	Total Toxins	Lead	Cadmium
Non-Hispanic Black	0.086**	0.203*	0.345***
	(0.029)	(0.090)	(0.073)
Hispanic	−0.015	0.091*	−0.044
	(0.027)	(0.043)	(0.062)
Other Race/Ethnicity	0.091	0.198*	0.394
	(0.057)	(0.094)	(0.239)
Education	−0.009	−0.039	−0.061*
	(0.011)	(0.026)	(0.027)
Employed	−0.024	−0.009	−0.036
	(0.028)	(0.042)	(0.064)
Income	−0.050*	−0.060	−0.141*
	(0.022)	(0.079)	(0.057)
Age	−0.001	0.004***	0.013***
	(0.001)	(0.001)	(0.001)
Female	−0.048*	−0.218***	0.036
	(0.024)	(0.045)	(0.051)

Notes: National Health and Nutrition Examination Surveys (2007–2008). Shown are unstandardized coefficients (b), standard errors (in parentheses), and two-tailed significance tests (***$p < 0.001$; **$p < 0.01$; *$p < 0.05$). Reference groups include: unemployed, male, and non-Hispanic white.

approach and the Sobel test (Sobel, 1982) of statistical significance because this approach is more commonly used and requires information for each link in the proposed mediation process (X → M and M → Y). In supplemental analyses (not shown), we replicated our mediation analyses using the coefficient change approach and the statistical test developed by Clogg and colleagues (1995). These results were substantively identical to our reported indirect effect tests.

RESULTS

Toxin Exposures

According to Table 2, non-Hispanic black respondents tend to exhibit *higher* levels of heavy metals in their urine specimens than non-Hispanic whites. This general pattern can be seen for total toxins, lead, and cadmium, even with adjustments for age, gender, education, employment status, and income. Race and ethnic differences are more sporadic when Hispanics and other races and ethnicities are compared with non-Hispanic whites. Although respondents who identify as Hispanic and other races and ethnicities tend to exhibit *higher* levels of lead, no differences were observed for total toxins or cadmium. Taken together, these results highlight the unique environmental burden of non-Hispanic blacks.

Table 3. Ordinary Least Squares Regression of Self-rated Physical Health ($n = 1{,}792$).

	Model 1	Model 2	Model 3
Total toxins	−0.115		
	(0.061)		
Lead		0.019	
		(0.028)	
Cadmium			−0.134***
			(0.028)
Non-Hispanic Black	−0.238***	−0.250***	−0.204***
	(0.059)	(0.059)	(0.059)
Hispanic	−0.332***	−0.333***	−0.332***
	(0.062)	(0.062)	(0.062)
Other Race/Ethnicity	−0.206	−0.215	−0.207
	(0.144)	(0.145)	(0.142)
Education	0.130***	0.131***	0.127***
	(0.025)	(0.025)	(0.025)
Employed	0.264***	0.267***	0.258***
	(0.061)	(0.062)	(0.061)
Income	0.209***	0.217***	0.192***
	(0.046)	(0.046)	(0.046)
Age	−0.004*	−0.004*	−0.002
	(0.002)	(0.002)	(0.002)
Female	−0.075	−0.066	−0.062
	(0.052)	(0.053)	(0.052)

Notes: National Health and Nutrition Examination Surveys (2007–2008). Shown are unstandardized coefficients (b), standard errors (in parentheses), and two-tailed significance tests (***$p < 0.001$, **$p < 0.01$, *$p < 0.05$). Reference groups include: unemployed, male, and non-Hispanic white.

Self-rated Physical Health

Table 3 reveals predictable race and ethnic differences in overall self-rated physical health. Non-Hispanic black and Hispanic respondents tend to report *poorer* self-rated physical health than their non-Hispanic white counterparts. These patterns are consistent across models with adjustments for environmental toxins. The embodiment of toxins overall and lead in particular are both unrelated to self-rated health. However, cadmium is inversely associated with self-rated health. This suggests that respondents who exhibit *higher* levels of cadmium in their urine also tend to report *poorer* overall self-rated physical health. These results persisted with adjustments for age, gender, education, employment status, and income.

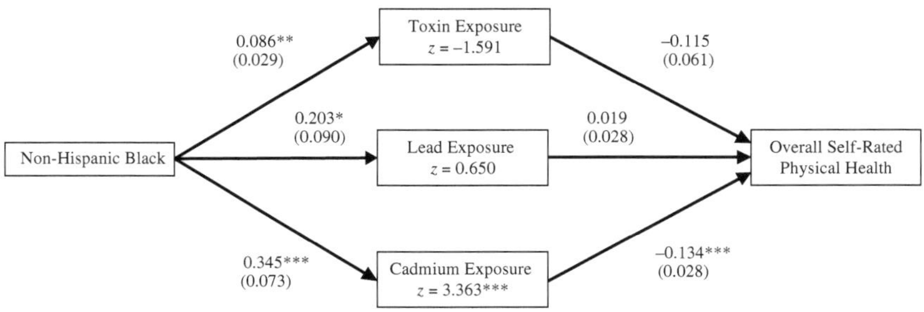

Fig. 1. Unstandardized Coefficients and Sobel Tests (*$p < 0.05$; **$p < 0.01$; ***$p < 0.001$) for Statistically Significant Indirect Effects (NHANES 2007–2008).

Mediation Analyses

Given that the Sobel test of indirect effects requires that each link in the proposed process be statistically significant, we can rule out total toxins and lead as potential mediators of any race or ethnic difference in self-rated physical health. Although non-Hispanic blacks tend to exhibit *higher* levels of lead and total toxins, these outcomes are unrelated to self-rated health. This leaves us with cadmium. Fig. 1 presents our mediation analyses, including unstandardized path coefficients, standard errors, and formal Sobel tests (z). We observe statistically significant indirect effects for black race through the embodiment of cadmium ($z = 3.363$, $p < 0.001$). Taken together, our mediation analyses suggest that non-Hispanic blacks may exhibit poorer physical health than non-Hispanic whites because they tend to embody *higher* levels of cadmium. There is no evidence to support total toxins or lead as mechanisms of race or ethnicity.

Supplemental Analyses

In supplemental analyses (not shown), we replicated our mediation analyses by replacing self-rated physical health with several diagnosed chronic disease conditions, including liver disease, heart disease, heart attack, congestive heart failure, stroke, cancer, and arthritis. There was no evidence of mediation for any of these outcomes. These supplemental analyses confirm that overall self-rated physical health may be especially sensitive to the potential mediating influence of environmental toxins.

DISCUSSION

Although established theoretical models suggest that race inequalities in physical health are at least partially explained by exposures to environmental toxins, there is little empirical evidence to support these processes. We aimed to extend previous work by formally testing whether black–white differences in self-rated physical health are mediated by the embodiment of environmental toxins.

Our first hypothesis stated that non-Hispanic blacks would tend to embody higher levels of environmental toxins than non-Hispanic whites. This hypothesis received consistent support.

Our analyses showed that non-Hispanic black respondents tend to exhibit *higher* levels of total toxins, lead, and cadmium in their urine than non-Hispanic whites, even with adjustments for age, gender, and SES. These associations are generally consistent with previous research (Brulle & Pellow, 2006; Bullard, 1993, 2000; LaVeist, 2005; Mohai et al., 2009).

Our second hypothesis stated that people who embody higher levels of environmental toxins would tend to exhibit poorer overall self-rated physical health. Evidence for this hypothesis was inconsistent. Overall toxin exposure and lead exposure were unrelated to self-rated physical health. However, cadmium was inversely associated with self-rated health. Our results for cadmium tend to support previous work (Ciesielski et al., 2012; Gallagher et al., 2008; Hecht et al., 2013; Järup, 2003; Larsson et al., 2015; Lin et al., 2009; Mendy et al., 2012; Peters et al., 2010; Rokadia & Agarwal, 2013; Tellez-Plaza et al., 2013; Wallia et al., 2014). However, our results for lead exposure are inconsistent with previous research (ATSDR, 2007; Järup, 2003; Navas-Acien et al., 2005; Schober et al., 2006; Schwartz, 1991).

Our third hypothesis stated that non-Hispanic blacks would tend to exhibit poorer overall self-rated physical health than non-Hispanic whites and that this association would be at least partially mediated or explained by the embodiment of environmental toxins. This hypothesis received moderate support. We observed that non-Hispanic black respondents tended to report poorer physical health than their non-Hispanic white counterparts, which is consistent with previous scholarship (Dressler et al., 2005; Ferraro & Farmer, 1996; Hayward et al., 2000; Kelley-Moore & Ferraro, 2004; Williams & Collins, 1995; Williams et al, 1997). Although we were able to rule out total toxins and lead as potential mediators, we observed a statistically significant indirect effect through the embodiment of cadmium. This evidence suggests that non-Hispanic blacks may exhibit poorer physical health than non-Hispanic whites because they tend to embody *higher* levels of cadmium. Our results for total toxins and lead confirm previous work showing no mediation via air toxins (Ard, 2016). To the best of our knowledge, this is the first study to directly test and show support for the mediating influence of embodied cadmium.

Our analyses are limited in several respects. First, the cross-sectional nature of the data do not allow us to assess short-term or long-term changes in toxin exposure and health. Longitudinal data are required to make stronger causal inferences. Second, our measurement of SES omits important measures like wealth and alternative indicators of income like the income-to-poverty ratio. It would be important for future research to replicate our results using additional indicators of financial status. Third, our measurement of employment status is relatively crude. More detailed assessments of occupational sectors and work-related environments are clearly required. For example, the Agency for Toxic Substances and Disease (2012) notes that cadmium is often found in the manufacturing of pesticides, batteries, glass, and PVC.

CONCLUSION

Despite these limitations, our results suggest that broader race inequalities in physical health may be at least partially explained by the embodiment of environmental toxins. This line of research points to the potential health consequences of further deregulation of environmental protections, especially for black Americans who already face higher rates of morbidity and mortality relative to their non-Hispanic white counterparts. Although this chapter contributes to previous work by bridging the fields of social epidemiology and environmental inequality and by formally testing established theoretical models, the veracity of our results is contingent upon replication using longitudinal data, other measures of physical health and environmental inequality, and more comprehensive assessments of SES. Additional research is also needed to explore race and ethnic variations in toxin exposure and physical health in different national contexts and at different levels of analysis (Ard, 2015, 2016; Ard et al., 2016) and in connection to income and wealth inequality (Hill & Jorgenson, 2018; Jorgenson, Schor, & Huang, 2017). Research along these lines would advance our collective understanding of the environmental processes linking race and health.

REFERENCES

Ademuyiwa, F., Gao, F., Hao, L., Morgensztern, D., Aft, R., Ma, C., & Ellis, M. (2015). US breast cancer mortality trends in young women according to race. *Cancer*, *121*, 1469–1476.

Agarwal, S., Zaman, T., Tuzcu, E. M., & Kapadia, S. (2011). Heavy metals and cardiovascular disease: Results from the national health and nutrition examination survey (NHANES) 1999–2006. *Angiology*, *62*, 422–429.

Agency for Toxic Substances and Disease Registry. (2005). *CERCLA priority list of hazardous substances*. Retrieved from http://www.atsdr.cdc.gov.cercla.

Agency for Toxic Substances and Disease Registry (ATSDR). (2007). *Public health service*. U.S. Department of Health and Human Services, Atlanta, GA.

Agency for Toxic Substances and Disease Registry (ATSDR). (2012). *Toxicological profile for cadmium*. U.S. Department of Health and Human Services, Atlanta, GA.

Ard, K. (2015). Trends in exposure to industrial air toxins for different racial and socioeconomic groups: A spatial and temporal examination of environmental inequality in the U.S. from 1995 to 2004. *Social Science Research*, *53*, 375–390.

Ard, K. (2016). By all measures: An examination of the relationship between segregation and health risk from air pollution. *Population and Environment*, *38*, 1–20.

Ard, K., Colen, C., Becerra, M., & Velez, T. (2016). Two mechanisms: The role of social capital and industrial pollution exposure in explaining racial disparities in self-rated health. *International Journal of Environmental Research and Public Health*, *13*, 1025.

Bailey, Z., Krieger, N., Agénor, M., Graves, J., Linos, N., & Bassett, M. (2017). Structural racism and health inequities in the USA: Evidence and interventions. *The Lancet*, *389*, 1453–1463.

Brailsford, J., Hill, T., Burdette, A., & Jorgenson, A. (2018). Are socioeconomic inequalities in physical health mediated by embodied environmental toxins? *Socius*, *4*, 1–9.

Brulle, R., & Pellow, D. (2006). Environmental justice: Human health and environmental inequalities. *Annual Review of Public Health*, *27*, 103–124.

Bullard, R. (1993). Race and environmental justice in the United States. *Yale Journal of International Law*, *18*, 319–335.

Bullard, R. (2000). *Dumping in Dixie: Race, class, and environmental quality*. Boulder, CO: Westview Press.

Christensen, K. (2013). Metals in blood and urine, and thyroid function among adults in the United States 2007–2008. *International Journal of Hygiene and Environmental Health*, *216*, 624–632.

Ciesielski, T., Weuve, J., Bellinger, D., Schwartz, J., Lanphear, B., & Wright, R. (2012). Cadmium exposure and neurodevelopmental outcomes in US children. *Environmental Health Perspectives, 120*, 758–763.

Clogg, C., Petkova, E., & Haritou, A. (1995). Statistical methods for comparing regression coefficients between models. *American Journal of Sociology, 100*, 1261–1293.

Collins, M., Munoz, I., & JaJa, J. (2016). Linking 'toxic outliers' to environmental justice communities. *Environmental Research Letters, 11*, 015004.

Curtin, L., Mohadjer, L., Dohrmann, S., Kruszon-Moran, D., Mirel, L., Carroll, M., ... Johnson, C. (2013). *National health and nutrition examination survey: Sample design, 2007–2010*. Hyattsville, MD: National Center for Health Statistics.

Cushing, L., Morello-Frosch, R., Wander, M., & Pastor, M. (2015). The haves, the have-nots, and the health of everyone: The relationship between social inequality and environmental quality. *Annual Review of Public Health, 193*, 193–209.

Date, A., & Gray, A. (1989). *Applications of inductively coupled plasma mass spectrometry*. London: Chapman & Hall.

DeMaris, A. (2002). Regression models. In M. Wiederman & B. Whitley (Eds.), *Handbook for conducting research on human sexuality* (pp. 255–287). Mahwah, NJ: Lawrence Erlbaum.

De Palma, G., Manini, P., Sarnico, M., Molinari, S., & Apostoli, P. (2010). Biological monitoring of tungsten (and cobalt) in workers of a hard metal alloy industry. *International Archives of Occupational and Environmental Health, 83*, 173–181.

Downey, L., & Hawkins, B. (2008). Race, income, and environmental inequality in the United States. *Sociological Perspectives, 51*, 759–781.

Dressler, W., Oths, K., & Gravlee, C. (2005). Race and ethnicity in public health research: Models to explain health disparities. *Annual Review of Anthropology, 34*, 231–252.

Evans, G., & Kantrowitz, E. (2002). Socioeconomic status and health: The potential role of environmental risk exposure. *Annual Review of Public Health, 23*, 303–331.

Evans, G., & Kim, P. (2010). Multiple risk exposure as a potential explanatory mechanism for the socioeconomic status–health gradient. *Annals of the New York Academy of Sciences, 1186*, 174–189.

Farmer, M., & Ferraro, K. (2005). Are racial disparities in health conditional on socioeconomic status? *Social Science & Medicine, 60*, 191–204.

Ferraro, K., & Farmer, M. (1996). Double Jeopardy, aging as leveler, or persistent health inequality? A longitudinal Analysis of White and Black Americans. *The Journals of Gerontology Series B: Psychological Sciences and Social Sciences, 51*, S319–S328.

Ferraro, K., Kemp, B., & Williams, M. (2017). Diverse aging and health inequality by race and ethnicity. *Innovation in Aging, 1*, igx002.

Gallagher, C., Kovach, J., & Meliker, J. (2008). Urinary cadmium and osteoporosis in US women ≥ 50 years of age: NHANES 1988–1994 and 1999–2004. *Environmental Health Perspectives, 116*, 1338–1343.

Hayward, M., Miles, T., Crimmins, E., & Yang, Y. (2000). The significance of socioeconomic status in explaining the racial gap in chronic health conditions. *American Sociological Review, 65*, 910–930.

Hecht, E., Landy, D., Ahn, S., Hlaing, W. W., & Hennekens, C. (2013). Hypothesis: Cadmium explains, in part, why smoking increases the risk of cardiovascular disease. *Journal of Cardiovascular Pharmacology and Therapeutics, 18*, 550–554.

Hill, T., & Jorgenson, A. (2018). Bring out your dead! A study of income inequality and life expectancy in the United States, 2000–2010. *Health & Place, 49*, 1–6.

Hummer, R. (1996). Black-White differences in health and mortality: A review and conceptual model. *The Sociological Quarterly, 37*, 105–125.

Hummer, R., & Chinn, J. (2011). Race/ethnicity and US adult mortality. *Du Bois Review: Social Science Research on Race, 8*, 5–24.

Idler, E., & Benyamini, Y. (1997). Self-rated health and mortality: A review of twenty-seven community studies. *Journal of Health and Social Behavior, 38*, 21–37.

Järup, L. (2003). Hazards of heavy metal contamination. *British Medical Bulletin, 68*, 167–182.

Jorgenson, A., Schor, J., & Huang, X. (2017). Income inequality and carbon emissions in the United States: A state-level analysis, 1997–2012. *Ecological Economics*, *134*, 40–48.

Kelley-Moore, J., & Ferraro, K. (2004). The black/white disability gap: Persistent inequality in later life? *The Journals of Gerontology Series B: Psychological Sciences and Social Sciences*, *59*, S34–S43.

Krieger, N., Jarvis, T. C., Waterman, P. D., Rehkopf, D. H., & Subramanian, S. V. (2005). Painting a truer picture of US socioeconomic and racial/ethnic health inequalities: The public health disparities geocoding project. *American Journal of Public Health*, *95*, 312–323.

Krueger, W. S., & Wade, T. J. (2016). Elevated blood lead and cadmium levels associated with chronic infections among non-smokers in a cross-sectional analysis of NHANES data. *Environmental Health*, *15*, 16.

Larsson, S., Orsini, N., & Wolk, A. (2015). Urinary cadmium concentration and risk of breast cancer: A systematic review and dose-response meta-analysis. *American Journal of Epidemiology*, *182*, 375–380.

Lasfargues, G., Wild, P., Moulin, J., Hammon, B., Rosmorduc, B., du Noyer, C. R., … Moline., J. (1994). Lung cancer mortality in a French cohort of hard-metal workers. *American Journal of Industrial Medicine*, *26*, 585–595.

LaVeist, T. (2005). Disentangling race and socioeconomic status: A key to understanding health inequalities. *Journal of Urban Health*, *82*, iii26–iii34.

Lin, Y. S., Rathod, D., Ho, W. C., & Caffrey, J. J. (2009). Cadmium exposure is associated with elevated blood C-reactive protein and fibrinogen in the US population: The third national health and nutrition examination survey (NHANES III, 1988–1994). *Annals of Epidemiology*, *19*, 592–596.

Linder, S., Marko, D., & Sexton, K. (2008). Cumulative cancer risk from air pollution in Houston: Disparities in risk burden and social disadvantage. *Environmental Science & Technology*, *42*, 4312–4322.

Mendy, A., Gasana, J., & Vieira, E. R. (2012). Urinary heavy metals and associated medical conditions in the US adult population. *International Journal of Environmental Health Research*, *22*, 105–118.

Mirowsky, J., & Ross, C. (2003). *Education, social status, and health*. New York, NY: Aldine de Gruyter.

Mohai, P., & Bryant, B. (1992). Environmental racism: Reviewing the evidence. In B. Bryant & P. Mohai (Eds.), *Race and the incidence of environmental hazards: A time for discourse* (pp. 163–176). Boulder, CO: Westview Press.

Mohai, P., Pellow, D., & Roberts, T. (2009). Environmental justice. *Annual Review of Environmental Resources*, *34*, 404–430.

Morello-Frosch, R. (2002). Discrimination and the political economy of environmental inequality. *Environment and Planning C: Government and Policy*, *20*, 477–496.

Morello-Frosch, R., & Lopez, R. (2006). The riskscape and the color line: Examining the role of segregation in environmental health disparities. *Environmental Research*, *102*, 181–196.

Moulin, J., Wild, P., Romazini, S., Lasfargues, G., Peltier, A., Bozec, C., … Perdrix, A. (1998). Lung cancer risk in hard-metal workers. *American Journal of Epidemiology*, *148*, 241–248.

Mulligan, K. J., Davidson, T. M., & Caruso, J. A. (1990). Feasibility of the direct analysis of urine by inductively coupled argon plasma mass spectrometry for biological monitoring of exposure to metals. *Journal of Analytical Atomic Spectrometry*, *5*, 301–306.

Navas-Acien, A., Silbergeld, E., Sharrett, A. R., Calderon-Aranda, E., Selvin, E., & Guallar, E. (2005). Metals in urine and peripheral arterial disease. *Environmental Health Perspectives*, *113*, 164–169.

Pastor, M., Sadd, J., & Hipp, J. (2001). Which came first? Toxic facilities, minority move-in, and environmental justice. *Journal of Urban Affairs*, *23*, 1–21.

Peters, J. L., Perlstein, T. S., Perry, M. J., McNeely, E., & Weuve, J. (2010). Cadmium exposure in association with history of stroke and heart failure. *Environmental Research*, *110*, 199–206.

Rokadia, H., & Agarwal, S. (2013). Serum heavy metals and obstructive lung disease: Results from the national health and nutrition examination survey. *Chest*, *143*, 388–397.

Schober, S., Mirel, L., Graubard, B., Brody, D., & Flegal, K. (2006). Blood lead levels and death from all causes, cardiovascular disease, and cancer: Results from the NHANES III mortality study. *Environmental Health Perspectives*, *114*, 1538–1541.

Schwartz, J. (1991). Lead, blood pressure, and cardiovascular disease in men and women. *Environmental Health Perspectives*, *91*, 71–75.

Shiue, I. (2015). Urinary arsenic, heavy metals, phthalates, pesticides, polyaromatic hydrocarbons but not parabens, polyfluorinated compounds are associated with self-rated health: USA NHANES, 2011–2012. *Environmental Science and Pollution Research International*, *22*, 9570–9574.

Sloan, F., Ayyagari, P., Salm, M., & Grossman, D. (2010). The longevity gap between Black and White men in the United States at the beginning and end of the 20th century. *American Journal of Public Health*, *100*, 357–363.

Sobel, M. (1982). Asymptotic intervals for indirect effects in structural equation models. In S. Leinhart (Ed.), *Sociological methodology* (pp. 290–312). San Francisco, CA: Jossey-Bass.

Szasz, A., & Meuser, M. (1997). Environmental inequalities: Literature review and proposals for new directions in research and theory. *Current Sociology*, *45*, 99–120.

Tellez-Plaza, M., Guallar, E., Howard, B., Umans, J., Francesconi, K., Goessler, W., … Navas-Acien, A. (2013). Cadmium exposure and incident cardiovascular disease. *Epidemiology*, *24*, 421–429.

Wallia, A., Allen, N. B., Badon, S., & Muayed, M. E. (2014). Association between urinary cadmium levels and prediabetes in the NHANES 2005–2010 population. *International Journal of Hygiene and Environmental Health*, *217*, 854–860.

Weidemann, D., Kuo, C.-C., Navas-Acien, A., Abraham, A., Weaver, V., & Fadrowski, J. (2015). Association of arsenic with kidney function in adolescents and young adults: Results from the national health and nutrition examination study 2009–2012. *Environmental Research*, *140*, 317–324.

Williams, D. (2012). Miles to go before we sleep: Racial inequities in health. *Journal of Health and Social Behavior*, *53*, 279–295.

Williams, D., & Collins, C. (1995). US socioeconomic and racial differences in health: Patterns and explanations. *Annual Review of Sociology*, *21*, 349–386.

Williams, D., & Mohammed, S. (2013). Racism and health I: Pathways and scientific evidence. *American Behavioral Scientist*, *57*, 1152–1173.

Williams, D., & Sternthal, M. (2010). Understanding racial-ethnic disparities in health: Sociological contributions. *Journal of Health and Social Behavior*, *51*, S15–S27.

Williams, D., Yu, Y., Jackson, J., & Anderson, N. (1997). Racial differences in physical and mental health: Socio-economic status, stress and discrimination. *Journal of Health Psychology*, *2*, 335–351.

Zwickl, K., Ash, M., & Boyce, J. (2014). Regional variation in environmental inequality: Industrial air toxics exposure in US cities. *Ecological Economics*, *107*, 494–509.

AUTISM SPECTRUM DISORDERS AND THE HEALTHCARE EXPERIENCES OF AGING ADULTS

Karen E. Joseph-Kent

ABSTRACT

Purpose – *This study illuminates the experiences of adults diagnosed with autism spectrum disorders (ASDs) and intellectual disabilities (IDs) and their challenges and successes in receiving quality healthcare services. Individuals with developmental disabilities often experience health issues associated with aging at earlier ages and at higher rates than the general population. This population has a higher incidence of chronic health conditions that require regular medical attention.*

The intent of this project was to learn directly from adults and their caregivers how well healthcare providers understand autism, explore their experience with how well their care is coordinated between primary healthcare and other specialty services, and identify factors which could impact access to care and to discover what other barriers which may potentially influence health outcomes for ASD adult.

Method – *A qualitative study conducted with semi-structured interviews with 12 adults diagnosed with ASD and/or their guardians/caregivers.*

Findings – *Some of the adults interviewed experienced negative health outcomes and suboptimal relationships with healthcare providers; others seemed to have positive relationships. Clinical and communications accommodations were necessary to make healthcare provision more comfortable. Barriers to accessing healthcare services existed in many forms.*

Underserved and Socially Disadvantaged Groups and Linkages with Health and Health Care Differentials
Research in the Sociology of Health Care, Volume 37, 87–117

ISSN: 0275-4959/doi:10.1108/S0275-495920190000037010

Implications/Limitations – *The healthcare needs of the growing population adults diagnosed with ASD/ID are anticipated to be significant. This challenge is further exacerbated given there are few trained healthcare providers who are prepared or dedicated to serve this population. Continuing to build awareness of the health needs of the ASD/ID adult population is critical.*

Originality – *This project is highly innovative as it is the first attempt to understand how the adult autism population accesses care and perceives their healthcare interactions. This study serves as a starting point to suggest new opportunities for further research for this growing population.*

Keywords: Autism spectrum disorders; aging; healthcare providers; health disparities; intellectual disabilities; access to healthcare; accommodations; exploratory research in ASD

INTRODUCTION

Autism spectrum disorder (ASD) is a lifelong neurodevelopmental disorder and is among the most common of the identified developmental disabilities (Volkmar, Paul, Rogers, & Pelphrey, 2014). ASD is associated with intellectual disabilities (IDs), problems with motor coordination, difficulties with social interaction, sensory impairments, and attention challenges. In addition to the characteristics of autism, nearly half of those diagnosed with ASD have major physical and mental health comorbidities that require regular medical attention, such as epilepsy, diabetes, falls, sleep disturbances, depression, sedentary lifestyle, and gastrointestinal problems (Happé & Charlton, 2011; Nebel-Schwalm, Worley, & Ollendick, 2014). Individuals with developmental disabilities, such as ASD, often experience health issues associated with aging at earlier ages and at higher rates than the general population (Haveman et al., 2010; Heller & Sorensen, 2013). This higher risk is due to the combination of biological factors, suboptimal access to adequate healthcare, and lifestyle and environmental issues (Heller & Sorensen, 2013). Often people with ASD are underdiagnosed with chronic illnesses because of the impediments they face with respect to identifying and communicating symptoms of ill health (Mouridsen, Rich, & Isager, 2016a, 2016b; Tregnago & Cheak-Zamora, 2012). Many of these conditions could be better managed and perhaps prevented through more effective screening and prevention services provided by healthcare professionals.

Autism is often portrayed by advocacy groups and the media as strictly a childhood disorder. In fact, over 400 million dollars are spent annually in the United States on autism research, which is primarily focused on autism prevalence, potential etiologies, early identification strategies, and possible treatments in children (Nicolaidis et al., 2015). The prevalence of ASD significantly increased since 2002, when rates were 1:150, to rates as high as 1:59 children and 1:102 in adults (Baio, Wiggins, & Christensen, 2018; Cheak-Zamora & Teti, 2014). Over the next ten years, nearly half a million children diagnosed with

ASD will turn 18 (Roux et al., 2013) and will begin transitioning to adult healthcare providers. The numerous and complex needs of this growing adult population are not well understood, in particular their healthcare needs (Piven & Rabins, 2011). The combined impact of an aging population in Western countries, an increasing rate of diagnosis of ASD, and the escalating use of healthcare services for ASD will impose special and significant demands on our already strained healthcare system.

Based on the limited literature, it seems reasonable to conclude that aging adults with ASD experience health disparities and may also experience challenges in navigating the complex healthcare environment (Nicolaidis et al., 2013). One recent study on 45 adults diagnosed with ASD and their informal and formal caregivers by Mukaetova-Ladinska and Stuart-Hamilton (2015) found 60% of all respondents felt ASD adults age differently than people without autism and require a different approach to care provision. This lack of research and knowledge regarding aging in ASD adults was recognized as one of the major barriers in delivery of quality care for people aging with ASD. The societal and healthcare financial costs of adults with ASD/ID are growing and are anticipated to be significant, while there are few trained healthcare providers who are prepared to serve this population. It is critical to research the experiences and concerns shared by adults with ASD and their families in order to find methods that facilitate communication, decrease patient anxiety, improve care and medication compliance and ultimately improve patient satisfaction, and perhaps, positively impact patient outcomes.

In order to better understand the needs of adults, this study focused on the population of adults with ASD who were also diagnosed with ID. The presence of ID in ASD is estimated to be 50%–60% (Baird et al., 2006); this population is challenged by a triple jeopardy of age, ID, and social/behavioral challenges. According to the most recent literature on adults with an ID diagnosis, there is a lack of a coordinated response to ensure the best possible health and social care is provided to this special population in later life (Lin, Lin, & Hsu, 2016). In addition, premature deaths are recognized in the ID population (Shavelle, Strauss, & Pickett, 2001). Heslop et al. (2014) conducted a study in England which found that nearly one quarter of people with ID died prior to the age of 50 and the median age of death for men and women was 64 years old. This was 13–20 years younger than in the general population. Most importantly, Heslop et al. found that good quality healthcare could prevent these deaths in 37% of adults with ID (as compared to 13% of the general population). Through proper identification of disease and more effective management of illness, we might achieve reduced mortality and improve quality of life during old age.

The role of the physician is key in early recognition and evaluation of ASD and associated comorbidities and in effective disease management of these chronic disorders (Tyler, Schramm, Karafa, Tang, & Jain, 2011). The primary goals of medical treatment for this population are to maximize functional independence and quality of life by minimizing the core ASD features, facilitating development and learning, promoting socialization, reducing maladaptive behaviors, and educating and supporting families (Myers & Johnson, 2007).

The studies on healthcare providers thus far report a lack of self-perceived competency by primary care providers (PCPs) in treating and diagnosing adults with ASD (Bruder, Kerins, Mazzarella, Sims, & Stein, 2012; Golnik, Ireland, & Borowsky, 2009). There is very limited literature on best practices for optimal compliance and enhanced comfort in the clinical setting for adults with ASD/ID. Therefore, it is essential to identify innovative and individualized ways to serve this population in the clinical setting and to remove barriers to care. Because so much focus has been on children with ASD, transitioning effective techniques proven in the pediatric environment to the adult care delivery setting needs to occur, thus enabling a seamless and successful transition of care. It is important for adult medical providers to understand the clinical experience of their patients with ASD/ID special needs in order to reach these previously mentioned goals for medical treatment.

RESEARCH PURPOSE

The purpose of this exploratory study is to describe the experiences of adults with ASD and their caregivers in navigating the healthcare system to receive healthcare services.

- to understand how well their healthcare providers understand autism, including the sensory, behavioral, social, and communication needs required of an adult with autism;
- to explore their experience with how well their care is coordinated between primary healthcare and other specialty or ancillary services and to identify factors which could impact access to care; and finally,
- to discover what other barriers (e.g. access to available health services, policy concerns, such as health insurance and residency location, advocacy, aging guardians, and others) can potentially influence the health for ASD adults.

RESEARCH METHODS

This project relied on qualitative data gathered through interviewing a purposive sample of adults with ASD/ID and their parents/guardians, as well as residential caregivers, when appropriate. A qualitative approach of enquiry was needed to learn about the specific aims and to meet the objectives outlined above; it was determined direct interviews were the most sensitive and direct methods to gain this information. The strength of this method was that it offered depth and detail to create a constructive understanding of the healthcare experiences of this population. This exploratory, descriptive method provided a straightforward look at the phenomenon, which was required due to the lack of information on the subject (Lambert & Lambert, 2013). Exploratory qualitative interviews allow for detailed exploration and deep understanding of the research questions and allow the voice and story of the participants to be told (Patton, 2002; Perry & Parmenter, 2004). An exploratory approach is suggested when a topic has not been researched extensively and a deeper understanding of an issue is desired (Patton, 2002).

Utilizing qualitative interviews as a research method enabled a richer and more descriptive understanding of adults with ASD/ID and their caregivers' shared relationship and life journey. Also, as a relatively unexplored area of research, interviews allow the interviewee to respond from their own experiences and provide context and explanation to their responses (Coyle, Kramer, & Mutchler, 2014; Silverman, 2008). This method of data collection allowed for deeper insights into their reality and lays a rich foundation of data for future research.

Sampling Strategy

The goal was to interview enough people to reach a point of credibility in describing the uniqueness of this population. Given this, achieving true "data saturation" (Lambert & Lambert, 2013) would be difficult given the diversity of IDs, health status levels, and ASD severities. The strength of this method is it yields the depth and detail to create a holistic understanding of the healthcare experiences of this population. Exploratory research is used when problems are in a preliminary stage, which is exactly where research on ASD adults is in many respects. This research method is flexible, provides a rich and detailed report on a small number of participants, and can address research questions of all types (what, why, how) (Shields & Tajalli, 2006).

The dyadic model, supported by disability studies (CDC) discipline, allows the individual with ASD/ID the opportunity to make the choice to answer the question or have the support person to answer for the person with ID (if in their best interest). The perspectives and experience of how caregivers support their loved ones with autism in utilizing healthcare services are also important to understand. The goal of this method was to capture in greater clarity the emergent and intrinsic properties of "healthcare experiences" that are shaped by a unique complexity of health conditions and health status. Based on other qualitative research conducted on people with learning disabilities (Finlay & Lyons, 2001; McCarthy, 1998), flexibility and the ability to offer follow-up questions is needed for this special population.

Accordingly, weight was given to the person with ID as the primary source of information. The data collected from the key support person function as a secondary source that parallels their supportive role and is contextualized accordingly during analysis. The goal of this project was to involve adults with ASD/ID in a way that participation is not only done in accordance with ethical practices but is also meaningful and representational. The researcher's role was to facilitate people with ID in sharing their experiences and having their perspectives and voices heard, when possible. For those ASD/ID adults who were not comfortable or able to participate in the interview process, the guardian or caregiver served as the voice for the ASD adult. The challenge in the population under study is that some possess very limited oral communication abilities, and some were nonverbal, thus eliminating the opportunity to fully participate in the interview. Additionally, if the guardian suggested a social service caregiver participated in the interview, instead of, or in addition to the guardian, that served as the additional voice of the ASD adult.

Ethical Issues: Human Subject Issues

Choosing the appropriate method is not only a methodological concern but also an ethical concern when interviewing people with special needs and their caregivers. Finlay and Lyons (2001) recommend that interviewers must be acutely aware of the tendency for individuals with ID/ to acquiesce during interviews. Questions were carefully crafted to avoid creating situations that may promote agreement and acquiescence to statements or questions, regardless of the content of the items. To further help to mitigate this concern, a focus group of ASD professionals and parents assisted in crafting these questions.

Morse (2003) suggests other concerns regarding bias, including the setting and the abilities of participants, need to be considered when developing a qualitative study. Home settings or other very familiar, convenient, and comfortable locations were utilized for the comfort and convenience of the ASD and guardian participants. Participants (parents/guardians) were asked to confirm the ID level and the diagnosis of ASD. The interview appointment allowed for breaks as needed and lasted a length that was comfortable for both the adult and their guardian.

Accommodations for Participant Recruitment

Participants were offered further accommodations, including using innovative disclosure methods such as a YouTube video (Capron, 1999; Dresser, 1996). A short video was prepared specifically for the adults with ASD. In the video, the researcher explained the goals of the project, any risks, or challenges they might encounter, the understanding that they could stop the interview at any time, and any benefits they may receive from the interview. This video was listed on all flyers and was attached to any promotional or recruitment emails. The video was very helpful for participants, both ASD adults and caregivers, so they could "meet" the researcher prior to the actual meeting time. The link to the video is https://youtu.be/F-FrCUAh5BE.

FINDINGS

Informant Characteristics

Informants fell into three categories: adults with ASD/ID, family members/guardians, and caseworkers/caregivers who support them in their residence. For those adults with ASD/ID who possessed the social and communication skills to participate in interviews, those individuals were included as active participants. There were four adult participants diagnosed with ASD/ID. All ASD/ID adults were interviewed along with their family member/guardians. There were six cases where individuals who were not willing or able to be active in the interviews. Based on the CDS discipline, family members/guardians were utilized as the primary source of information. In some cases, caseworkers/caregivers were suggested to be part of the interview in order to give a complete picture of the healthcare experiences. In particular in group home situations, caseworkers/caregivers are the individuals who often accompany ASD/ID adults to their physician or hospital visits.

In total, 12 ASD/ID adults ($n = 12$) were studied as part of this analysis, with an average age of 41.5 years. All 12 adults included interviews with their parent or sibling guardian. The four individuals with ASD/ID who participated in the study were identified by family as those with mild to moderate IDs. Those adults with severe IDs were either nonverbal or lived with significant communication challenges which made inclusion in the interview difficult. All parents or guardians were offered the opportunity to include their ASD/ID adults in the interviews, if they so desired.

Table 1 provides details on the ASD/ID adults enrolled in the study. Ten men and two women were included in the study. All participants reported their race as white. As ASD is identified in 20% of females, and less frequently in older aged cohorts, fewer women were anticipated to be enrolled in the study. There was a wide range of ID from mild to profound, most diagnosed with an ID at an early age, as reported by their family member. Several were not identified with ASD until an older age (often diagnosed with other labels such as mentally retarded, emotionally disturbed, "limp baby," and other disabilities), even into adulthood. This is not a surprise given the changing criteria for diagnosis over the last 40 years. Most in this study reported being in good to fair health. Two cases included adults who were deceased, with their parents reporting their healthcare experiences.

Table 1. Characteristics of ASD/ID Subjects under Study.

Informant ID	Current Age	Sex	Age of ASD Diagnosis	Level of ID (Reported)	Health Status (Reported)
Subject 1	40	M	5	Medium	Good
Subject 2	32	F	5	Medium	Good
Subject 3	53	M	Adult	Severe	Fair
Subject 4	45	M	42	Mild	Good
Subject 5	31	M	3.5	Medium	Good
Subject 6	53	M	5	Mild-Med	Good
Subject 7	25	M	4	Severe	Good
Subject 8	34	M	1	Severe	Good
Subject 9*	24	F	3	Mild	Deceased
Subject 10*	41	M	4	Severe	Deceased
Subject 11	59	M	10	Severe	Fair
Subject 12	61	M	4	Severe	Good

Note: *Deceased.

Table 2 offers more details regarding additional social attributes of the adults who were enrolled in the study. All participants had medical coverage either under Medicare, Medicaid through a state waiver program or through their parents' medical coverage, while several participants who had employment also had access to commercial insurance to supplement their healthcare coverage at some point in their lives. All reported they had "just enough" financial resources to get by in life. Participants were nearly split in terms of their residence. Half lived independently with various levels of support while the rest lived in a group home setting. Most reported being in relatively good health, yet all reported at least three chronic concerns, most often psychiatric/behavioral, gastric and weight/dietary issues. Other significant reported diseases included epilepsy, vertebrae, and other orthopedic challenges, sleep disorders, diabetes, dental, and hyperlipidemia. Nearly all individuals in the study were hospitalized at least once in their lives, if not more than once. Finally, all reported a relationship with a PCP, although all had some difficulties in maintaining that relationship at times due to challenges with finding a physician who accepts Medicaid patients. Most notably, five of the 12 participants reported using the same PCP as a family member which allowed for a longer relationship with that provider than those who did not have a familial relationship. Very few held a high school diploma, and as a result, few had sustainable employment. A few participants were covered by Medicare, which makes the dual eligible. Those who had a high school diploma did have some successful employment and at times, medical benefits through their employer, which allowed them broader access to medical care as they did not have to find physicians who would accept Medicaid.

Table 3 offers information regarding the guardians who participated in each interview. Guardians' demographic data and information were collected on both their lifestyle and healthcare status. Parent participants who actively supported their adult children ranged in ages from 49 to 94, with an average age of 67. As most were reaching older ages, many not only supported their adult child but also attended to their own chronic illnesses. All participants had a higher level of education with a college degree and some with advanced or terminal degrees. All reported to be in relatively good health ranging from good to fair. Some were also caregiving to other adult children, some with special needs and some were caregiving to spouses. Three adults with ASD/ID had siblings who were very involved in supporting their needs as guardians. These guardians ranged in age from 49 to 60 with an average age of 56.

SPECIFIC AIM 1

To understand the perception of patients and their caregivers about how well their healthcare providers understand autism, including the sensory, behavioral, social, and communication needs required of an adult with autism.

The first aim of this study was to learn, in the words of ASD/ID adults and their caregivers, how well their healthcare providers worked to accommodate their needs. There were many stories of positive impressions of healthcare providers having a complete understanding of autism and the needs that come with

Table 2. Social Characteristics of ASD/ID Adults.

Informant ID	Residence Status	Educational Attainment	Ever Hospitalized	See Same Physician as Family?	Medical Needs
Subject 1	Independent with support	No HS Diploma	Yes	Yes	GI, dietary, weight concerns
Subject 2	Independent with support	No HS Diploma	Yes	Yes	Diabetes, weight, mental health
Subject 3	Group home	No HS Diploma	Yes	No	GI, dietary, dental
Subject 4	Independent	Some College	Yes	No	GI, dietary, weight, dental, mental health, vertebrae
Subject 5	Group home	No HS Diploma	Yes	No	Epilepsy, mental health, diet
Subject 6	Family home	HS Diploma	Yes	Yes	Club feet, orthopedic, speech
Subject 7	Group home	HS Diploma	Yes	No	Epilepsy, sleeping, history of GI surgery, mental health
Subject 8	Group home	No HS Diploma	Yes	Yes	Food intolerance, mental health
Subject 9*	Group home	No HS Diploma	Yes	No	GYN, GI, mental health, sleep, weight, ear infections
Subject 10*	Group home	No HS Diploma	Yes	No	GI, prolapsed rectum, sleep, diabetes, weight issues, dental
Subject 11	Group home	No HS Diploma	Yes	No	GI, weight, dental, dietary restrictions
Subject 12	Group home	No HS Diploma	No	No	Spinal, cardiac, mental health

Note: *Deceased.

Table 3. Guardian Characteristics.

Informant ID	Current Age	Guardian?	Relationship	Accompany ASD/ID Adult to Doctor's Visits?	Caregiving for Other Family Members?	Health Status (Reported)
Guardian 1	65	Yes	Mother	Yes	No	Good
Guardian 2	49	Yes	Brother	No	No	Good
Guardian 3	94	No	Mother	No	No	Fair/Poor
Guardian 4	75	No	Father	Sometimes	Yes	Good
Guardian 5	66	Yes	Mother	Yes	Yes	Good
Guardian 6	60	No	Sister	Yes	No	Good
Guardian 7	66	Yes	Father	Yes	Yes	Good
Guardian 8	68	Yes	Mother	Yes	No	Good
Guardian 9*	49	Yes	Mother	Yes	Yes	Good
Guardian 10*	73	Yes	Mother	Yes	No	Good
Guardian 11	79	Yes	Mother	Yes	No	Fair
Guardian 12	60	Yes	Brother	No	No	Good

Note: *Adult with ASD is now deceased.

it. However, there were other stories that explained less than positive or suboptimal experiences. The healthcare environment can be a very distracting and sensory stimulating experience. As a result, ASD/ID adults may need additional customer service attention, special treatment in the clinical setting and extra time to have procedures explained to them. Communication and physical approach to examinations must be planned in a careful way, as not to startle or upset the patient. Also, a feeling of respect toward the adult with ASD/ID is important to both the adult and their caregivers. Behavioral needs were significant care management challenge, as well as dental needs were often cited as one of the most challenging areas for providers to understand the needs for an adult with ASD/ID. A variety of accommodations, clinical decision-making, and communication methods were reported and could be identified in five major categories of needs. These include clinical accommodations, environmental adjustments, communication practices, transitioning on psychotropic medications, specific social needs requirements, and the double jeopardy stigma of ageism/disability.

Clinical Accommodations

Clinical accommodations run a gamut of sensory and behavioral concerns, including changing the clinical room arrangements, adapting the typical patient flow process, shortening the interactions in waiting and examination rooms, and utilizing pediatric providers. All of these accommodations are adaptations to allow the adult with ASD/ID to successfully handle the medical environment with the least amount of stress possible, for them, the providers of care and for the family.

Clinical Accommodations: Sensory Needs

As mentioned in the literature review, pediatric providers have access to helpful literature and training opportunities to help ASD/ID children in the clinical setting. Developmental pediatric physicians are trained to accommodate disabled individuals in the clinical setting. Adult healthcare providers are not provided the same level of training. Often, the clinical environments are not friendly to people with ASD and family/guardians must serve as the primary advocates for accommodations in the clinical setting. A major source of frustration is the waiting room experience. For adults with ASD/ID, especially those with behavior challenges, waiting can add to anxiety, heighten frustration and result in negative physical or verbal behavior. Several families shared their frustration with long waits in waiting rooms.

Mrs J who mentioned her son saw the only PCP in the area who specialized in seeing adults with developmental disabilities. She acknowledged the special needs community was lucky to have this professional in the marketplace; however, this was not a good match for her son because of the crowded environment and long waits times:

> Mrs. J: We waited for long periods in a large waiting room to see him. Our waits were usually at least two hours, just too long for anyone with autism. I just decided that wasn't a good match. So we went to (her PCP) instead.

Nearly all of the participants expressed environmental concerns, such as waiting room environments, the length of wait times, and the exam room environment, make a difference to adults with ASD/ID. Guardians of lower functioning adults with ASD/ID noted the challenge of needing advocacy and supervision in the clinical settings. For those adults, most needed their guardians or representatives from their group home accompany them to the office. Here is a story of why that supervision is so important, and it also indicates the challenges clinical staff may have in serving this population:

> Mrs. W: One time, I remember when (the doctor) was on our board of directors, and we had a meeting this one evening and I'm on the board. He said well, (your son) destroyed my office today. His caregiver had taken him and she told (him) to "stay right here, I have to go to the bathroom, OK." So out the door she goes and he just trashed everything. Just smashed the place up.

Often, people with ASD will destroy objects when they are anxious and uncomfortable. This story illustrates the need for extra support which is needed in the clinical environment, especially for adults who have significant disabilities.

Clinical Accommodations: Environmental Adjustments

Clinical accommodations are welcomed by families to ensure the best experience possible for their loved one. Mrs J, who developed several effective strategies for her son with the assistance of her son's physician, offered several suggestions for PCPs who serve adults with ASD/ID:

> Mrs. J: They need to find more ways to conduct tests more comfortably and less invasively. For example, using finger sticks instead of blood draws. Also, be sure to work with speech therapists so that those with weak communication skills can identify pain through pictures or other descriptions. Also, it is essential to have community supports, like service coordinators, to enable access to care and good coordination of care.

All of these examples point to the need for special accommodations to meet the behavioral and sensory needs of the adult ASD/ID population. Long waits in exam rooms, lack of supervision, and other distracting environments should be avoided to ensure a successful healthcare encounter. Also, creativity in allowing for special accommodations, including bending the usual rules of visitors or the common way of conducting examinations, should be considered.

Clinical Accommodations: Utilizing Pediatric Providers

Some of the younger participants continued to see pediatric providers, as the choices for adult practitioners were very limited. Most children "age out" of pediatric providers between the ages of 18 and 22. For the ASD population, this transition time can be very challenging to find adult providers who understand ASD needs. A limited choice of clinical providers is a concept that will be discussed at a later point; however, clinical accommodations are often made by pediatric providers to ensure continuity of care in an environment which is sensitive to ASD/ID needs. Pediatric providers have more training in serving those with developmental disabilities

Some specialty providers, like dentists, will continue to see adults on the autism spectrum. In this case, the parent was told there were no general dentists in their area they could refer to, and as a result, the pediatric dentist was willing to continue to see her as a patient. This option is not always available to all patients, leaving many in a quandary where to go for services. Whether this will be an accepted practice in the field of medicine remains to be seen. Mrs K made the suggestion for pediatric providers to continue their relationship with adults with ASD/ID. After the inappropriate placement of her daughter in the adult inpatient psychiatric ward, she strongly indicated the need of the local pediatric hospital to take adults patients with ASD/ID :

> Mrs. K: Well my first thing would be that they need to have a different wing at (their local) children's hospital for adults with autism because it is not appropriate to put a person who thinks like a 3 year old in with 40 or 50 year olds in a psychiatric setting. Their needs are not the same. For example you go to the (adult academic medical center); they don't have Disney videos in the adult psychiatric unit. I think they just need some place to serve these people and not in an adult setting. That would be a solution for so many of us. Other parents have horror stories about, out of desperation, having to admit their adult child into a hospital and it is just horrid. They are just mistreated and not understood.

Pediatric hospitals are facing increasing pressure to serve adults who have a gap in service once they leave the pediatric specialists, especially related to all developmental disabilities because of the lack of expertise in adult medicine.

Pediatric health providers may be an option for many who find those physicians who are willing to accommodate the needs of an adult. Some specialty physicians, such as dentists and psychologists, seemed to be more willing to accommodate these adult requests from the people interviewed in this study. However, as adults age, pediatricians may not be the most appropriate medical providers, given the expertise needed for adults.

Communication Practices

Communication in the Clinical Environment

Mrs S. mentioned the importance to approach her son with a calm and deliberate approach. Although her son has expressive language issues, his receptive language is well developed and he is compliant with directions if approached by medical professionals in the right way. Mrs S offered the following comment:

> Mrs. S: Well he has gone to different doctors, you know, and he is not a guy you can go to and say "hi how are you doing"? It startles him when someone is really loud. You have to explain in detail this is what we are going to do, now you give me your finger and we will get a little blood out of it [...] The funny thing of it is, he does not initiate a conversation but if anybody asks him a question, he knows exactly what the person is saying; he knows everything that I say to him. I can tell him things that I would think he would never do [...].

This comment should serve as reminder to healthcare providers that many people with ASD do have receptive language skills, even when their expressive skills are modest. It is best when the parent/guardian or residential caregiver clearly explains the communication skill level to the healthcare worker. In fact, many adults with ASD/ID expect clear explanations. Many parents and siblings mentioned the need for their loved ones to understand what is happening in the healthcare environment. Compliance improved when adults with ASD/ID were given clear descriptions of what to expect, not only did it provide instruction but also offered a level of respect which is palpable to them.

Nancy, an adult with ASD/ID also reiterated the importance of clear explanations and for written instructions:

> Nancy: Yeah, he tells me what is going to happen and he writes things down so I can look at it later. He tells me what I need to do. You know, some people scream when they go to the doctor, they do not like shots (mentioning something that bothers her).

Nancy's comment, as someone with ASD/ID, indicates she appreciates the effort her doctor takes to explain things and to give her a written document to remind her of important directions. Also, she indicates her frustration in the environment, at the same time. Her brother, her guardian, echoes his appreciation for her physician's approach for communications:

> Nancy's guardian: Yes, (Nancy's doctor) does all of that and he tries to teach her things that will help her health and so does the team. They will tell her behavioral stories to encourage her in certain behaviors, when she is not being cooperative or she doesn't understand why it is helpful, so they do that too, one of the people on the staff, so that is good.

The story of Nancy reinforces the importance of utilizing "teaching moments" and having appropriate educational information and directions for people with ASD/ID. Obviously, these materials need to be at a level which can be understandable and useful to the patient.

Communication with Guardians and Residential Caregivers

Communication with guardians and residential caregivers (group home and supported living situations) is also key in order to develop an integrated plan with healthcare providers. In particular for guardians who live a distance from their loved one, the coordination between the guardian, caregiver, and medical professional is essential to ensure proper consent and coordinated care planning. Nancy's brother, who serves as her guardian, lives about 200 miles from Nancy. Both he and his wife have been integral to communicating with providers and attempting to reduce her psychotropic medications, increasing her physical activities, changing her diet, and providing her with more social interaction. However, it has taken a great deal of patience and time to achieve this level of care and health for his sister:

> Wife: They have seen a tremendous change in her because we are working together because we really want her to have a full life.

> Nancy's Guardian: They have, over time figured out what she likes and what she doesn't like. Right now things are fairly status quo for her and pretty much everything she is doing she is comfortable with […] it has taken five years.

Nancy's guardian also shared his concerns regarding communications from the medical professionals. Consent was not received for some of the procedures during visits. In addition, medication changes were always made without his input.

> Nancy's Guardian: The main problem I have with the healthcare professionals is making decisions without consulting us. I mean, I have never gone the legal route because it has never got to that point, but that has been very hard. I mean they all have letters, they all have the information, but they just don't think about it.

This example illustrates how important it is for healthcare providers to clearly understand the legal relationship of the adult diagnosed with ASD/ID and their guardian. Particularly in group and supportive living situations, residential caregivers are not allowed to consent for medical procedures.

Patient Social/Behavioral Requirements

An interesting thing to note for two of the ASD/ID participants was their reluctance to be recognized as having a disability. They did not view themselves as "autistic" and one adult indicated he "grew out of it." It is not clear if they avoid the diagnosis because of the stigma associated with it, or the adult feels they live a fine life without having the label of "autistic." Others who received the ASD diagnosis as an adult recognized the ASD diagnosis with a sense of relief (as it explained and verified their behavior and feelings which were not understood previously). This presents challenges to healthcare providers to know how to approach each ASD/ID client about their developmental diagnosis. The role of the caregiver is very helpful in interpreting these perspectives to healthcare providers. In order to develop a trusting relationship, this psychosocial approach to the patient's disability is quite important. The neurodiversity movement may change the view of the disability, for those with the diagnosis and for those who serve them.

Related to communications is the challenge of understanding how the person with ASD/ID expresses their feelings of pain or discomfort. Working with this population is challenging in ascertaining how they experience or identify illness symptoms. Some interviewed were very capable of managing their health and asking questions. However, for lower functioning ASD/ID individuals, it is their caregiver who must serve as the interpreter to the clinician. Each individual with ASD/ID should be evaluated for their capabilities of expressing their understanding of their health:

> Mrs. J: The difficult thing is (her son) cannot explain what his symptoms are, he cannot tell us how he feels. Now that he had that experience (he was hospitalized for gut pain), whenever he does not feel well, he tells us it his stomach, but often, it is not. This is the words he has learned to describe not feeling well.

This mother, who is also a healthcare professional, developed innovative tactics for improving her son's healthcare experiences and accomplished this in concert with the PCP. This exemplifies a successful approach to managing her son's stress in clinical and other life situations. Each of the stories in this section illuminates the need for communication between the healthcare provider and the parent/guardian (as well as the residential caseworker) to ensure providers have the best preparation to serve the adult with ASD/ID.

Transitioning On/Off Psychotropic Medications

All participants, including those adults with ASD/ID, expressed serious concerns regarding the medical management of ASD with psychotropic medications. All but one participant was taking at least one, if not more, psychotropic medications. The balancing act of the right medications and the right dosage is something that is a lifelong challenge for every individuals interviewed. Several spoke of the need to start medications at very young ages, especially in order to function in the educational environment. Many of these medications have not been tested on children; thus, the medical literature has little information on the long-term use of these medications. Every parent/guardian discussed the early use of medications; the most striking stories are shared here:

> Mrs. K: In about the third grade she just started, you know, terrible sleeper, tons of anxiety and nothing you could do would make her happy and she would just have these complete meltdowns. She developed these repetitive activities that disturbed other people. She would rub her face until it was red and raw, she would bite herself and when she was really frustrated she would spit on people. So we started down a path of taking all of these wild medications.

> Mrs. W: Well when (my son) was young and he went to the (the children's hospital) psychiatric center, not even in school, I think he was about 3 years old they had him on Haldol.

These stories speak to several issues. Severe behavior problems, present for many of these individuals at young ages, gave many families the difficult choice to utilize some very powerful psychiatric medications. Behavioral therapy was not available for many of the adults that took part in this study, and prescription drugs were really the only option. These prescriptions are used "off label," meaning that their FDA approval is for other, related conditions such as attention deficit hyperactivity disorder (ADHD), sleep disturbances, or depression. Off-label use is common in nearly all areas of medicine and is usually done to relieve significant autistic characteristics in the absence of sufficiently large and targeted studies. These medications were not tested on children, and their long-term use is still not well understood. For many of these adults, the lifelong use of psychotropic medication is appearing to cause physical consequences as adults. In particular, the family of the adults who died prematurely attributed their many of their children's health problems to psychotropic medications. All family members/guardians shared their ongoing worries related to these medications, including issues around weight gain, drowsiness, gastrointestinal upset, elevated cholesterol levels, and diabetes. Mr Z expressed what he referred to as the "freaky balance" in ensuring his brother's behavior was well managed, in order to remain at the care facility which he has lived in for over 20 years. The medications offered an important relief to aggressive behavior, but it brought serious concerns regarding health implications to several guardians:

> Mr. Z: It is a very freaky balance really. Risperdal is very powerful anti-psychotic and you probably know what it is but it has been linked over time to shrinkage of brain volume. It is really a horrifying med but when I try to get them to reduce the dose, which they were happy to do because they don't like it either, to their credit, he flipped out. So yes, it is a choice made for keeping him there and relatively happy. It is a lousy choice but that is such a reality.

Among the frustrations related to medications was the mixed advice they received regarding safety and effectiveness. In the end, the families were hoping for relief for their loved ones:

> Mrs. S: Well anyway, it (the psychiatric admission) was a hideous experience. They put him in there and they started taking him off of his drugs. Because he was an adult they wouldn't talk to us because we weren't his guardians (the group home was the guardian). They would not even confirm that he was there and I said, look, I know he is here. He got so bad during that stay because of being off the medication and they couldn't deal with it. They didn't know what to do for him [...]. He cried the whole time. I mean he never cried [...] so when you hear him cry it was just heartbreaking. We had an experience where we took him to a doctor up in (city) who did the opposite. He just bombed him with medication [...] the poor guy was drugged his entire life for the most part because of his behavior.

As indicated by Mrs S in her comment above, several participants noted the challenge of changing medications or attempting to reduce high dosages. Often participants were hospitalized for a significant period of time, as they went through very difficult periods, which heightened anxiety and produced very challenging physical and emotional behaviors. This "balancing act" of ensuring socially appropriate behavior was articulated by Mr Z, as one that could impact the ability to live in the most desirable circumstances for his aging brother.

Thus, the management of medications was essential for his brother's all-around well-being:

> Mr. Z: It is a tough process. With my brother you are dealing with a terminal condition. He is not going to change; he is not going to get any better. He has reached that stage where all I really care about is that he stays at this place. It is the best place in the world [...] So I just can't allow that to happen. He is very happy overall and they love him very much. They show him a tremendous amount of affection, the staff does, but he is volatile and I don't want him to blow it.

Essentially, the use of psychotropic medications frustrated many and was seen as something of an inescapable issue for adults with ASD/ID.

Double Jeopardy Stigma of Ageism/Disability

As indicated in the literature review, stigma is a mark of disgrace that sets people and groups apart from the rest of society and often results in negative actions and discrimination. Rarely would stigma toward age and disability be overt in institutionalized settings; however, insidious discrimination exists in forms such as challenges in accessing services, difficulties in communicating needs, and expectations and subjective decision-making by healthcare workers. All three research questions shed light on the issues surrounding accessing services and difficulty in communicating needs. Subjective decision-making and judgments were experienced by all family participants; these experiences worried some parents and guardians to the real attitudes by some healthcare providers toward their loved one. The dual stigma of disability and age can potentially impact access to care based on the experiences shared by the informants. As a result, families often must maintain a protective and vigilant attitude to ensure their loved ones receive appropriate care.

SPECIFIC AIM 2

To explore ASD-impacted adults and their guardians' experience with the coordination between primary health, other specialty or ancillary services, and factors which could impact access to care.

The primary care physician (PCP) is often counted on to serve as the "gatekeeper" for specialist services and medication coordination. As examined in the literature review, pediatric literature is full of supporting data related to the value of medical homes for the special needs population, yet little evidence exists on patient-centered medical homes for adult patients with ASD. This specific aim wanted to better understand the degree of fragmentation and coordination of medical services received by ASD adults. Several of the adults with ASD/ID shared the same PCPs as other family members, and this "family doctor" scenario will be explored. It became clear from the interviews that it is often not a physician who coordinates services, but often the family is responsible for this coordination, with support (sometimes leading support) of caseworkers from residential settings [...].

There were several situations where coordination of care was challenging, in particular, in emergency rooms (ERs). Several stories will be shared of the challenge in this environment. In addition, preventive medical screenings, usually coordinated through the PCP, can also be a challenge for some adults with ASD/ID. Those stories are also shared in this section.

PCP Serving as Coordinator of Care/Services: Positive Experiences

All but one of the participants had a dedicated PCP, and most were followed by their physician for some time (greater than three years). Five of the 12 adults with ASD/ID had the same PCP as their family member. These five reported very strong and confident relationships with their physicians, often in more positive terms than those who saw different physicians than their family members. Perhaps the longevity, understanding of family history and combined relationships made that connection stronger. When the relationship is well coordinated and roles are clearly identified, the adult with ASD/ID benefits from well-planned healthcare delivery.

Mrs F explained the very special relationship her son has with his PCP. Her son transitioned to her (and her husband's) physician at the age of adult transition. This physician has cared for members of the family for 28 years. Their physician was instrumental in helping her son recover from malnutrition which happened in his mid-20s while in the care of a group home where he was physically and emotionally abused. This PCP facilitated all referrals to any specialty needed, including neurology, psychology, neuro-psychology, GI, and dentistry. Mrs F described this strong bond her son and his physician share:

> Mrs. F: (Her son has seen his physician) since he was 22 or 21. Like if I write down (her doctor's name), (her son) will whisper "that is my best friend" […]. He was so desperately sick for about a year and he saw (his doctor) all the time and he knew that (he) was helping him and saving him and he was worried about himself. He adores (him) […].

This quote indicates the bond of trust which exists between their PCP and Mrs F's family, in particular for her son with ASD/ID. Mrs F feels strongly their PCP saved her son's life when he got very ill from this traumatic experience.

Given multiple examples in this study of sharing the same PCP, there appears to be great value in this arrangement as it seems to enhance the understanding of the family medical history, while sharing a social connection. In addition, due to the closer relationship, there appears to be improved coordination with other providers of services. It seems this model appears to emulate some of the same structures as patient-centered medical homes (PCMH).

PCP Serving as Coordinator of Care/Services: Less Positive Experiences

Mr L, the parent of a 25-year-old son, earlier mentioned the continued use of a pediatric specialist for the management of his son's psychotropic medicine. His son sees an adult PCP, who would normally coordinate his prescription medications; however, Mr L did not seem concerned about the lack of coordination between the pediatric specialist and the adult PCP:

> Mr. L: I have no idea how they coordinate (his care). In fact I had to tell (his son's adult PCP) that his medications were going to be coordinated by (a pediatric ASD specialist) and I felt a bit awkward telling him.

Mr L presents a potentially challenging situation in terms of coordination of care and symptom monitoring. As many of the psychotropic medications may cause physical side effects, such as weight gain, gastric distress, elevated cholesterol, and blood pressure levels and more, effective information sharing is critical. In many cases, it is up to the parent of guardian to be the conduit between and among medical professionals.

Role of Family Members in the Coordination of Care

Typically, families must be actively involved in coordinating healthcare for their family members. Although a PCP can serve as a "gatekeeper" of referrals to specialists and oversee general health, the family must be actively engage in advocating for their loved one in the medical environment.

Jack is a higher functioning adult with ASD/ID and sees many specialty physicians, as well, have long-term relationship with his internist. However, Jack's sister is really the coordinator of a vast network of orthopedic surgeons who care for her brother's issues, which has ranged from club feet, a broken femur, broken ankle, Achilles heel repair, and fluid on the knee. Jack's sister maintains a meticulous notebook with her brother's medical history, and she serves as his medical historian and care coordinator.

> Sister: Yes, I have Jack on "My Chart" now.
>
> Researcher: (speaking to Jack) Yes and you can look at your records too. (To Jack's sister) Are you going to keep your book?
>
> Sister: Yes, I will keep it.
>
> Researcher: Yes, because you have copious notes before My Chart became available.
>
> Sister: Yes, we have folders and folders on him.

Given the complexity of Jack's orthopedic history, his sister is wise to maintain this important information and to continue to advocate for his needs. Jack is accompanied by his sister or his mother to every doctor's visit. She feels strongly advocacy is a necessary part of maintain her brother's active life.

Strong partnerships among family and healthcare practitioners are key to ensuring a good medical plan and ongoing health. Family members who are not always available to attend physician visits need caseworkers and other residential support to be involved in communications between the guardians and the physician.

Reliance on Caseworkers in Coordination of Care

For those aging adults with ASD/ID, many have failing or deceased parents who can no longer serve as their guardian. At this point in life, it is often a sibling who takes on that responsibility. Several sibling guardians participated in this study shared their reliance on group home caseworkers to assist in coordinating their medical care and visits. Nancy's guardian lives approximately 250 miles away from Nancy and counts on both her case coordinator and Nancy's PCP to keep him informed of Nancy's health status and healthcare management:

> Nancy's Guardian: Well, (the caseworker) is our eyes and ears. She is our advocate (there) because she is very devoted to (Nancy) and she is very professional. So the two combined, we asked her to be our eyes and ears and our advocate there so any time there needs to be a decision made we always involve her and we always copy her on everything because she spends a lot more time with Nancy than we can [...]. (Her primary care physician) keeps records on all of the medications. (Her doctor) is supposed to be the one making sure she isn't having any issues with her medicines.

As mentioned previously, Nancy's guardian worked diligently to improve communications among all of the physicians Nancy sees for her chronic illnesses. Her caseworker is integral to the success of this coordination, and her guardian has "let his guard down" on worrying about coordination issues now that her casework is so capable of managing Nancy's care.

Often, if a group home resident is hospitalized, a home worker accompanies the adult and serves as a "sitter" in order to make their hospitalization as smooth as possible. Mrs K's son was hospitalized and recuperating from a surgery, when a complication developed. Tragically, her son passed away due to the complication. Mrs K is left with many questions from her son's death; one concern she shared was the reliance on group home workers in the inpatient setting:

> Mrs. K [...]. Well, our provider at the time (group home) had someone there with him the whole time. So here is my question; did they rely on them more than they should have? I mean they are not medical professionals. It wasn't that they didn't see signs of his deterioration, I think he was throwing up blood or something.

As we learn from these examples, residential and supported living caseworker play an integral role in coordinating care and ongoing home treatments for adults with ASD/ID. Their role in conveying information is counted on by guardians and healthcare professionals. This last story brings concerns about their roles in the inpatient environment, as hospital employees seem to consider caseworkers to be "sitters" and may rely on them in ways which they are not properly trained to fulfill.

Coordination of Care Challenges: Emergency Rooms

Several informants mentioned the difficulty in using ER services where communication with the patient's PCPs is not a common practice. In both of these stories, adults with ASD/ID were referred to a pediatric ERs, as their PCPs thought they would find more "understanding" care for their loved one.

> Mrs. J: One area where we did have some difficulties when he was sick last year. He was very sick to his stomach with acute pain. She (his PCP) did not know where to send us for care. She suggested we go to a children's hospital! I said, I cannot take an adult man to a children's hospital! It concerns me that we did not know where to send him and if got very sick again, I am not sure what we should do. Other than that situation, we are very pleased with (their primary care physician).

ERs can be a daunting experience for any person, but especially those with significant ASD/ID sensory challenges. Some emergency departments are now designing designated spaces for geriatric patients, and this kind of environment, which has much less sensory stimulus, may be a better care environment for aging adults with ASD. Many of the participants noted their fear of taking their loved ones to ERs, as few emergency departments know how to accommodate adults with ASD/ID.

Coordination of Care Challenges: Preventive Health Services

Preventive health services are important to protecting, promoting, and maintaining health and well-being and to prevent disease, disability, and potentially death. For an adult visiting a PCP, common preventive health services include vaccinations, screening for several chronic concerns including blood pressure, hepatitis B and C, cholesterol, diabetes, obesity, colorectal cancer, depression, and diet counseling. For women, other preventive screening includes mammography, osteoporosis screening, and cervical cancer screening. As mentioned in the literature review, adults with ASD/ID may have difficulty in handling some of the more invasive testing and minor procedures. Some of the informants shared these challenges in receiving preventive care:

Earlier, we heard the story about Mrs K's daughter, who had a significant complication from the Depo Provera shot. Her daughter never received a GYN exam, as they assumed she would have to be sedated to undergo that type of examination. The other woman in the study, Nancy, did not receive GYN exams either, even though she received the same Depo shot to reduce her menstrual cycle.

> Nancy's Caregiver: No, she does not (have GYN exams). (Her brother) asked me about that too. She hasn't had any problems with that. I told (her brother) that if (the doctor) ever asked for it that I would take her, but I'm just not sure how she would do. I don't see that ending very well.

Mrs. S mentioned her son has high blood pressure, and his PCP ordered an EKG in order to monitor his heart function. Unfortunately, her son would not comply with the screening:

> Mrs. S: He has had a few primary care doctors throughout the years. I don't think he stayed too long, you know. There were certain things that he would not let them do, one of them is to have an EKG [...] I'm not sure what it was, but he was absolutely hysterical.

Preventative health services are essential in the management of chronic illness and needed as adults age. Unfortunately, for many people with ASD/ID, the invasive nature of some procedures, even things like blood draws and immunizations, can be quite traumatic. For many, they must be fully sedated to undergo most simple medical procedures. As mentioned by several interviewees, including Mrs J, there is a need to develop innovative ways to find less invasive ways to screen people for disease. As medical technology evolves to find less invasive testing, adults with ASD/ID will benefit from these innovations.

SPECIFIC AIM 3

To discover what other barriers (e.g., access to available health services, policy concerns, such as health insurance and residency location, advocacy, aging guardians, and others) can potentially influence the health for adults with ASD.

As indicated in the literature review, there are other potential barriers to providing optimal care which may impact healthcare outcomes and influence the determinants of health in the adult ASD/ID population. First, access to healthcare and the quality of health services impact health outcomes, especially in an acute episode. Access to care is challenging for ASD/ID adults and their caregivers, as so few providers are trained to serve people with special needs. In particular, since many of the adults interviewed were covered by Medicaid as an insurance payor, this can provide a first layer of access limitations for this population. Policymakers can make decisions that impact access to care, as well as influence other social service supports which ultimately impact determinants of health, including policy related to residential support. Residential living can also present challenges for many residents, as other residents may present physical aggression and caregivers may not live up to their responsibilities. Finally, the support received from aging parents and guardians, and their continued ability to advocate for their loved ones influences access to care and potentially healthcare outcomes.

Barriers to Health: Access to Available Services

For many, it is very challenging to find a PCP who is focused on the needs of those with ASD or ID, in addition to caring for a broader population of patients in their general practice. One informant discussed the only adult internist who devoted his practice to people with IDs in this mid-Western city.

> Mrs. M: I'm not sure he had control over the environment and there were so many people trying to get into see him [...] he was just slammed all the time. [...] I heard he had cut back (on appointments) and that is why he was going out to (a residential center) for a half day per month but I don't know. I know people are going to be really upset when he retires because there is no one else.

Another informant in this study, who was from one of the largest cities in the United States, mentioned there was only one adult psychiatric unit in the city that would admit people on the autism spectrum:

Mrs. F: The neurologist was at the only hospital in (the city) that would take an autistic person. It was the only psych ward (in the entire city that would take a person on the ASD spectrum).

Mrs M echoed the concern regarding the lack of access to specialty care devoted to adults with ASD/ID:

Mrs. M: We talked about this when I was on (a community leadership group for professionals serving the ASD population). I mean how do you train or get a doctor that is interested in developmental disabilities? Because once they leave (pediatric services) and age out of there, I mean the (local pediatric ASD center) has taken back a few adults, but that is not full medical care [...] I have a patient [...] (who) is mentally disabled and (he is going into) a medical home. And I said, awesome, perfect. Because if it is designed that way, then maybe that will work [...].

Every informant interviewed shared concerns about access to physicians. Some were concerned about the lack of access as a Medicaid patient (and some practices do not see Medicaid patients), some just found obstacles to care, as we saw in particular with Mrs F, who had one choice for a psychiatric facility in one of the largest cities in the United States. Very few adult PCPs have expertise in developmental disabilities and no participant was enrolled in a medical home.

Barriers to Health: Medicaid Coverage

Certainly, a major component of this access issue is the kind of health insurance coverage the individual possesses. Since the vast majority of those with ASD and ID are not gainfully employed with healthcare benefits, most are reliant on public support (Medicaid) once parental insurance is no longer available (now extended to the age of 26, based on the Accountable Care Act provisions). Two participants did have gainful employment in the past, with healthcare benefits. Alex, who was injured on his way home from work when he encountered ice on his bike ride, was especially challenged with Medicaid. He tells two stories here: the first related to dentistry (Medicaid only pays one visit per year) and the next with losing all benefits through no fault of his own:

Dad: You can tell her how you would go to dentists and they wouldn't work on you and stuff?

Alex: Yes I had one that had an office in xxxx and xxxx and for some reason they kept rescheduling my appointment and I would ride the bus only to find out my appointment was cancelled and I had a meltdown right in the lobby.

Researcher: What would be their reason for cancelling you?

Alex: They would say my insurance wasn't working.

Dad: From a perfect state he lost continuity.

This story speaks to the insurance problems in finding a dental practitioner who would accept Medicaid, but also speaks to the lack of communication, and in turn, respect for the patient (Alex took three different buses, totaling over two hours of travel to get to this dental office). Alex also experienced significant problems when he was disenrolled in Medicaid, for no apparent reason. This resulted in Alex being unable to visit a doctor for nearly a year while the applications were updated for his membership:

> Alex: […]. I have only seen him (his physician) one time because we had to change last year because I had a little problem. I got everything through Job and Family Services and we had a little debate with them. They took away my Medicaid for a few months and we finally got that straightened out. They said I forgot to renew one time and me and my case manager had to go through and get everything straightened out. So we just went through my schedule so I can get my dentist and doctor's appointments all caught up […] I haven't seen anyone in over a year.
>
> Alex's Dad: Even the caseworker said we did nothing wrong.

Insurance coverage is a significant concern for all Americans, and for this population, public programs are often utilized. Given the concern regarding the lack of access due to Medicaid, it speaks to the larger issue regarding public policy for adults with developmental disabilities. Several informants shared their concern that public policy decision-makers do not "get it":

> Mrs. J: I want them to appreciate what it is like to be him in this world that causes sensory challenges and these sensory challenges can sometime cause physical pain. I hope their staff will be willing to help. Medicaid does not fully support all of the needs of this special population, and that is scary to think about as we age.
>
> Mrs. F: Well the concern is he will never see a dentist. We have had quite an adventure at the dentist. He has to be sedated to sit in the chair […] In (their state) you can only see a dentist once a year and if anything is wrong. You can only have anesthetic if you break your jaw […]. We live in a very primitive world over here. It cost me $1400 to get anesthetic for him to get his teeth cleaned. Out of pocket.

These stories illustrate the frustration in insurance coverage for basic medical, dental, and psychiatric issues for this population. It is truly the "stroke of a pen" that can mean access to care for this special needs population.

Barriers to Health: Group and Supported Residential Living

Public policy matters go beyond health coverage issues and access to medical services, as it also includes issues related to residential funding. Mrs F told the story how a good placement for her son became a very dangerous situation due to a significant decrease in funding:

> Mrs. F: The funding was never strong. It was a small group home and we helped to found it […]. They were short funded here in (my state) […] now they are 10 to 15 people short staffed so the agency moved in 3 super low-functioning violent people to get extra funding so (my son) and his friend started getting hurt […] the staff became very lazy, they just wanted to sit around and watch Netflix and drug up the kids […] So all of these kids would just sit in their rooms and be sad and (her son) was getting severely hurt, I mean really bad injuries and they would say "oh he must have fallen out of bed" […] So he stopped eating because he was scared to eat with them. And the staff didn't do anything about it. He lost 65 pounds in two months.

Mrs M also worried about her son's treatment in his group home, as staff were sometimes shorthanded and turnover is high, due to low wages. Also, some of the staff was not as committed as they could be to the residents of the home, as described below by Mrs M. She also shared concern for the behavior challenges from other residents, who may be lacking appropriate supervision:

> Mrs. M: That is what we worry about for the future [...] that is why we wanted (name) as our provider, because they get it. But they have got to train their staff because they have high turnover and they don't pay well [...] Well, I walked in and the staff was asleep last week. I mean they were really asleep. They didn't hear me come in twice. [...] Yes, he (her son) could have been behind a locked door, and a seizure happens, so I reported her but, I hated to [...]. Group homes are wonderful and terrible because you know, there are roommates [...]. When you put people with autism together, you have a bunch of people with autism.

Mrs M's son was in a previous group home where gaps in care were very evident, actually harming her son's health:

> Mrs. M: He has head injuries from the seizures and falls and had to get stitches in his head. But that's because they were not giving him his medicine in (his group home) He had to be hospitalized (there) and when I arrived there he was having seizures and come to find out his blood level was zero for his seizure meds. So the doctor looked at me and said "I think there is only one answer for what's going on here". Somebody was stealing his medicine. That is when I brought him back (home).

Several participants shared these alarming stories about their adult's residential placement, while others had very positive stories. From these stories, we can sense the link between physical and emotional well-being and residential placement.

Advocacy: Influence on Ability to Serve

Many family participants talked about their continued advocacy for their loved ones, as they attempted to remove barriers to treatment and care. Even those parents who were at advanced ages continued this effort, such as Mrs S:

> Mrs. S: Well you know, no one taught us anything hardly. You know in the 50's they had nothing. We went through a lot. Fortunately or unfortunately we knew politicians. I think today it is the same way. It's not what you know, it's who you know. That will never end. When (my son) was growing up we were very close to a couple of local politicians and they did a lot to help us. To find places and whatever, you know. We were lucky in that respect.

As his brother's guardian Mr Z is very involved in advocating not only for his brother but also for other's with ASD, through volunteer work with the national advocacy organization, Autism Speaks. Here, he talks about his appreciation of his mother's dedication to his brother, as well as his new role of guardian to his brother:

> Mr. Z: Yes it is a real mess but I'm lucky because my mother did all of the heavy lifting. I just have to do all of the bureaucratic follow through and it is substantial. You have to become a guardian and a representative payee and all of those other things that is involved in taking over the life of someone who is disabled. But I'm glad that I am doing it to face the bureaucratic entity.

DISCUSSION

The goal of this exploratory study was to describe the experiences of adults with ASD/ID and their caregivers in navigating the healthcare system, bringing to light the successes, challenges, thoughts, and perspectives of the informants. Since limited research exists on the life events of these adults, it was unclear what would be learned about their lives, especially related to their health. The intention of this discussion is to sensitize readers to the experiences described by these adults, their family, and their caregivers and to consider how to improve the lives of this growing population. Some of the adults interviewed encountered negative health outcomes and suboptimal relationships with healthcare providers; others seemed to have very positive relationships, with good preventive care and monitoring of health. Clinical and communication accommodations were absolutely necessary to make healthcare provision more comfortable for this population. Coordination of care was seen as an imperative, with most family members taking on this responsibility, with support from residential caregivers and some primary care physicians. Several barriers to accessing healthcare services included finding appropriate services, managing sensory concerns, lack of healthcare professional training, and insurance limitations. The informants offered insights and suggestions to enhance clinical and patient care experiences, communication, and coordination improvements and advocacy strategies that could make a positive difference in their lives. The key to each adult's success will be to balance customization of their individual care needs with a broader system, designed to meet their emotional, sensory, social, behavioral, and coordination of care requirements. Creating partnerships with families, residential care providers, and healthcare professionals may offer opportunities to better serve and understand the health needs of these vulnerable adults. This study supports the critical need for more healthcare professionals to dedicate their practice to this expanding population and for many healthcare providers to gain training in working with adults with ASD, as well as ID. Of course, health policy must support these strategies; especially promoting training of physicians and other healthcare professionals and further expansion of medical homes through the Medicaid program. Perhaps some of the lessons learned in this study can offer novel ideas on how healthcare delivery systems, research organizations and public policy administrators might be more responsive to the needs of aging adults with ASD/ID.

Several key elements learned from this study deserve more in-depth discussion, including utilizing a life course perspective in studying aging adults with ASD/ID, issues related to access to care, utilization of family physicians, the residential location and its impact on health, the impact of communication challenges, and access to preventive healthcare services.

LIMITATIONS

This study was intended to work as closely with people with ASD/ID as possible, as suggested by the critical disabilities studies discipline. However, only four adults participated as active informants in the study. Parents and guardians were very interested in participating in the study, but the eight other participants indicated their adult children/siblings were unable to actively participate in an interview (two were deceased, but the other six declined the interview). The interview questions for adults with ASD/ID were shared in advance so that guardians could make informed decisions regarding their participation. This was disappointing, as the goal was to have their direct perspectives and voices heard. However, this is understandable, given the potential communications challenges between the researcher and the adults with ASD/ID. Good qualitative research demands we build on the strengths of people with disabilities, while understanding their (and our own) limitations (McCarthy, 1998). People with ID who are recruited as informants may be considered vulnerable if their ability to provide assent is compromised (Roberts & Roberts, 1999). Thus, the number of adult participants was limited.

A further limitation was the challenge in finding adults above the age of 40. The original design of this project was to find adults who were considered approaching the "older ages" of ASD. Initially, it was difficult to find this population, as many people in that age cohort were never given the diagnosis of ASD. In fact, several people expressed an interest in the project, but did not have the official diagnosis (although family and caregivers noted their assumption of the adult being on the autism spectrum). Also, once the study was announced, many of the family members of younger participants asked to have their voices heard. Since many of these individuals had other comorbidities and extensive experience in the healthcare environment, it was determined they should be included in the project.

The characteristics of the study informants may result in some limitations to a broad understanding of healthcare experiences. Interestingly, the guardians/family members in this study were all well-educated people, with both parents and guardians possessing at least a Bachelor's degree, and many who earned advanced or terminal degrees. It is unknown whether the healthcare experiences for those whose family have less education is different from this more highly educated set of informants. Finally, the study evaluated two women as part of the study. According to the emerging literature on women with ASD/ID, females seem to have more frequent incidence of chronic illnesses and have shorter life spans than men. It would also be interesting to do a more focused study on women as a single group, separate from men.

CONCLUSIONS AND FUTURE WORK

According to the most recent literature on adults with a combined ASD/ID diagnosis, there is a lack of a coordinated response to ensure the best possible health and social care is provided to this special population in later life (Lin et al., 2016). This study confirms there seems to be no coordinated planning, including the integration of residential, healthcare, and occupational services for this growing population. The opportunity for better understanding, planning, and intervention is upon us and must be pursued. Public policy is important to building this integration of services which impact well-being. Further research should guide and enhance public policy changes to create improved coordinated planning programs.

This study presents many opportunities for further research. Several areas warranting additional research include better understanding of the healthcare provider relationship (from the provider perspective) with the ASD/ID adults, sharing and spreading best clinical and environmental practices, assessing alternative care settings to prevent injury and reduce ER use, exploring expanded use of the medical home concept for adults which has been reasonably successful in pediatrics, conducting longitudinal studies of the impact in using psychotropic medications, and deepening our understanding of how the life course perspective and the neurodiversity movement may apply to the adult ASD/ID population.

The Provider Perspective and Sharing Best Practices

It would be very interesting to learn about the healthcare provider side of this relationship. The studies on healthcare providers thus far report a lack of self-perceived competency by PCPs in treating and diagnosing adults with ASD (Bruder et al., 2012; Golnik et al., 2009). There is very limited literature on best practices for optimal compliance and enhanced comfort in the clinical setting for adults with ASD/ID. Some individual physicians are becoming more creative on preventive medical procedures for this population; for example, Mrs J noted using finger sticks as an effective method for traditional blood draws. Sharing these kinds of approaches would be very helpful to adult medicine practitioners. As more evidenced-based data emerge on "best practices," finding effective ways to create a dialogue on the treatment of adults with ASD/ID to share these practices will be very helpful in starting this movement to enable improved patient care.

Alternative Care Settings to Prevent Injury and Reduce Emergency Room Use

Also, hospital settings must be better prepared for these adults, especially in the ER and in the operating room (OR). A recent study by Miller (2015) examined the extent of ASD knowledge among nurses working in an ER and found that about two-thirds of ER nurses surveyed reported having accurate knowledge, correctly identified causes of visit and co-occurring illnesses, and chose appropriate interventions for ASD cases. However, nurses still reported having limited knowledge and resources available to them and felt a need for ASD education early on in their training. In addition, adults with ASD are using the ER at higher rates, presumably as they are now entering older age and may have limited access to primary and preventive care. In a recent study by Vohra, Madhavan, and Sambamoorthi (2016), they found the rate of ER visits in the United States for adults with an ASD diagnosis more than doubled from 2006 to 2011 (2,549–6,087 per 100,000 admissions). Adults with ASD (all types) visited the ER most often for the following reasons: primary psychiatric disorder, primary non-psychiatric disorder, and injury. The study also found the mean total ER charges for adults with ASD were 2.3 times higher than for adults without ASD. As the majority (80%) of adults with ASD were covered by public health insurance, as compared to one-quarter (25%) adults without ASD, this finding reflects public payors account for the vast majority of adults with special needs. These special, stressful environments deserve more scrutiny to identify how to optimize treatment and enhance patient care experience.

Exploring the Medical Home Concept for Adults with ASD/ID

This study had no participants who were members of a medical home. As mentioned in the literature review, pediatric PCMH, originally organized to serve special needs children, are now considered the standard of care for all children. Providers who serve as a medical home have demonstrated more comprehensive and coordinated care and greater success at meeting needs when compared to the broader cohort of children and youth with special needs (Volkmar et al., 2014). It is surprising, as more Medicaid programs look for ways to reduce cost and improve care, that medical homes are not becoming more of a standard model for serving adults with IDs. This points to another intersection of opportunity for public policy and research to work together to improve healthcare delivery and potential healthcare outcomes for adults with ASD/ID.

Understanding the Long-term Impact of Using Psychotropic Medications

The pervasive use of psychotropic medication in the adults under study, and the concern conveyed by all of their caregivers is certainly an area of research which needs more attention. As we learned from our informants, many different drugs are utilized to manage anxiety, depression, and behavior for people with ASD/ID. Many participants utilized these medications for nearly their entire life, with very mixed results of improvement in autistic traits. Today, the only medications which are approved for children with ASD by the US Food and Drug Administration (FDA) for reducing agitation and irritability are risperidone (brand name Risperdal) and aripiprazole (abilify). However, both drugs commonly produce significant weight gain, as do many of the other medications our informants mentioned utilizing over time. What are the long-term effects of these medications (most never approved by the FDA for the treatment of ASD) over the decades? Funding is needed to conduct longitudinal studies to better understand the health impact of psychotropic medications.

REFERENCES

Baio, J., Wiggins, L., Christensen, D. L., Maenner, M. J., Daniels, J., Warren, Z., … Durkin, M. S. (2018). Prevalence of autism spectrum disorder among children aged 8 years – Autism and developmental disabilities monitoring network, 11 sites, United States, 2014. *MMWR Surveillance Summary*, *67*(6), 1. doi:10.15585/mmwr.ss6706a1

Baird, G., Simonoff, E., Pickles, A., Chandler, S., Loucas, T., Meldrum, D., & Charman, T. (2006). Prevalence of disorders of the autism spectrum in a population cohort of children in South Thames: the special needs and autism project (SNAP). *Lancet*, *368*, 210–215.

Bruder, M. B., Kerins, G., Mazzarella, C., Sims, J., & Stein, N. (2012). Brief report: The medical care of adults with autism spectrum disorders: Identifying the needs. *Journal of Autism and Developmental Disorders*, *42*(11), 2498–2504.

Capron, A. M. (1999). Ethical and human-rights issues in research on mental disorders that may affect decision-making capacity. *The New England Journal of Medicine*, *340*(18), 1430–1434.

Cheak-Zamora, N. C., & Teti, M. (2014). "You think it's hard now… It gets much harder for our children": Youth with autism and their caregiver's perspectives of healthcare transition Services. *Autism*, *19*(8), 992–1001. 1362361314558279.

Coyle, C. E., Kramer, J., & Mutchler, J. E. (2014). Aging together: Sibling carers of adults with intellectual and developmental disabilities. *Journal of Policy and Practice in Intellectual Disabilities*, *11*(4), 302–312.

Crabtree, B. F., & Miller, W. L. (Eds.). (1999). *Doing qualitative research*. Los Angeles, CA: Sage.

Dresser, R. (1996). Mentally disabled research subjects: The enduring policy issues. *JAMA*, *276*(1), 67–72.

Finlay, W. M., & Lyons, E. (2001). Methodological issues in interviewing and using self-report questionnaires with people with mental retardation. *Psychological Assessment*, *13*(3), 319.

Golnik, A., Ireland, M., & Borowsky, I. W. (2009). Medical homes for children with autism: A physician survey. *Pediatrics*, *123*(3), 966–971.

Happé, F., & Charlton, R. A. (2011). Aging in autism spectrum disorders: A mini-review. *Gerontology*, *58*(1), 70–78.

Haveman, M., Heller, T., Lee, L., Maaskant, M., Shooshtari, S., & Strydom, A. (2010). Major health risks in aging persons with intellectual disabilities: An overview of recent studies. *Journal of Policy and Practice in Intellectual Disabilities*, *7*, 59–69.

Heller, T., & Sorensen, A. (2013). Promoting healthy aging in adults with developmental disabilities. *Developmental Disabilities Research Reviews*, *18*(1), 22–30.

Heslop, P., Blair, P. S., Fleming, P., Hoghton, M., Marriott, A., & Russ, L. (2014). The confidential inquiry into premature deaths of people with intellectual disabilities in the UK: A population-based study. *The Lancet*, *383*(9920), 889–895.

Lambert, V. A., & Lambert, C. E. (2013). Qualitative descriptive research: An acceptable design. *Pacific Rim International Journal of Nursing Research*, *16*(4), 255–256.

Lin, J. D., Lin, L. P., & Hsu, S. W. (2016). Aging people with intellectual disabilities: Current challenges and effective interventions. *Review Journal of Autism and Developmental Disorders*, *3*(3), 266–272.

McCarthy, M. (1998). Interviewing people with learning disabilities about sensitive topics: A discussion of ethical issues. *British Journal of Learning Disabilities*, *26*(4), 140–145.

Miller, S. M. (2015). Nurses caring for adults with autism in an emergency department: A survey of knowledge. Doctoral projects, Paper 7. Retrieved from http://scholarworks.sjsu.edu/etd_doctoral/7

Morse, J. M. (2003). Principles of mixed methods and multimethod research design. In A. M. Tashakkori & C. B. Teddlie (Eds.), *Handbook of mixed methods in social and behavioral research* (pp. 189–208). Thousand Oaks, CA: Sage.

Mouridsen, S. E., Rich, B., & Isager, T. (2016a). Injury patterns among individuals diagnosed with infantile autism during childhood: A case-control study. *Scandinavian Journal of Child and Adolescent Psychiatry and Psychology*, *4*(2), 88–95.

Mouridsen, S. E., Rich, B., & Isager, T. (2016b). Diseases of the circulatory system among adult people diagnosed with infantile autism as children: A longitudinal case control study. *Research in Developmental Disabilities*, *57*, 193–200.

Mukaetova-Ladinska, E. B., & Stuart-Hamilton, I. (2015). Adults with autism spectrum disorder (ASD): Service user perspective on ageing transition (s). *Journal of Autism*, *2*(1), 1–11.

Myers, S. M., & Johnson, C. P. (2007). Management of children with autism spectrum disorders. *Pediatrics*, *120*(5), 1162–1182.

Nebel-Schwalm, M., & Worley, J. (2014). Other disorders frequently comorbid with autism. In T. E. Davies, III, S. B. White, & T. Ollendick (Eds.), *Handbook of autism and anxiety* (pp. 47–60). New York, NY: Springer International Publishing.

Nicolaidis, C., Raymaker, D., McDonald, K., Dern, S., Boisclair, W. C., Ashkenazy, E., & Baggs, A. (2013). Comparison of healthcare experiences in autistic and non-autistic adults: A cross-sectional online survey facilitated by an academic-community partnership. *Journal of General Internal Medicine*, *28*(6), 761–769.

Nicolaidis, C., Raymaker, D. M., Ashkenazy, E., McDonald, K. E., Dern, S., Baggs, A. E., ... Boisclair, W. C. (2015). "Respect the way I need to communicate with you": Healthcare experiences of adults on the autism spectrum. *Autism*, *19*(7), 824–831.

Patton, M. Q. (2002). Fieldwork strategies and observation methods. In M. Q. Patton (Ed.), *Qualitative research and evaluation methods* (pp. 259–338). Thousand Oaks, CA: Sage.

Perry, J. (2004). Interviewing people with intellectual disabilities. In E. Emerson, C. Hatton, T. Thompson, & T. Parmenter (Eds.), *The international handbook of applied research in intellectual disabilities* (pp. 115–132). Chichester: John Wiley & Sons.

Piven, J., & Rabins, P. (2011). Autism spectrum disorders in older adults: Toward defining a research agenda. *Journal of the American Geriatrics Society*, *59*(11), 2151–2155.

Roberts, L. W., & Roberts, B. (1999). Psychiatric research ethics: An overview of evolving guidelines and current ethical dilemmas in the study of mental illness. *Biological Psychiatry*, *46*(8), 1025–1038.

Roux, A. M., Shattuck, P. T., Cooper, B. P., Anderson, K. A., Wagner, M., & Narendorf, S. C. (2013). Postsecondary employment experiences among young adults with an autism spectrum disorder. *Journal of American Academy Child Adolescent Psychiatry*, *52*(9), 931–939.

Shavelle, R., Strauss, D., & Pickett, J. (2001). Causes of death in autism. *Journal of Autism and Developmental Disorders*, *31*(6), 569–576.

Shields, P. M., & Tajalli, H. (2006). Intermediate theory: The missing link in successful student scholarship. *Journal of Public Affairs Education*, *12*(3), 313–334.

Silverman, C. (2008). Fieldwork on another planet: Social science perspectives on the autism spectrum. *BioSocieties*, *3*(3), 325–341.

Tregnago, M., & Cheak-Zamora, N. (2012). Systematic review of disparities in healthcare for individuals with autism spectrum disorders in the United States. *Research in Autism Spectrum Disorders*, *6*(3), 1023–1031.

Tyler, C., Schramm, S., Karafa, M., Tang, A., & Jain, A. (2011). Chronic disease risks in young adults with autism spectrum disorder: Forewarned is forearmed. *American Journal on Intellectual and Developmental Disabilities*, *116*(5), 371–380.

Vohra, R., Madhavan, S., & Sambamoorthi, U. (2016). Emergency department use among adults with autism spectrum disorders (ASD). *Journal of Autism and Developmental Disorders*, *46*(4), 1441–1454.

Volkmar, F. R., Paul, R., Rogers, S. J., & Pelphrey, K. A. (Eds.). (2014). *Handbook of autism and pervasive developmental disorders: Diagnosis, development, and brain mechanisms* (Vol. I). Hoboken, NJ: John Wiley & Sons.

HEPATITIS C AND SUPPORT GROUPS IN RURAL COMMUNITIES

Atsuko Kawakami, Juyeon Son and Charley Henderson

ABSTRACT

Purpose – *This study aims to better understand the key factors that affect the quality of care that patients with Hepatitis C are likely to receive in rural communities and to consider how to build a more effective health support system for the rural residents.*

Methodology/Approach – *This qualitative study with a grounded theory approach allowed us to draw a conceptual map of the occurrence while informants had the opportunity to contemplate and share their thoughts on the issues, which led into new understandings of the subject matter.*

Findings – *The local leaders held a romanticized view toward rural life while the disadvantaged reported a sense of powerlessness to bring about the needed changes to help them battle Hepatitis C.*

Research Limitations/Implications – *Although describing a single social setting provides in-depth description, generalizability to other settings is always a limitation. If one wishes to start a support group, he/she may have to start asking the clergy of different churches to be the cofounders of the support group organization.*

Underserved and Socially Disadvantaged Groups and Linkages with Health and Health Care Differentials
Research in the Sociology of Health Care, Volume 37, 119–135

ISSN: 0275-4959/doi:10.1108/S0275-495920190000037011

Originality/Value of Paper – *Churches may have the most potential to bring about the needed changes in rural settings by fostering a supportive heath care environment in their communities.*

Keywords: Rural community; Hepatitis C; privacy; stigma; religion; support groups

BACKGROUND

A number of studies have examined how the Hepatitis C virus (HCV) is contracted, its effect on the patient's health, and the treatment of the symptoms that are a result of the HCV (i.e., American Liver Foundation, 2015; Centers for Disease Control [CDC], 2016; Holmberg, Spradling, Moorman, & Denniston, 2013; Mintz, 1992). For example, medical procedures such as blood transfusions and dental surgeries or other procedures such as tattooing can be the source of the HCV contraction. Medical professionals were not aware of the infection risk prior to the late 1980s; thus, the baby boomers who had such procedures when they were young have the highest risk of having Hepatitis C (CDC, 2016; Conrad, Garrett, Cooksley, Dunne, & MacDonald, 2006; Holmberg et al., 2013).

Because intravenous drug use and homosexual activities can be possible sources for contracting Hepatitis C (CDC, 2016), the HCV has often been linked to the image of socially perceived deviant behavior. If such negative perceptions are pervasive, it is likely to form a stigma toward those infected with HCV. As a result, the patients and their families may not receive timely diagnosis, adequate treatment, and sufficient support out of a fear of stigmatization. There is not an HCV vaccine available yet and the treatment is still limited. Since antiviral HCV treatment is not only expensive and burdensome but also toxic and ineffective for those patients who tried the therapy, Rich and Taylor (2010) suggest that it is imperative to develop strategies to prevent HCV transmission.

The Effect of Hepatitis C on Social Class and Social Life

Although HCV epidemiology and pathology of as well as treatments for managing the virus have been the main focus for many researchers, the social aspect on how it affects one's life has been also examined. Awofeso (2001, p. 184) describes HCV as "a disease of poverty" since the significantly higher exposure of HCV is observed in developing countries as well as in the lower socioeconomic classes within a given community. A study shows that HCV-related mortality is disproportionately higher among non-Hispanic black men and elderly men of all ethnicities (Wise, Bialek, Finelli, Bell, & Sorvillo, 2008). However, regardless of their socioeconomic status or age, many individuals with HCV reported that they felt socially rejected due to their internalized shame that led to a change in everyday life (Zacks et al., 2006).

Marinho and Barreira (2013) also reported that many individuals believe that Hepatitis C is "deserved" because the virus's contraction can be from drug use or sexual promiscuity. This stigma contributes to the patients' sense of self-worth and social isolation such as the prevention of diagnosis or withdrawal of treatments. The CDC (2016) maintains their concern for social isolation of individuals with HCV since it is detrimental to their health. One of the elements that may help prevent social isolation and promote the emotional well-being is one's religious affiliation. For example, Sherkat and Reed (1992) reported a positive effect of one's religiosity on people's sense of well-being as it assists with coping with stressors; the level of religiosity is found to have a negative correlation with deviant behaviors. In this sense, it is possible that religiosity plays an important role for individuals to avoid social isolation when they are dealing with viral infectious diseases. This leads us to further consider the role of the religious institutions at the societal level, more specifically, the role of religious institutions to improve the social environment for the patients and their family members. It is also possible, however, that religiosity can be a double-edged sword; once individuals found they were infected, they could also be isolated spiritually from their belief and/or withdraw from the religious affiliation due to a sense of shame and fear of stigmatization.

Social Environment in Rural Community

A patient with HCV may be physically absent from his/her work, school, or social gatherings due to extreme fatigue. When this becomes chronic behavior, the patient may easily fall into social isolation lacking a sense of social connection. It is clear that in addition to the pathological experience of the illness, considering the illness as experienced by people situated in various social environments is crucial when evaluating the patients' quality of life.

The focus of previous studies has been on the patients and their families in urban areas and in a hospital setting (i.e., CDC, 2016; Conrad & Schneider, 1992; Zacks et al., 2006). For example, the Chronic Hepatitis Cohort Study collected data from over 13,000 patients with Hepatitis C in Detroit, Danville, Portland, and Honolulu; the study shows a consistent result with other studies that only 32%–38% of those who would qualify to receive therapy have been identified and referred for appropriate care (Holmberg et al., 2013).

Even in the urban settings where care facilities and support groups are available, there are a considerable number of patients not utilizing the health care services. Then, one has to wonder about the situation in many rural areas where the services and support systems are not readily available. It is well documented that rural communities are often disadvantaged in terms of health care and social services. Since less than 10% of physicians actually practice in rural areas (Ricketts, Hary, & Pirani, 2000), rural residents have higher morbidity and mortality rates in general compared to those in urban areas (Gamm, Hutchison, Dabney, & Dorsey, 2003). In addition to the shortage of health care providers, the limited types of employment in rural areas often leave residents without employer-paid health insurance coverage. Rural areas' limited health care access and lack of transportation contribute to the difficulties of those in poverty (Pistella & Bonati, 2000). Humble, Lewis, Scott, and Herzog (2013) point out the necessity of using a social worker's personal connections such as neighbors, church members, and colleagues; however, utilizing those connections can be a source of social workers' burnout due to constantly being "on duty" as well as resilient for rural community members dealing with their life circumstances.

Purpose of This Study

There is a need to examine how a rural community can provide necessary support for the patients and their family members. Given that rural communities differ significantly from urban areas, this study examines the social conditions in a rural community in order to (1) identify whether there is a distinctive barrier in a rural setting to providing sufficient care and support for Hepatitis C and (2) gain insight into how a rural community can better provide social supports for the patients regarding whether there is a barrier to developing support groups.

In order to foster a healthy rural community environment, it is essential to gain a good understanding of the relationship between the social structure and characteristics of a rural community and their effects on building a more efficient and supportive environment for patients with HCV. This study focused on better understanding the key factors that affect the quality of care of patients with HCV are likely to receive in rural communities so that ways to building a more effective health support system for the rural residents can be identified.

METHODS

Selecting Qualitative Inquiry

Our focus of this study was to examine the conditions that affect the development of support groups for Hepatitis C in a rural community. We aimed to identify the common themes from the responses of the residents in a rural community related to their social support systems. This study used an inductive approach in order to obtain holistic, profuse, and detailed qualitative knowledge, as it could better reveal the study subject's complexity in real contexts (Miles & Huberman, 1994). This was the most suitable approach in order to identify the common themes in the complex society. Furthermore, grounded theory approach allowed us to draw a conceptual map of the occurrence while informants were given the opportunity to contemplate and share their thoughts on the issues, which led into new understandings of the subject matter (Glaser, 1998). This approach facilitated our study's goal of proposing how to enhance rural communities' support systems through identifying the residents' views on the support systems for patients with Hepatitis C and their families.

Institutional Review Board

We received each study participant's written consent before he or she answered any questions. All participants received a copy of the informed consent form in accordance with the Institutional Review Board (IRB). None of the participants received monetary or any other compensation but they gave us generous amounts of their time answering the questions. Their participation was voluntary and they received the contact information of the researchers in case they had questions or concerns about this study. The risk of conducting this study might have included occasional discomfort to talk about health issues or their own community's problems, but those risks were considered minimal. No serious reactions such as anxiety, anger, or discomfort of talking about issues on health and community were reported during or after the interviews.

Selecting Location

As described above, the majority of the previous studies focused on the perspectives of urban communities on the issues of Hepatitis C. Therefore, we selected a rural, pseudonymous city, Riverside, as our study site. Riverside was a rural community remotely located from any big cities in one of the southern states in the United States. The main industries of this community were in the tertiary sector such as locally owned shops and a couple of chain restaurants as well as the primary sector such as farming. The median income of the household was approximately US$24,000. The median age was 40.3 years old. The mean and mode averages of income and age were not available. The population of this community at the time of data collection were roughly 4,500 people; Caucasians comprised 85% of the population and the rest of the 15% were Hispanic/Latino, African American, Native American, Asian, others, and biracial or multiracial.

Although no official data were available to indicate the residents' religious affiliations, it was safe to assume that the majority of residents held a Christian faith and churches play a major role as a social institution in Riverside since there were 28 churches in this 6.2-square-mile community. That means there was one church in every 0.22 square miles in this community; this number did not include 15 other churches that were located outside of, but adjacent to, its city limit.

Collecting Data

All of our study participants were residents of Riverside at the time of data collection; some of the study participants had experiences of interacting with people with Hepatitis C and some did not. Some of them had knowledge about the disease and some did not. Previous studies suggested that the majority of the patients with Hepatitis C were middle-aged or above (Wise et al., 2008); therefore, we purposefully did not include minors for this study. We asked our personal acquaintances to start the snowball sampling and recruited other participants by asking their referral for potential participants. We discontinued recruiting new participants when no more new themes and concerns sprang up from the participants. The participants had the option of a face-to-face interview format or written survey format. Some participants preferred answering in written form but most participated in face-to-face interviews. The questions consisted of a few themes such as the participants' general understanding of Hepatitis C, their views on how the community members treated the patients and their family, and what they thought about their own community's readiness to support the patients and their family members. Additionally, demographic information was collected such as participants' age, gender, length of residency in the community, occupation, and income. Since Riverside was a very small community, protecting participants' privacy while encouraging them to participate in the study was the main concern for the IRB. For that reason, some demographic inquiry was considered too sensitive to ask one's education level. Likewise, we had to ask participants' age, income, and length of residency in categorical form instead of asking in the numerical form. To ensure confidentiality, pseudonyms replaced all individuals' names, places, and organizations.

Although the list of the questions was semi-structured, some participants took the conversation in its own direction. With the open-ended questions, we encouraged the participants to expand the topics and express their opinions freely. We audiotaped all face-to-face interviews, transcribed verbatim within a week after the interview, and kept the data electronically in password-protected computers to read multiple times. The average length of interview time was about 30 minutes, ranging from 15 minutes to 2.5 hours. The interviews were conducted from May 2016 to August 2016. The interview data were read, coded, categorized, and analyzed as follows: First, we used open coding to identify similar themes such as community's views on viral infections, opinions about their own community, and perspectives on religion and church followed by using axial coding with consistent terminology such as support groups/system, patients with Hepatitis C and their family members, lower/upper class, and gossip in the community. Finally, we used selective coding to support our analysis with the participants' direct quotes.

Composite Descriptions of Study Sample

A total of 30 participants shared their personal experiences and opinions on the topics of Hepatitis C and their community. Gender distribution of the sample was seven males and 23 females. There were 27 Caucasian/White participants and three Hispanic participants. All of the study participants lived in Riverside at the time of data collection. Table 1 shows the distribution of participants' age, income, and length of residency as well as their occupation.

Compliant with IRB approval, we were only allowed to ask participants' age categorically, instead of numerically. The sample's ages ranged from 31 to 70 years. With the assumption that samples of each age category were distributed equally, the estimated median age was 49 years, the mean age was 48.66 years, and the mode age category was 31–35 years. With IRB approval, the income distribution was described with eight different categories, including "refused to answer." Therefore, it was unsuitable to estimate the mean, median, and mode averages since the category of "Over US$60,000" could be any number. Likewise, estimating the mean, median, and mode of the participants' length of residency in the community would be inappropriate since the category of "More than 30 years" could be any number. However, it clearly displayed one of the characteristics of this community; most people in Riverside have lived in the

Table 1. Descriptive.

Age Distribution (years)	
31–35	8
36–40	1
41–45	3
46–50	4
51–55	2
56–60	7
61–65	3
66–70	2
Over 70	0
Refused to answer	0
Total	30
Income Distribution (US$)	
Under $10,000	1
$10,000–19,999	2
$20,000–29,999	4
$30,000–39,999	3
$40,000–49,999	6
$50,000–59,999	2
Over $60,000	9
Refused to answer	3
Total	30
Length of Residence (years)	
Less than one year	0
1–5	2
6–10	1
11–15	2
16–20	3
21–25	6
26–30	3
More than 30 years	13
Refused to answer	0
Total	30
Job Distribution	
Church Secretary/Pastor	2
Heavy equipment operator/maintenance foreman	2
Housewife/Homemaker/Mother	3

Table 1. (*Continued*)

LVN/RN/Nurse/Hospital Administrative	4
Office/Shop Manager	2
Rancher	2
Service (Barber/Casher/Postal Employee)	3
Small Business Owner/Self Employed	3
Educator (retired and active)/Administrative in Education	5
Waitress/Cook	2
Retired (none specified)/No answer/Refused to Answer	4
Total*	32

Note: *The total number exceeds 30 because some participants held more than one occupation.

community for a long time as the category of "More than 30 years" had the highest number in all categories.

FINDINGS

One of the major themes identified was how the rural community's characteristics affected the residents' perceptions on the possibility of starting HCV support groups or educational programs. After inductively detecting this theme, we used the selective coding to identify underlying cases for the unsupportive environment for HCV and other viral infectious diseases in a rural community. Contrary to the common belief that a tight-knit rural community has a supportive environment for their members, a rural community's characteristics appeared to make it more difficult for patients to feel comfortable to seek help and to find a supportive environment for themselves and their families. However, some rural community characteristics could be utilized to effectively fight against the spread of viral infectious diseases such as Hepatitis C or to start a support group. In the following section, we presented the findings from this case study and illustrate how rural community characteristics are related to illness experience of patients with HCV as well as to their implications for building the community support system.

Community Members' Perception of the Social Structures in Riverside

The notion of leadership in Riverside was not purely based on their financial resources. Many participants described retired teachers, ranchers, and business owners as the opinion leaders. Some participants said that the city and chamber of commerce committee members were the community leaders because they defined what the community's problems were and how to deal with the issues in Riverside. When asked who was considered upper class in the community, study participants pointed to the people involved in community organizations such as the members of the city, hospital, and chamber of commerce committees. For example, a participant described the community leaders as the individuals who "basically run the town" by serving "for boards of things […] [and] boards of organizations." More specifically, individuals that played an active role in the community's decision-making processes whether through private or public channels were considered as an influential "clique" of people. It is worthwhile to mention that those members of "boards of things" and "boards of organizations" tended to be the elderly individuals that often displayed their Christian faith and voiced their concern for the loss of traditional family values. In contrast, people that received financial assistance from the government were often considered to be in the lower socioeconomic status.

Changes in the Community

Increased Number of Patients with Hepatitis C

A nurse at a local hospital in the community discussed an increasing number of individuals who were carrying the HCV as "a huge, huge increase in Hep C [...], at least two new [patients] a month." In terms of the ability to treat Hepatitis C and other viral infectious diseases at the local hospital, another nurse sounded agitated with the fact the local hospital was being viewed as better prepared than it actually was. She said, "Obviously [...] We're not, you know, a specialist. We don't do that."

Another participant who worked at the hospital mentioned how the community needed educational programs to create a better supportive environment for those with viral infectious diseases and to stop the spread of the diseases. She said:

> I don't think our community is that aware of the Hepatitis things [...] yeah they are gonna be very prejudice against that. But I don't think they are that aware of it. Like, um, [sigh] it's like it's a big monster to them. [...] I think if they had more education, [...] they would be more accepting [...].

Since this nurse had experience working in a bigger city, she could confidently say that in the urban area, people were more open about discussing their diseases in a constructive way with "no hesitation at all." Of course, it is dangerous to take this comment at face value, but at least this nurse thought a bigger city had more accepting attitudes and support systems for individuals with Hepatitis C compared to a rural community. Those who were in the health care industries, patients with Hepatitis, their friends, and families in Riverside were well aware of the increasing number of Hepatitis incidences. However, there was no notion of putting an effort into stopping the spread of the disease or establishing support systems for those infected in the community so far.

Increased Number of Low-income Families

While the increased number of Hepatitis C was noticed by some community members, other residents were concerned about the increased number of low-income families in relation to the disease. They described Riverside as the "welfare pit." Some of the opinion leaders in the community such as retired teachers, farmers, and business owners tended to see this trend unfavorably and that it continued to attract more low-income families because of "how easy it is to gain welfare" in this community. This community's attitude toward the low-income residents was attributed to a perceived connection between the disease and unsavory characteristics of how it was contracted. Hepatitis C was often stigmatized since it was associated with drug usage and sexual promiscuity; patients were at risk of withdrawal of treatments, prevention of diagnosis, and social isolation (Marinho & Barreira, 2013).

Additionally, when patients could no longer work or maintain their daily activities because of extreme fatigue, people saw them as just "lazy welfare recipients who avoid working" as one participant stated. This was true whether the patients were actually welfare recipients or not. The increased number of Hepatitis C cases was understood as the result of the increase in low-income families in Riverside. Hence, Hepatitis C was viewed as a disease of those with lower socioeconomic status in the community.

"We Don't Just Have Hepatitis": Intentional Ignorance as a Way of Categorizing Undeserving People

The socioeconomically well-off community members did recognize that there were many financially struggling individuals and families in the community as one of the participants voiced her concern. "It's just there is a lot of [them in the community]." This decisively middle-class participant did not think one's economic predicaments were due to his/her personal fault as she said "[…] it's not by any means the lower economic people's fault"; however, it was obvious that she did not see those struggling individuals and families as positive community members.

Some individuals, especially those who were financially comfortable elderly individuals, tended to intentionally overlook any serious problems in the overall community and minimize certain problems. One such participant illustrated this thought pattern when she bluntly said, "We don't just have Hepatitis." The reason for her to make such a comment was "because we are […] an older community" as if older populations were automatically protected from Hepatitis C.

Another participant, a retired educator, said she did not see any intolerance against one's religion, socioeconomic status, race/ethnicity, sexuality, or health status in the community because she did not "get much further than this right here." Her logic was that since she was retired, she did "not have to know a lot of things." She described herself as "the ostrich in the sand [that] keep[s] [her] head buried." She was content within her small geographical and social territory such as her house and a few of her neighbors; she did not want to know what was going on in larger community. Keep in mind that Riverside was already a very small community, but for her, Riverside was too large "to know a lot of things."

This type of intentional blindness among the well-off residents about the issue was creating the notion that patients with Hepatitis and their families did not need help in the community. In fact, many recognize that the community had a large number of struggling individuals and families due to various illnesses, lack of employment opportunities, and other intergenerational cases of poverty, but they saw no obligation for the community to help those individuals and families.

Instead, community leaders opted to improve the community by hiring an artist at considerable cost to decorate the downtown facades.

However, one of the participants who acknowledged her lower socioeconomic status in the community said, "They (the community) don't help people like they should." Another participant also disagreed with the way the community spent their budget for the beautification project in the downtown area instead of spending money establishing educational or support programs for youth and struggling individuals. In a sense, residents who acknowledged their lower status indicated how they were ignored or invisible in the community. One participant expressed her frustration about how the community seemed to ignore the problem. When she was asked about the spread of Hepatitis C, she rolled her eyes and said sarcastically, "It (Hepatitis C) doesn't exist (in the eyes of the community leaders)!"

It was clear that the well-off residents tended to view the Hepatitis C issue in the community as not "theirs." Their lack of sense of ownership of this issue appeared to be associated with the negative notion that patients with Hepatitis C and their families were often regarded as low income and undeserving to receive any assistance from the community.

Barriers to Forming a Support Group

Discrepancy on the Views of the Community's Support System

Although the number of patients with Hepatitis C was increasing, there were no social support groups or educational programs to stop the spread of Hepatitis C or any viral infectious diseases in the community. When participants were asked if they knew any support groups of any kind in the community, the most frequent response was, "I doubt there are any support groups here" or "I don't know any."

Those ones who spoke of favorable characteristics in the community as "tender," "caring," or accepting other "individuals with a [...] second chance" tended to be financially secure, elderly residents. They had lived in Riverside for more than a few decades. One of those participants spoke highly about the community as caring; she spoke of the community residents providing assistance to those in need by holding bake sales and other charity events as evidence. Since they tended to perceive the community as already providing support for those in need, efforts to establish a new formal support system to help patients with HCV or to develop educational programs to stop the spread of HCV were considered unnecessary.

Contrary to this idealistic view of this rural community held by the upper "clique" of Riverside residents, one middle-aged female participant whose husband was diagnosed with Hepatitis C gave a very different picture of the community. According to this woman, people who used to greet them and frequently enjoyed events with the entire family started to distance themselves or even excluded the entire family from the community after her husband's diagnosis with the disease. For instance, her teenaged daughter who worked at a local restaurant at that time was told by a customer, "You should not be working here." Baffled by the comment, the daughter asked why. The customer continued, "You can give everyone what your father has." Clearly, this indicated the community's culture toward the people with the disease. In addition, despite the belief that the small community was like a big family, her family's experience in battling her husband's disease did not comply with the image. Because her husband did not qualify for government assistance, she and all of their teenaged children had to find multiple part-time jobs to make ends meet while the husband was battling with the disease. During this hardship, the family did not receive any financial assistance from community fundraising efforts to help with his medical bills or expenses after his death.

Lack of Anonymity and Privacy

One reason behind the lack of support for those with Hepatitis C in this rural community appeared to be closely related to the lack of anonymity and privacy. One of the nurses in Riverside said:

> You can't have […] anything without anyone knowing about it. You can't have one of these [viral infectious] diseases without somebody knowing it. So I think you have this constant fear if you are trying to live with it you know in privacy over the condition, you know it is hard to get privacy here. It is hard to deal with it without everyone knowing.

Due to Riverside being a small community geographically isolated from any big cities, it would be easier for health care providers and personnel at the hospital to recognize their patients at the individual level such as personal friends, neighbors, and acquaintances in their personal life. This was an important issue for the health service utilization of people with stigmatized diseases, which might not be as much of a concern in bigger cities. One of the nurses interviewed said:

> I would not take my daughter […] or son to the local hospital […] they [the hospital staff] don't follow HIPPA (Health Insurance Portability and Accountability Act of 1996) and everyone would find out what happened.

It was clear that the lack of anonymity in a small town could hinder access to the local health care facilities as well as their ability to address disease issues in a constructive way. This resulted in greater difficulty to create support groups.

One participant described the characteristics of how Riverside residents spread rumors:

> If […] somebody hears […] that somebody is cheatin' on somebody when they don't know for a fact, they are still willing to spread that. […] Whether they are learning facts or rumors you're going to have to decide there! [laugh] 'cause everyone is going to talk, so most of what they know is going to be based on rumors.

The gossip culture could seem innocuous gossip on what was going on with other residents' private lives but it also had negative implications on the lives of those gossiped about. For example, a story shared by Anne, a resident in the community, showed how the community's gossip actually impacted her entire family. When Anne and her husband stopped attending local and school events due to his illness, the community members started spreading rumors that Anne and her husband were going through a divorce. When this false rumor eventually reached one of their teenaged children, Anne and her husband had to come out to their children and the rest of the community about his illness. The fastest way to avoid becoming a victim of the community's gossips might be leaving the community. All of Anne's children left Riverside as soon as they graduated high school because of unpleasant experiences they went through as teenagers. It was understandable why Riverside residents seemed to hesitate to start a support group in the community for any illnesses or behavioral problems that might be associated with deviant behaviors.

However, even if the residents intentionally disassociated themselves from anything that might incur gossip, it was almost inevitable that their private lives were gossiped about in the community. Actually, some of participants who were aware of the HCV issues hoped to be more constructive, talking openly about the illness in a support group or spreading accurate knowledge about the illness such as infection routes, treatments, or presentations in an educational program in the community to eliminate unnecessary fear or discrimination.

DISCUSSION

Despite that there was an increasing incidence and prevalence of HCV in the community, which the local health professionals were well aware of, the members of the area tended to share the perception that it wasn't really happening nor was affecting them. In part, it was because they considered HCV as a disease of only the poor and rather "of the newcomers," thus, not "their" problems. This attitude was exacerbated by the recent inflow of low-income families into the area and how they were perceived by the community. One local church member's comment about "how easy it is to gain welfare" in this community captured this attitude toward the newcomers. The community culture played an important role in adding more difficulty to espouse a supportive environment. The rural community's practice of spreading rumors and gossip as "concerning for the community members" as our study participants described and interpreting "everyone knows everybody else's personal business" as a "family-like environment" were, undeniably, their way of romanticizing the rural living. It was true especially when inconvenient truths such as lack of support system for the increasing number of patients with Hepatitis C were intentionally ignored as the "caring [...] community [is already] providing [enough] assistance [...] [by holding] bake sales and other charity events." Those commonly observed, romanticizing practices in a rural community were preventing them from become a supportive community. Unless the opinion leaders and community leaders stopped minimizing or intentionally ignoring the problem of widespread Hepatitis C, it would not be regarded as the community's problem. The stigma toward HCV was readily adapted into the community as the newer residents were considered to be fitting the profiles of those that were known to contract the disease: the poor. It is significant to understand, then, how the existing community culture could boost the spread of stigma as facts.

The people in lower class were more aware of the spread of Hepatitis C; however, their responses also revealed a sense of helplessness as they felt they were not in the position to start a support group in the community based on their perceptions about the power they possessed. Lacking the influence in their own community made it difficult to start support groups or educational programs. One of the community members, who admitted her lower socioeconomic status in the community, said that the support group and support system were needed but she thought it was dependent upon who "will pull together to do something for you" in order for them to succeed. The sense of powerlessness observed in her interview made it seem as if it would be impossible to start support groups or educational programs unless the upper "clique" people initiated them. Given the extent and amount of power the small number of community members tended to play in rural areas, it made sense that the residents who lacked resources in Riverside were doubtful about the feasibility to pull resources together without the support of the leader group members.

Although some of the social conditions discussed tended to hinder for the rural community to create and utilize support groups, we could also turn our attention to the very same characteristic in small communities such as Riverside to make it work to their advantage. Because their geographical and social proximity was limited, the interactions with the upper hierarchical members in a rural community were relatively easy for individuals from various social classes when compared to lobbying upper hierarchical members' support in urban areas. For example, we observed that a group of community leaders and opinion leaders, such as business owners, retired educators, and farmers who were financially secure, congregated for lunch at a local restaurant after church services at least six times during the data collection period. One of the employees at a local restaurant attested that she usually saw some of the community leaders at least 15–20 times a month since they congregated almost every day or every other day at the same restaurant after church as well as for some other occasions to discuss a variety of community issues. Since they had lived in Riverside for more than a few decades or even a few generations and kept their religious affiliation, they were seen as the opinion leaders and the source of trusted opinions in the community.

We also observed the community leaders casually talking with wait staff and other restaurant employees on a first name basis, which indicated relatively easy access to talk to those opinion leaders, especially at their church or at the restaurant after church services. It did not have to be a professional lobbyist to get the rural community's opinion leaders interested in starting an educational program for viral infectious diseases in their community. Therefore, it might be constructive to get church leaders' consensus to promote the awareness of viral infectious diseases in the community.

Local churches and clergy seemed to have the greatest potential to be the most effective and powerful focal center to change the picture. The residents overwhelmingly had a positive image of Christianity and believed in the church's willingness to help the community members in general even though there were not any church-based (or any organized) support groups currently existing for those with viral infectious diseases. When participants were asked if patients with viral infectious diseases could receive support from church, they answered,

"I think they could if they came to church and wanted to be a part of it. They definitely could get support." "If they (church) find out that [people] really need, there, this church that I am talking about – are always willing to help with even financial needs for things of that order." However, one participant was quick to mention:

> There has to - as far as the church that I know - has to kind of ask a lot of questions and dig into some of their personal life so that they know that they are not just out there going from church to church to church to try to live off of the churches.

As this comment indicated, anonymity was difficult to keep in the rural community even with getting help from churches. If anonymity was the most difficult issue to resolve, openly discussing illnesses with the help of church members might be more effective than avoiding the discussion to help those in need. This would be successful only when local church members and the leaders were supportive of patients with viral infections diseases. Humble et al. (2013) mentioned the possibility of social workers being threatened by residents to reveal who had the disease as well as the possibility of non-participation among the patients due to their fear of being identified and stigmatized by the community when starting a support group. However, if the support group was formed and supported through the local churches, then the patients and their family members could expect more sympathetic views and cooperative attitudes due to the authority, respect, and trust the local churches hold in the community.

Riebschleger (2007) found that social workers in rural communities utilized neighbors and church members as possibilities to improve a client's situation within the help process. As discussed earlier, religiosity could be a double-edged sword. Patients could be isolated spiritually from their belief or withdraw from their church activities due to a sense of shame and fear of stigmatization. However, one could also expect the positive effect of religiosity to cope with stressors (Sherkat & Reed, 1992). Recognizing this double-edged nature of religiosity, we argue that expanding the role of a church may lead into organizing and forming substantive action plans for patients with HCV and their families in rural communities. If one wishes to start a support group, he/she may have to start asking the clergy of different churches to be the cofounders of the support group organization. The clergy's regular attendance of the meetings and events would be crucial in order to minimize the risk for the patients and their families being ostracized by the community. Priests, preachers, pastors, or ministers may not need to use the support group for themselves, but their presence may be more effective than social workers or the local government's welfare department personnel. With the symbolic interaction approach, what is morally right or wrong is dependent on the culture, time, and setting as well as the actors in society. In fact, what is defined as moralistic behaviors is the byproduct of the beliefs of the community leaders (Conrad & Schneider, 1992). In that sense, educating and persuading the clergy maybe the first and most effective step to establish a more supportive environment in a rural community.

CONCLUSION

We have illustrated the social structures of Riverside and how residents of this small community saw their own community. We found that some common characteristics in rural communities had important implications on dealing with the HCV and that it was important to give attention to the contextual interplay of the community perception, reception, and treatment of the disease. We also showed that the mechanism of a close-tied rural community tended to be a hindrance to the constructing a supportive environment for those impacted by the Hepatitis C. In order to care more effectively and accurately for the people affected by the disease, it was crucial to fully understand the local dynamics. People's perception of the disease as well as the behavioral tendencies had a rather immediate and direct impact on those with Hepatitis C seeking support from the community. Gossip and rumors tended to be shared more freely and rapidly among the members in small communities, which tended to have greater impact on one's personal life in a rural area. The lack of anonymity and confidentiality combined with the preexisting prejudicial climate in the community seemed to be closely linked with a total lack of support groups. The patients were not the only ones affected by it but their family members also had to face extra burdens when they sought help. The leaders of the community openly idealized and romanticized their rural living in general. They ironically also appeared to actively turn a blind eye to the increasing need of addressing HCV in the community. This issue was exacerbated in part by the sense of powerlessness among the disadvantaged to initiate change such as organizing new support groups.

While we found that the close-knit rural community might not indicate an ideal supportive place for all, due to its rural characteristics, we could have a strategic approach to improve the effectiveness of intervention efforts to better treat HCVs. This could be accomplished through utilizing one of the most crucial social institutions in small rural communities: the churches. Systematically targeted programs to help start an inter-church support group in rural areas can have a significant contribution to encouraging the community's participation as a whole rather than initiatives through other major venues such as hospitals and government agencies. We argue that using the authority and respect that clergy at local churches hold is a great asset to develop a more supportive environment in rural communities.

This study is a case study rather than multi-site, qualitative research as the data are collected from one rural community. Although describing a single social setting provides in-depth description, generalizability to other settings is always a limitation. The study sample is small, and thus, the distribution of age, gender, income, and residential length are somewhat polarized. Although we were able to talk to many church members, only two individuals whose occupations were involved with a church participated in this study. Further study is needed to assess the feasibility of creating inter-church support organizations by surveying the various churches in a rural community.

REFERENCES

American Liver Foundation. (2015). *How is Hepatitis C transmitted or spread?* Retrieved from http://hepc.liverfoundation.org/diagnosis/how-hep-c-is-spread/

Awofeso, N. (2001). Hepatitis C virus infection: A disease of poverty. *Tropical Doctor*, *31*(3), 184–184. doi:10.1177/004947550103100329

Centers for Disease Control and Prevention (CDC). (2016). *Viral Hepatitis-Hepatitis C information*. Atlanta: U.S. Department for Health and Human Services. Retrieved from http://www.cdc.gov/hepatitis/hcv/cfaq.htm

Conrad, P., & Schneider, J. W. (1992). *Deviance and medicalization: From badness to sickness*. Philadelphia, PA: Temple University Press. Retrieved from https://books.google.com/books?hl=en&lr=&id=hYpZjDD67dkC&oi=fnd&pg=PR13&dq=how+does+the+level+of+education+affect+views+of+deviance&ots=GJsG7-AFc4&sig=G_GjWG7b7HugknOJ1x86MjrU6Aw#v=onepage&q&f=false

Conrad, S., Garrett, L. E., Cooksley, W. G. E., Dunne, M. P., & MacDonald, G. A. (2006). Living with chronic Hepatitis C means: "You just haven't got a normal life anymore. *Chronic Illness*, *2*(2), 121–131. doi:10.1177/17423953060020020701

Gamm, L. D., Hutchison, L. L., Dabney, B. J., & Dorsey, A. M. (Eds.). (2003). *Rural healthy people 2010: A companion document to healthy people 2010* (Vol. 2). College Station, TX: Texas A&M University Health Science Center, School of Rural Public Health, Southwest Rural Health Research Center.

Glaser, B. G. (1998). *Doing grounded theory: Issues and discussions*. Mill Valley, CA: Sociology Press.

Holmberg, S. D., Spradling, P., Moorman, A. C., & Denniston, M. M. (2013). Hepatitis C in the United States. *New England Journal of Medicine*, *368*(20), 1859–1861. doi:10.1056/NEJMp1302973

Humble, M. N., Lewis, M. L., Scott, D. L., & Herzog, J. R. (2013). Challenges in rural work practice: When support groups contain your neighbors, church members, and the PTA. *Social Work with Groups*, *36*(2–3), 249–258 doi:10.1080/01609513.2012.753807

Marinho, R. T., & Barreira, D. P. (2013). Hepatitis C, stigma and cure. *WTG: World Journal of Gastroenterology*, *19*(40), 6703–6709. doi:10.3748/wjg.v1.i40.6703

Miles, M. B., & Huberman, A. M. (1994). *Qualitative data analysis: An expanded sourcebook* (2nd ed.). Newbury Park, CA: Sage.

Mintz, P. D. (1992). Transmittal of Hepatitis C. *American Association for the Advancement of Science*, *255*(5044), 516. Retrieved from http://www.jstor.org/stable/2876796

Pistella, C. L., & Bonati, F. A. (2000). Social work practice in a rural community collaborative to improve perinatal care. *Social Work in Health Care*, *30*(1), 1–14.

Rich, J. D., & Taylor, L. E. (2010). The beginning of a new era in understanding Hepatitis C Virus prevention. *The Journal of Infectious Diseases*, *202*(7), 981–983. doi:10.1086/656213

Ricketts, T. C., Hary, L. G., & Pirani, M. (2000). How many rural doctors do we have? *Journal of Rural Health*, *16*(3), 198–207.

Riebschleger, J. (2007). Social workers' suggestions for effective rural practice. *Families in Society: The Journal of Contemporary Social Services*, *88*(2), 203–212.

Sherkat, D. E., & Reed, M. D. (1992). The effects of religion and social support on self-esteem and depression among the suddenly bereaved. *Kluwer Academic Publishers*, *26*(3), 259–275. doi:10.1007/BF00286562

Wise, M., Bialek, S., Finelli, L., Bell, B. P., & Sorvillo, F. (2008). Changing trends in hepatitis C-related mortality in the United States, 1995–2004. *Hepatology*, *47*, 1128–1135. doi:10.1002/hep.22165

Zacks, S., Beavers, K., Theodore, D., Dougherty, K., Batey, B., Shumaker, J., & Fried, M. W. (2006). Social stigmatization and Hepatitis C Virus infection. *Journal of Clinical Gastroenterology*, *40*(3), 220–224. doi:10.1097/00004836–200603000-00009

"I KINDA LOOK UNHEALTHY, BUT I'M NOT UNHEALTHY" – EXPLORING RURAL CHILDREN'S PERSPECTIVES ON HEALTH, WELL-BEING, AND NUTRITION

Anne Scheer

ABSTRACT

Purpose – *The purpose of this study is to explore rural children's own perspectives on health, well-being, and nutrition to better understand how they approach, navigate, and make sense of these topics.*

Methodology/Approach – *This study uses a qualitative ethnographic research design theoretically informed by the "new" Sociology of Childhood and methodologically informed by constructivist grounded theory. This ongoing study with fifth-grade students in an elementary school in a small rural school district in central Illinois consists of ethnographic observations conducted at the school, in-depth interviews with students, and participatory tools that seek to involve students more fully in the process of data collection.*

Findings – *Preliminary findings of this pilot study suggest that many aspects often discussed in the context of childhood obesity, especially in rural settings, including knowledge or education about healthy eating, increasing physical activity levels, or access to healthy foods, are complex and multifaceted and do not easily lend themselves to standard interventions. Findings also indicate that children's ideas about healthy eating deviate from their own eating practices.*

Underserved and Socially Disadvantaged Groups and Linkages with Health and Health Care Differentials
Research in the Sociology of Health Care, Volume 37, 137–162

ISSN: 0275-4959/doi:10.1108/S0275-495920190000037012

Research Limitations/Implications – *Conceptualized as a grounded theory study, the research is not intended to be generalizable or reproducible. Instead, the study seeks to develop hypotheses directly from the field and study participants' views and voices. These perspectives will inform a more in-depth study of childhood obesity in rural settings planned for 2019.*

Originality/Value of Paper – *Findings from this pilot study will inform innovative, informed interventions that are guided by children's own experiences and perspectives. Study findings will also be of benefit to practicing pediatricians and other child health professionals as they understand how to better think about and address challenges of health and weight management of patients and their families.*

Keywords: Childhood obesity; rural children's health; Sociology of Childhood; children's perspectives on health, well-being, and nutrition; informed interventions

INTRODUCTION

This chapter presents preliminary findings of a qualitative pilot study designed to explore rural children's perspectives on health, well-being, and nutrition. This ongoing study with fifth-grade students in an elementary school in a small rural school district in central Illinois consists of ethnographic observations conducted at the school, in-depth interviews with students, and participatory tools that seek to involve students more fully in the process of data collection. Findings from this pilot study will identify topics that arise directly from the views of the populations served by Southern Illinois University School of Medicine (SIU SOM), hoping that this will allow us to create more successful, informed interventions that are guided by children's own experiences and perspectives.

Childhood obesity has long been and continues to be an issue of concern inside and outside the medical community. An estimated 13.7 million or 18.5% of US children and adolescents were considered obese in 2015–2016 (Hales, Carroll, Fryar, & Ogden, 2017). In addition, there is a rural-urban disparity in childhood obesity and research suggests that rural children are 26% more likely to be obese than their urban counterparts (Johnson & Johnson, 2015). Despite the ongoing efforts to prevent and treat childhood obesity, rates in the United States continue to grow (Hales et al., 2017). As a qualitative childhood sociologist at a medical school, I have partnered with stakeholders from our pediatrics department who are planning to create new interventions to address childhood obesity. Together, we have decided that our first step should be to learn about the views and voices of those we are trying to serve. This study is the product of an ongoing collaboration between myself (the principal investigator) and Merrie Fairfield (with the exception of SIU SOM, all names of people and places in this chapter are pseudonyms), a quality improvement nurse at SIU SOM, who is actively involved in obesity-related initiatives in the Pediatrics Department.

Following a series of conversations about childhood obesity in rural settings, we agreed that future efforts to address this issue should be more informed by the views and voices of those we are trying to serve: the children themselves. This includes questions such as: What are the children's own views about health and well-being? What do they think of when it comes to "healthy" versus "unhealthy" eating or activity patterns? What factors influence them to engage in certain behaviors and refrain from others? As a long-standing resident of Midwest Town – a small rural village and the location of Midwest Elementary School, the research site of this study – Merrie was instrumental in connecting me to the school and securing the administration's support for this research. The study began in late August 2018 and is ongoing. Data collection will be completed by February 2019.

Purpose of the Study and Research Questions

The purpose of this study is to explore children's own perspectives on health, well-being, and nutrition to better understand how they approach, navigate, and make sense of these topics. The primary research question guiding this study is: How do fifth-grade students in a small rural elementary school view health, well-being, and nutrition – their own as well as that of children in general? The following questions are designed to help explore this primary research question: (1) How do children *define* health and well-being? (2) What does being "healthy" or "unhealthy *mean* to them? (3) How and in what ways does children's understanding of health and well-being relate to their perception of an individual's personality, physical appearance, activity levels, and nutritional practices? (4) To what extent and in what ways do children's own nutritional practices correspond to or deviate from their ideas of a "healthy" diet? And (5) What other factors, such as peer pressure or social identity, affect children's ideas and practices around health and well-being?

Theoretical Framework

This study uses a qualitative ethnographic research design theoretically informed by the "new" Sociology of Childhood and methodologically informed by constructivist grounded theory as described by Charmaz (2014). The "new" Sociology of Childhood views children as active agents who are not passive recipients of adult values and expectations and should be treated as competent commentators on their own experiences (Corsaro, 1997; Prout, 2002; Prout & James, 1997). In contrast to older sociological approaches to childhood, the "new" Sociology of Childhood insists that research must view children as active social *beings* and not conceive of them merely as *becomings* (Prout & James, 1997). At the most general level, this "new" Sociology of Childhood places children's experiences and perspectives at the center of academic inquiry. In line with this conviction, the "new" Sociology of Childhood emphasizes that children are competent social actors and capable informants about their own lives.

Grounded theory is a systematic research method that aims to develop theory directly from the data: theory is grounded in the data, rather than validated through hypothesis-testing as in deductive research. Grounded theory is interested in actions and interactions, focuses on processes rather than structure, and considers the ways in which actors interpret and make sense of their experiences (Charmaz, 2006, 2014, pp. 14–15; Thornberg, Halldin, Bolmsjö, & Petersson, 2013, p. 311). In contrast to the classic version of grounded theory developed by Glaser and Strauss (1967) which aims at the "discovery" of grounded theory, constructivist grounded theory treats research acts as constructed, not given (Charmaz, 2014, p. 13) and argues that we, as researchers, "construct our grounded theories through our past and present involvements and interactions with people, perspectives, and research practices" (Charmaz, 2014, p. 16). In line with the "new" Sociology of Childhood's perspective on children as active agents, this approach is ideal to study children's views and voices (Corsaro, 1997; Prout, 2002; Prout & James, 1997).

State of the Research: What Do We Know?

Classic grounded theory, as developed by Glaser and Strauss (1967), explicitly advocates to delay the literature review until the analysis is finished, lest extant ideas and theories impact on the study, which is believed to hinder the development of original theory. In this view, researchers' own ideas – not preconceived notions or disciplinary paradigms – are supposed to guide theory development. Over the years, this approach has increasingly been rejected, partially because a lack of familiarity with the state of research about a subject risks reinventing the wheel: the scholar might think (s)he stumbled upon something new and insightful, only to then discover that this aspect has long been the subject of scholarly debate (Thornberg, 2012). Other scholars point out that it is neither likely nor desirable that a scholar is entirely unfamiliar with the relevant literature (Clarke, 2005; Dunne, 2011; Goldkuhl & Cronholm, 2010; Henwood, & Pidgeon, 2003, r2009; Lempert, 2012; Thornberg, 2012; Tummers & Karsten, 2012; Walls, Parahoo, & Fleming, 2010). According to this perspective, it is inevitable that scholars have opinions or views that are influenced by their respective discipline or prior scholarly experience (cf. Charmaz, 2014, p. 306). Charmaz points out that most studies require some type of permission or approval and that the process of preparing the necessary proposals already requires a high degree of familiarity with the current state of research (p. 307). To overcome the dilemma between the need to stay as conceptually uncontaminated as possible and what he calls "naïve empiricism", Thornberg (2012) suggests that grounded theory researchers "use the literature as a possible source of inspiration, ideas, "aha!" experiences, creative associations, critical reflection and multiple lenses" (p. 249). He calls this approach "informed grounded theory" which:

> refers to a product of a research process as well as to the research process itself, in which both the process and the product have been thoroughly grounded in data by GT methods while being informed by existing research literature and theoretical frameworks. There is, as Dey (1993) highlights, "a difference between an open mind and an empty head" (p. 63). In contrast

> to the classic GT tradition, but in accordance with the constructivist GT tradition, an informed grounded theorist sees the advantage of using pre-existing theories and research findings in the substantive field in a sensitive, creative, and flexible way instead of seeing them as obstacles and threats. (Thornberg, 2012)

The use of literature in this study is guided by this approach. As recommended by Thornberg (2012), I apply the logic of theoretical sampling to the identification and review of relevant literature and treat the literature search as an ongoing process that is an integral part of the overall iterative nature of this research (pp. 251–252).

While children's health and well-being have been studied from various perspectives in the social and health sciences (Brady, Lowe, & Olin Lauritzen, 2015), much of this research has been conducted *for* or *on* children and has focused on diagnosing and treating diseases and their causes or improving health outcomes more generally (Brady, Lowe, & Olin Lauritzen, 2015). Although these certainly have made and continue to make children's lives better, there is also a need to more fully understand the meaning of health and well-being from children's own perspectives (Brady, Lowe, & Olin Lauritzen, 2015). Furthermore, as Brady et al. (2015) emphasize, "there is a need to explore the social and cultural contexts of child health that frame the lived experiences of children and their parents" (p. 173). Particularly rural children's own views on health and well-being are underresearched and undertheorized. Regarding children's health, we, as adults, too often assume that educating about health and health risks, offering programs designed to promote healthy behaviors, and facilitating access to such programs are sufficient efforts to improve children's health outcomes. A widespread assumption inside and outside the medical community suggests that if we could just communicate emphatically enough how "bad" fast food is, for example, people will not eat it. While such rationales are appealing and convincing in theory, they rarely hold up to mundane practices. Children may well know, for example, that certain habits or behaviors are bad for them and yet engage in these behaviors as a result of peer pressure (Michell, 1997; Pavis, Cunningham-Burley, & Amos, 1996; Pavis, Cunningham-Burley, & Amos, 1997). Regarding food choices of children aged 13–15, for example, Stead, McDermott, MacKintosh, and Adamson (2011) found that "it was emotionally and socially risky to be seen to be interested in healthy eating" because:

> the social and symbolic meanings associated with healthy eating conflicted with processes and values which are of crucial importance in adolescence, such as self-image and fitting in with the peer group. (Stead et al., 2011, p. 1131)

Insights such as these underline the need to listen to children's own voices to gain an in-depth understanding of their perspectives on health.

Significance of the Study

The holistic picture of the health and well-being of children in rural communities this study hopes to help paint adds value in two key ways: (1) It will offer valuable insights into children's own views on health and the ways they do (or do not) navigate available knowledge and resources. (2) These insights can, in turn, inform frameworks to promote children's health that are more sustainable than traditional approaches, which often operate on an adult-centric and one-size-fits-all logic that fails to do justice to the complex matter of children's health in rural communities.

In line with principles guiding grounded theory research, this pilot study is designed to generate hypotheses for a larger, more in-depth follow-up study in 2019 directly from the field, rather than from the literature alone (Thornberg, 2012). More specifically, the study hopes to identify topics that arise directly from the views of the populations our medical school serves, hoping that this will facilitate more successful, informed interventions that are guided by children's own experiences and perspectives. In addition, study findings will be of benefit to practicing pediatricians and other child health professionals as they understand how to better think about and address challenges of health and weight management of patients and their families.

Midwest Town and Midwest Elementary School

Midwest Elementary School, the research site for this pilot study is located in Midwest Town – a small rural village in central Illinois. Located between two small urban centers, at the intersection of two central Illinois counties, Midwest school district boundaries encompass the three rural towns of Midwest Town, West Midwestern Town, and East Midwestern Town. Together, these rural towns have a population of just under 3,000 residents. No pediatricians are located in the district. Median household incomes are US$54,091 (Midwestern Town), US$54,165 (West Midwestern Town), and US$62,059 (East Midwestern Town). Child poverty rates are 3.1% (West Midwestern Town), 3.3% (East Midwestern Town), and 7.2% (Midwestern Town). Unemployment rates range from 4.4% (East Midwestern Town) to 12.1% (West Midwestern Town) and 12.6% (Midwestern Town). The district meets the USDA's definition of a food desert as an area "vapid of fresh fruit, vegetables, and other healthful whole foods" (American Nutrition Association, 2015): Since the last grocery store in Midwestern Town closed in the summer of 2018, there is no grocery store in the entire school district, making access to healthy and nutritious foods a challenge for district families. The closest grocery stores are located in the two small urban centers, translating to travel distances between eight and 30 miles.

In 2017–2018, Midwest school district had a student population of 724: 93% white, 3% "two or more races," 2.2% Hispanic, 0.8% Asian, 0.7% American Indian, and 0.3% black. The four district schools are located in the three communities that comprise the district: the elementary school (pre-KG – second grade) is located in East Midwestern Town, Midwestern Town houses the intermediate (3–5) and middle schools (6–8), and the high school (9–12) is located in West Midwestern Town. With 46.4% of district students classified as "low-income" in 2017–2018, poverty appears disproportionately concentrated in the public schools.

In the school year 2018–2019, Midwest School housed 158 students in grades 3–5. The school predominantly serves white students (96.8%) and only 3.2% of students identify as two or more races. 62% of students are classified as low-income ("families receiving public aid, living in substitute care, or eligible to receive free or reduced price lunches," Illinois State Board of Education, 2018), compared to 46.6% at the district and 49.9% at the Illinois state level.

METHODS

Methodological Considerations in Research with Children

Scholars in the "new" Sociology of Childhood emphasize that research methods in the study of children do not necessarily have to be different from those used to study adults (Christensen & James, 2008; James & Prout, 1997). However, even though child-centered studies can employ similar methodological strategies as research with adults, observing and interviewing children is not the same as using these methods with adults. It is important, for example, to be aware of the unequal distribution of power between adults. While power always plays a role in research, Christensen and James (2008) argue:

> that the inherent power relations between researcher and researched in childhood studies must be seen as reinforced by more general cultural notions of the power relations which exist between children and adults (p. 6)

Similarly, Corsaro and Fingerson (2006) caution that "the power imbalance between the researcher and respondent is heightened because of the age and status difference" between adults and children (p. 132). Adults have authority over children in most institutionalized settings – or, in any case, claim to have authority. At the same time, children are often highly skilled at resisting, avoiding, or otherwise undermining adult claims to power and authority (Greene & Hogan, 2005, p. 10). For the adult researcher working with children, it is important to be mindful of these considerations and avoid taking advantage of the power differentials between children and adults. The unequal distribution of power between adults and children must also be considered in designing and conducting interviews. It is possible that "children may give answers that are determined more by their desire to please than their desire to be truthful" (Greene & Hogan, 2005, p. 9). While this is certainly a possibility, it is not more likely in interviews with children than in adult interviews. As Scott (2008) points out:

> [c]hildren's responses will also be subject to the standard biases that have been relatively well researched in the question and answer process for adults – things like context effects, [...] [or] social desirability. (p. 98)

Researchers interviewing children should be mindful of these aspects, as well as of the possibility that children "deliberately set out to lie and deceive" (Greene & Hogan, 2005, p. 7). At the same time, it is important to understand that these factors also influence interviews with adults – they are not necessarily more likely because the interview partners are minors. On the contrary, Scott

(2008) points out that "it has been claimed that children may be less susceptible than adults to social desirability bias" (p. 98; emphasis added).

Participants

Participants for this study are recruited from the school's two fifth-grade classrooms. Altogether, there are 52 fifth-grade students (27 girls and 25 boys) at Midwest Elementary (classroom A: 14 girls and 12 boys; classroom B: 13 girls and 13 boys). In close collaboration with the two homeroom teachers and the school principal, I introduced myself to students in both classrooms at the beginning of the research. I told them who I was, why I was there, and what I hoped their role in my research would be. I explained my position as a researcher and Sociologist and proceeded to clarify these terms in a way I hoped was meaningful to the kids. I emphasized that I was most interested in their views – what they liked and disliked and what kinds of things mattered to them inside and outside of school. I informed them that I would take part in their daily routines for a while before we would start interviews on a volunteer basis. I pointed out that I would be very happy if they chose to help me with my work, but that no negative consequences awaited those who did not want talk to or interact with me during my fieldwork. We also talked about the interviews I planned to conduct: I showed them my tape recorder and told them that I would record the interviews so that I could remember everything that was said afterwards. I emphasized that I was neither a teacher nor a counselor or social worker. I made a particular effort to underline that interview participation was entirely voluntary that I would neither be mad nor would they get a bad grade in case they chose not to participate. I stressed that I wanted to learn about their views and opinions and about the ways they usually do things. And finally, we discussed the terms "anonymity" and "confidentiality" and I assured them that all names would be changed in any presentations or publications so that nobody could know who they were. Based on previous research I conducted with students in a similar age group (Scheer, 2017), I emphasized that I am a mandated reporter and explained that this limits the confidentiality I can promise: should students tell me that someone is hurting them or they are planning to hurt themselves or others, I would have to inform other adults.

In all my conversations and interactions with students I tried to avoid, as much as possible, to approach the kids from a position of authority. In the literature, this approach has been referred to as the "least adult role" (Mandell, 1988) or the "least possible adult" (Thornberg, 2008, p. 420). These concepts describe a situation in which the social distance and difference between the adult-as-researcher and the child-as-researched are minimized to the utmost extent, especially regarding the position of superior authority adults otherwise occupy vis-à-vis children.

Doing interpretive qualitative research with children in a school setting means entering the social world of the school for the duration of the study. In all qualitative research but especially so in studies with children, it is very important to respect research participants. According to Charmaz (2014), one way to express this respect is through efforts to establish rapport with participants (p. 33). She emphasizes that "for many projects [rapport] is a prerequisite to gaining solid data and maintaining access for collecting further data" (Charmaz, 2014). One important way to establish this rapport is to give students the opportunity to get to know the researcher before conducting any interviews. In this study, I tried to facilitate this by being present at the school on as many days as possible for the first two weeks in which I did not actively collect any data but merely participated in students' daily routines: I sat in their classrooms and watched their lessons, accompanied them to special area classes such as Music or PE, gave them an opportunity to approach me and talk to me during breaks, had lunch with them in the cafeteria, and went outside for recess with them. As a researcher, this is an important period of any study for me, because it allows students to become familiar with my presence and get to know me before I ask them to share their views and experiences with me during interviews.

Data Collection

This study employs a combination of data collection methods including ethnographic observations, interviews, and a series of games I designed specifically to collect data for this study.

Ethnographic Observations

On-site research is conducted using ethnographic observations of daily routines of fifth-grade students in the classroom and school. Observations are recorded in a field journal and later transferred into an electronic word-processing document. While some of my participation – especially at the beginning of the study – was not designed to collect data, I have continued to participate in lunch sessions whenever I am at the school. As of late November 2018, I have eaten lunch with students on 15 of the 16 days I have spent at the school.

Games and Exercises

To explore students' own views on health, well-being, and nutrition, this study uses whole-class games or exercises. The first of these activities, "*This is what I usually have for* [...]" is a whole-class exercise designed to explore what individual students usually have for breakfast, lunch, dinner, and snacks and what students think a healthy/unhealthy child usually has for each of these meals. More specifically, it is designed to explore what kinds of foods students *report* to usually consume: "What people say might not be what they do, have done, and would do in the future." (Charmaz, 2014, p. 78). Similar to interviews, self-reports are also "performances that research participants give for particular purposes." (Charmaz, 2014) This exercise was voluntary and students could opt out by not participating. Students were asked to put their name on the top of each worksheet only if they are willing to be part of a follow-up interview in which we discuss their responses. Alternatively, students could participate in this activity without including their names. Students could choose to write down names of foods and drinks, or draw pictures of their choices for each worksheet. Of the

52 students in both classrooms, all 47 who were present the day the exercise was administered completed the worksheets. 24 girls and 18 boys returned the worksheets with their names included and five students returned theirs anonymously.

The second activity, *"This is what a* […] *child eats and drinks – a three-part exercise"*, was designed to explore the relationship between food and social identity (cf. Stead et al., 2011) from the children's own perspectives by involving students directly in identifying and naming which the social groups exist in their classrooms, instead of using adult-/researcher-defined groups. In the first part, students in both classrooms were asked to write the names of any social groups they could think of on post-it notes and place these on the whiteboard in their classroom. This first part was anonymous but all students present for the exercise participated actively. Of the hundreds of post-it notes both classes produced, I selected nine groups that were named most frequently for part II of the exercise: (1) athletic/sporty, (2) gamer, (3) popular, (4) unpopular, (5) band, (6) nerd/nerdy, (7) bad, (8) good, and (9) happy. In part II, students were asked to either draw and/or write what they thought a child in each of these nine groups usually eats or drinks. Each student was given a total of nine of these sheets – one for each group – and asked to fill out information for as many groups as possible. Before conducting this part of the exercise, I again emphasized that participation in the activity was voluntary and students could either opt out entirely or they could choose not to put their names on the worksheets. Altogether, 43 of the 52 students in both classrooms participated in this activity, with four students being absent that day. Of the 43 students who participated, nine returned completed sets in which they had filled out responses for all of the nine groups. The remaining 34 students returned incomplete sets, ranging from returned sets with only one group filled out to sets in which all but one category was completed. Twenty-three of the 43 returned sets were filled out by girls (out of 27 girls in both classrooms) and 18 were filled out by boys (out of 25 boys in both classrooms). Two sets were returned anonymously. Follow-up sessions for both exercises are scheduled for December 2018 and January 2019.

Student Interviews

The most important data source for this pilot study are student interviews, not least because they facilitate the exploration of research participants' experiences and perspectives and have long been used as a successful method in qualitative research (Hopf, 2008, p. 349). Interviews with students are conducted on a volunteer basis. So far, individual interview sessions have lasted between 15 and 70 minutes, depending on how much time was available. Some students have been interviewed multiple times, because one session did not cover everything I wanted to address. Interviews are tape recorded and later transcribed for analysis. As of late November 2018, I have conducted 16.5 hours of interviews in 33 sessions with 22 students (11 girls and 11 boys).

Heeding the methodological considerations in research with children outlined above, this study uses a mix of unstructured interviewing and semi-structured interviewing as a method for student interviews (Bernard, 2002, pp. 204–206).

While semi-structured interviews rely on an interview guide comprising certain questions that generally must be covered in a particular sequence, the interview guide for this study serves more as a backup than a formal guide (p. 205). Which questions are addressed in each interview session and in what order depends on individual students and contexts. In this regard, my approach more closely resembles unstructured interviewing which is "based on a clear plan that you keep constantly in mind but [is] also characterized by a minimum of control over people's responses." (Bernard, 2002) Unstructured interviews are not to be mistaken with informal conversations. As Bernard (2002) puts it:

> [t]here is nothing "informal" about unstructured interviewing, and nothing deceptive either. You sit down with another person and hold an interview. Period. Both of you know what you're doing, and there is no shared feeling that you're just engaged in pleasant chitchat. (pp. 204–205)

Informed Consent

In any classroom-based research that also involves observations, it is not possible for an individual student to opt out of the study entirely and refuse to be part of the observation. While this can certainly be seen as problematic from an ethical standpoint, it comes with the methodological territory. Although students consequently could not give or deny consent for participation in the study itself, informed consent was sought and obtained verbally from students for all interviews. Following IRB recommendations, I did not seek written consent from students or parents in order to avoid creating a written record of names. Instead, I sent a letter to each family, informing them of my background, research, objectives, and possible roles their children might play in my study and gave families an opportunity to deny consent by contacting either the school principal or emailing me directly. Because no family made use of this opportunity, all students were included in all observations and interviewees have been recruited from the entire group of 52 students. In line with the "new" Sociology of Childhood's perspective on children as competent actors in their own right, I placed particular emphasis on obtaining verbal informed consent for the interviews from students themselves (Prout, 2002). Viewing children as active agents, capable of making their own decisions about most matters affecting them, also means allowing the children to decide for themselves whether or not they want to be interviewed. While allowing their parents to deny consent can be seen as an important prerequisite for children's participation in this study, it is my responsibility as a researcher to make sure that children do not feel compelled to participate in interviews because their parents expected this.

At the beginning of the interview phase, I asked for student volunteers and interviewed only those who actively expressed their interest. As the interview phase progresses, I have started selecting students more deliberately to ensure that interview materials reflect gender distribution in the two classrooms. In addition, I also approach individual students whose perspectives and views present themselves as particularly relevant or valuable to the themes that are beginning to surface in the emerging analysis. Whenever I wish to speak to a particular student, I approach these individuals several days in advance to give them time to think about whether or not they want to be interviewed. At the beginning of each interview, I remind each student that their participation is voluntary and that they will face no negative consequences if they choose not to participate. In addition, I inform them that we can skip any question or topic they do not want to talk about, or end the interview at any time.

Data analysis

Rather than gathering all data first based on a set of fixed hypotheses and analyzing them afterwards in two distinct stages, grounded theory envisions a simultaneous process of data collection and analysis (Charmaz, 2014, p. 14). The main stages in this iterative process are coding, constant comparison, memo-writing, and theoretical sampling (cf. Charmaz, 2014; Glaser & Strauss, 1967). In contrast to other types of qualitative analysis, coding of data in grounded theory begins early on in the research process and is conducted in multiple phases: initial coding, focused coding, and theoretical coding (Charmaz, 2014). Throughout these phases, codes and categories become increasingly abstract and theoretical. Data collection in grounded theory is informed by theoretical sampling: categories that emerge from initial coding guide what additional data are collected over the course of the research process (pp. 197–198). The objective of theoretical sampling is to advance the construction of theory by developing and elaborating analytical categories (pp. 192, 198). The link between data collection and analysis that facilitates the iterative process characteristic of grounded theory is memo-writing (p. 162 ff.). Memos are analytical notes in which ideas about codes, categories, the relationships among and between them are explored, developed, and refined (p. 162). Memos can reveal contradictions that must be resolved, identify areas to be further scrutinized, or help clarify categories and thereby advance the emerging theory (Charmaz, 2014). Memos are written at any point in the research process and are so central to the construction of theory that Charmaz argues they "will form the core of your grounded theory" (p. 191). Through multiple rounds of coding the data, writing memos, theoretical sampling, and constant comparison, initial codes are used to construct focused codes which are later raised to conceptual categories. Ultimately, the objective is to achieve theoretical saturation of the core concepts which represent the central building blocks of the grounded theory constructed from the study (pp. 213, 299, 345). Following these guidelines, data collection and analysis for this pilot study are iterative and non-linear to the extent possible. Theoretical sampling and constant comparison play key roles in my fieldwork and memo-writing forms an integral part of my research: I record all ideas, questions, or theoretical considerations in a notebook I always take with me. As the analysis is progressing, I also create diagrams, tables, and conceptual maps to visualize relationships or overcome conceptual deadlocks.

As indicated above, interviews are the main data source for this study. Before they can be subjected to formal analysis, all interviews have to be transcribed.

All transcriptions for this study are being done by a professional transcription service. Of the 33 interviews I have conducted so far, I have received 16 completed transcripts. All interview transcripts are saved as Microsoft Word Documents, printed out for initial coding, and then uploaded into MAXQDA 2018 for further coding and analysis. MAXQDA is a qualitative data analysis software produced and distributed by Berlin-based software firm VERBI GmbH. This software allows sections of a text to be highlighted, coded, and linked to one another. According to Charmaz (2014), grounded theory coding means to "take segments of data apart, name them in concise terms, and propose an analytic handle to develop abstract ideas for interpreting each segment of data" (p. 113). The objective of coding, even more so in grounded theory than in other types of qualitative coding, is always the development of theory: codes are created "to explicate how people enact or respond to events, what meanings they hold, and how and why these actions and meanings evolved" (p. 112). It is important to note that codes are *constructs*, not accurate or fixed depictions of some kind of objectively existing reality. They are shaped by the unique perspective of each researcher and reflect what (s)he deems important or relevant and the interpretations (s)he affixes to participants' words and actions (p. 114). According to Charmaz, grounded theory coding, at minimum, consists of two phases: an "initial phase" in which small parts of the data are named and a "focused, selective phase" during which the most important initial codes are employed to further sort and arrange the data (p. 113). Currently, I am finalizing this initial phase to be able to move on to the focused, selective phase in which I will collect additional data to expand and get a better understanding of themes that are emerging from the initial phase. In the following section, I will outline and illustrate the most important initial codes that have emerged from the analysis so far.

PRELIMINARY RESULTS

In line with Charmaz's understanding of an "interview guide as a flexible tool to revise" (2014, p. 62), this document is evolving over the course of the research and is adapted as needed. Questions that prove to be confusing to students are reworded or omitted entirely. Informed by theoretical sampling and working toward theoretical saturation, questions are added as relevant themes surface or emerging categories require elaboration. I address relevant themes with students as interviews progress and try to include those students in interviews whose perspectives may be particularly relevant to certain emerging themes. Against this background, the following initial codes also include themes that were not part of the initial interview guide and include facets not originally considered as part of the research questions.

Knowing the Difference

The most consistent finding across all means of data collection used so far is that study participants seem to know the general difference between "healthy" and “unhealthy” foods and drinks (i.e., items students themselves have listed as examples of “healthy” or “unhealthy”). In their drawings or verbal responses to the “this is what a (healthy/unhealthy) child usually has for breakfast/lunch/dinner/snack”, as well as in interviews and informal conversations, students consistently list fruits, vegetables, certain meats (such as chicken), some grains (such as rice or pasta), and water or milk as examples for “healthy” food and drink choices. In comparison, fast food or junk food is consistently used as examples of “unhealthy” choices. Many students name popular fast food restaurant chains as examples of fast or junk food. Others mention deep fried foods, other high-fat foods, sweets, or candy as “unhealthy” examples. Unhealthy drink choices consistently include soda or “pop” and other sugary drinks. Several participants identified “balance” and “moderation” as important aspects, emphasizing that all or most foods are okay if and when they are consumed in moderation and no single food or drink is entirely “off limits”.

These initial findings contrast beliefs I repeatedly encounter in the clinical realm regarding a perceived “need” to fundamentally educate patients (in this case children and their families) about healthy vs. unhealthy dietary choices. Preliminary data suggest that study participants already possess a good working knowledge of this basic difference. However, the extent to which children are able to *act* on this knowledge – for example, how much control they have over the types of food that are purchased and consumed in the family – or the extent to which, given the opportunity, children actually choose healthy over unhealthy foods, is a matter of practice. Exploring dietary *practices* is beyond the scope of this preliminary study and subject to a different set of methods, for example, food diaries or visual methods such as photo voice (Daly, Foote, & Wadsworth, 2017).

Knowledge vs Choice

While it is important to learn that most study participants seem to know the difference between “healthy” and “unhealthy” foods and that they are aware of the role that balance and moderation play in selecting certain foods and drinks, findings that fall into these categories tell us anything neither about actual *choices* that are made and nor about the reasons for these choices. The fact alone that someone knows that certain foods or drinks are less healthy than others does not yet mean they consistently refrain from consuming these. In fact, interviews as well as the exercise “*This is what I usually have for breakfast/lunch/dinner/snack*” indicate that several students “usually” consume foods and drinks they would otherwise describe as unhealthy, including items such as pop tarts, candy bars, or fast food items.

Time Constraints and Convenience

When asked in which situations such items are consumed, student responses indicate that time constraints play an important role. One participant, for example, reported that her family often eats pop tarts for breakfast on the weekends because several of the children in the family play different sports and the various games that occur on weekends translate into a time crunch to get everyone ready, fed, and out of the house in time.

Closely related to "time constraints", participants also described situations in which less "healthy" meal choices are preferred over "healthy", freshly prepared meals because they are faster and more convenient. While some participants ascribed such choices to time constraints (e.g., not enough time left to cook after work or extra-curricular activities), some recounted situations in which these choices were made because there was no desire to cook, for example, because a parent "doesn't like to cook".

What's Cooking?

Another issue that has emerged underlines how important it is to collect as much information, in as much detail as possible about what each family's specific food practices are. While many adults in my personal and professional life tend to associate a "home-cooked" meal with generally "healthier" choices, this is not consistently reflected in the responses I have collected from students so far. Two interview questions ask "Who usually cooks in your house?" and "What does this person usually cook when they cook?" While several students describe well-balanced meals, including soups, stews, crockpot meals, or roasts, some participants list "biscuits and gravy" or "mac and cheese" as their family's "usual" home-cooked meal. This is not to suggest that such choices are inherently "bad" or should be subject to any moralizing judgment in and of themselves. Nevertheless, it is important to be mindful that different ideas, definitions, and concepts surrounding "cooking" or "home-cooked" meals exist – especially when such topics are addressed in surveys which do not allow for probing or follow-up and could consequently produce misleading results if related questions contain the implicit bias that "home-cooked" equals "healthy" or "healthier" than other possible meal sources. More data needs to be collected about this particular issue to more fully comprehend whether grouping it within the "knowledge versus choice" system adequately reflects different families' realities. It is possible that the extent to which families make less "healthy" choices surrounding cooking could indicate that there is a kind of "grey area" between knowing which foods are "healthy"/"unhealthy" and understanding the need for a "balanced" diet, however, and instances when families consume certain types of foods or consume them often, on the other: Families' understanding of the exact meaning of "balanced" or "in moderation" may well deviate from what would be recommended as a daily intake. In other words, while there might be consensus or general agreement that deep fried foods are "unhealthy" and salad greens are "healthy", certain foods, including "biscuits and gravy" or "mac and cheese", may not fall into these binary categories as neatly or in the same way for all families. Alternatively, it is possible that we use the same terms or concepts such as "balanced" or "in moderation" to differentiate a "healthy" from an "unhealthy" diet, but what exactly those concepts mean in practice may be very different.

Does Skinny Mean Healthy?

Another initial code is "Does skinny mean healthy?" Two main observations feed into this code: (1) While several of the "bigger" students in my study are very physically active – many play various sports – several of the "skinny" participants report little or no physical activity and describe very sedentary life styles. (2) My observations indicate that school lunches sent from home (i.e., students who do not eat the school lunch but instead bring their own) often include various "unhealthy" items, including candy bars, cookies, cakes, sugary drinks, or foods high in fat and sodium (such as "Lunchables", pre-packaged peperoni/salami snacks, or packaged crackers filled with cheese or peanut butter). Some lunches consist exclusively of such items and it seems to be primarily students within the range of a "normal" body mass index (BMI) who bring such foods to school.

Research about overweight or obese children as well as medical/clinical practice, primarily focus on children above a certain BMI, not least because excess weight places them, in the aggregate, at a higher risk for certain metabolic conditions such as diabetes or cardiovascular diseases (Baker, Olsen, & Sørensen, 2007; Centers for Disease Control [CDC], 2016; Freedman, Khan, Dietz, Srinivasan, & Berenson, 2001; Krebs et al., 2007; Lobstein, Baur, & Uauy, 2004; Must & Strauss, 1999; Singh, Mulder, Twisk, van Mechelen, & Chinapaw, 2008). However, my observations indicate that we may need to expand our conceptual focus if our main concern is children's health, as I argue it should be. An image that is as widespread as it is popular is that skinny children (or adults for that matter but they are not the focus of this study) are healthy or at least healthier than overweight or even obese individuals. While a growing literature surrounding a concept described as "healthy obesity" in adults suggests that as many as 50% or even 75% of obese adults are metabolically healthy (Rey-López, de Rezende, Pastor-Valero, & Tess, 2014), my study suggests at least a note of caution in two regards: (1) Metabolic health issues attributed to excess weight tend to be cumulative and often do not materialize until later in life. Regarding the idea of "healthy obesity", this means that even though "bigger" children might be physically active in the present, this does not necessarily prevent later metabolic issues. (2) Children's bodies and minds are constantly growing and developing. As such, they have unique nutritional needs above and beyond caloric intake itself. Their bodies and minds require certain macro- and micronutrients for optimal development. Observing that many "skinny" students regularly consume large amounts of highly processed, high-sugar, high-fat, and/or high-sodium foods and knowing that their "normal" BMIs, by default, exclude these students from many academic and clinical perspectives, at the very minimum calls for a reevaluation of our current paradigm. After all, if we want to improve and/or safeguard children's health, then any diet that does not contain the macro- and micronutrients necessary for optimal growth and development should be a cause for concern. Of course, observations at this point are limited to selected lunch periods and neither reflect what else these students consume on a regular basis nor do they permit any large-scale, generalizable conclusions. Nevertheless, these observations suggest a need to collect more, broader, and deeper information about the dietary habits of *all* students. Creating interventions that would go beyond mere weight/BMI measures to include a focus on health and developmentally relevant nutrients may also reduce the stigma attached to interventions that single out only students above a certain BMI and could possibly have unintended consequences detrimental to these children. There is a lot of rich and important exploration surrounding statements such as "I kinda look unhealthy but I'm not unhealthy" made by one of the girls I interviewed. Similarly, it is worth exploring if those students who look "healthy" are, in fact, as healthy as their BMI suggests.

Family-specific Codes

Two themes have emerged as important initial themes addressing students' home and family lives: the rules in place in each family regarding food and the size and structure of different families.

Family Food Rules

During our interviews students identified different types of what I call "family food rules", including: (1) Are kids allowed to select certain food or drink items when the family goes grocery shopping? If so, what items can they pick and who controls the timing and amount of consumption? (2) Does the family have a designated snack cabinet, box, or similar location in which snacks are stored? If so, what kinds of snacks are available? What kinds of snacks are permissible for children to have? Who controls access to these places? Are children allowed to help themselves to whatever is in these places whenever they would like or do they have to ask for adult permission? How else is the timing and amount of consumption regulated? Can kids eat as much of a certain item as they would like? (3) Does the family regularly consume meals together or do family members eat at different times and in different locations? What are the reasons for these practices? (4) What alternatives are available to children if and when they do not like what is served as the family meal (if a family meal is available)? Can they help themselves to any other type of food that is available or do parents limit alternatives to certain foods/types of food?

These are all questions that have emerged from the interviews and my conversations with students – they were not part of the initial interview guide. The next phase of data collection will focus on these questions in more detail to explore the role they play in children's food practices and help create specific questions and hypotheses for the in-depth study that is planned to follow this preliminary project.

Family Size and Structure

Another initial code that has emerged from the data is family size and structure. Several students describe rather complex arrangements: They may live with, for example, one biological parent for part of the week or month and with their other biological parents for the rest of the time. Children often share these households with their biological siblings, half-siblings, and step-siblings, resulting in large household sizes of five or more children at various times of the week or month (as half- and step-siblings also live in different households at different times). Any study hoping to explore children's or families' food rules or perspectives consequently also has to explore if and how these are different in each of the households children regularly spend large amounts of time in. What is of particular interest here is less the size or structure of each family itself, but the extent to which food rules are related to these variegated living arrangements. In addition, it will be important for future research to explore if and how food is used as a reward or social control mechanism. For example, is one parent of a formerly cohabitating but now separated or divorced couple, more permissible regarding certain "unhealthy" foods or snacks in an effort to be seen as the more desirable parent? Alternatively, it would be important to explore the role of the non-biological, now cohabitating adult and how food rules are negotiated for the various biological or step-children.

Physical Activity

Nutrition and caloric intake are only one aspect of any discussion surrounding children's weight. It is also important to consider the level and intensity of physical activity. In a study of rural children's weight status, Daly et al. (2017) found, for example, that:

> [f]ruit and vegetable consumption was not related to BMI or access to fruits and vegetables. [but instead] that children's physical activity and sedentary behavior impacts weight status of children residing in a rural environment.

As part of the interviews, I ask students whether they play any organized sport, what sport or sports they are involved in, and what they usually do in their free time. While these questions allow me to collect data about how many participants engage in regular physical activity, student responses to these questions also revealed the following initial themes that will be explored in more detail in the upcoming weeks and months.

Performance as a Health Incentive

Being engaged in an organized sport itself can be beneficial to cardio-vascular health: All the organized sports my participants have listed (football, basketball, soccer, and baseball) involve running as part of the sport itself. However, in addition to additional calories burned or other health benefits immediately linked to the physical activity itself, several participants indicated that being involved in an organized sport also brings additional health benefits because wanting to be better or achieve their personal best causes them to choose certain foods that are healthier than others and/or forego foods students otherwise view as tasty and desirable because they could limit performance. These students described a "need" to eat "well" so they can be their personal best or become better, faster, or stronger and explicitly described fast or junk food as detrimental to their performance.

The Blessing and Curse of Extra-curricular Activities

While physical activity during extra-curricular activities certainly comes with many important health benefits, study participants also indicate that being involved in such activities can come at the expense of making healthy food choices. Strongly related to the codes "time constraints" and "convenience" above, several students involved in extra-curricular activities reported that their activities can be so time-consuming that they and their families do not have time to eat together, eat at home, or eat "healthy". This is particularly true for families with multiple children who play sports, especially when different family members are involved in different sports. According to the kids' narratives, practice schedules, timing, and location of games frequently result in meals purchased at popular fast food chains and consumed in the car because there simply is not time to cook or eat at home.

Self-exclusion from Recess and PE

Many public schools struggle to make regular recess and PE available to their students. Reasons include staffing or time constraints or the need to give priority to instructional time in order to prepare for high-stakes testing. Other schools use recess as a disciplinary tool and make it available only as a "privilege" that must be earned by the good behavior of the entire class and is quickly lost when a few individuals do not exhibit desired behaviors (Scheer, 2015). Midwest Elementary School is a laudable exception in this regard and students are scheduled to have PE and recess every day of the week.

One of the strengths of qualitative research is the ability to observe and identify where and in what ways theory and practice diverge, and the ways in which recess/PE is used in practice at Midwest Elementary illustrates this strength well: While recess and PE are both *available* to students on a daily basis, my observations show that some students exclude themselves from any actual physical activity during these times. This self-exclusion can take the form of individual students sitting on the bench during recess instead of playing on the playground with their peers, or it can take the form of students walking around the track when they are supposed to be running. While walking is certainly better than no activity at all, it does not have the same cardiovascular benefits as running. While self-exclusion during recess generally appears to be unmediated by adults – I have not observed an adult telling a student to sit during recess, except for brief "time-outs" or other disciplinary exclusions which appear to be rare – self-exclusion from moderate-to-vigorous physical activity (MVPA) during PE appears to happen with full knowledge and at the discretion of the PE teacher. When the activity technically involves running, students are given an alternative that is much less physically challenging, such as walking around the track instead. Further exploration of the reasons and rationales for giving students such options is needed in the remainder of this study.

> We used to play outside but then the new video game came out.

Another initial code that has emerged from the analysis so far and seems to be particularly worthy of further inquiry is the role that watching TV and playing video games play in students' lives and in their perceptions of "healthy" vs. "unhealthy" life styles and individuals. In the "food and social identity" exercise, the vast majority of students listed "unhealthy" food and drink choices when asked to list what they thought a "gamer" eats and drinks. Examples included large amounts of fries and other fried foods, chips, candy, and "lots of soda". When asked to describe an "unhealthy" child in the interview, students described an individual who "plays video games and stares at the TV all day", "probably watches TV all the time [...] and plays video games", or "just wants to stay home and play video games and take naps and watch TV". One participant told me about several places in his neighborhood he and his friends used to play outside and then clarified "Well, we used to play there until the new "Madden" [*a popular American football video game developed and published by EA Sports, my comment*] came out". Similar to "family food rules", these preliminary findings highlight a need for further inquiry into something that could be called "family free time rules": Who controls access to the video game console? What, if any, rules regulate the time kids can spend playing video games? Can they access the console(s) in their house whenever they want to and play for as long as they would like? Alternatively, do parents set time limits and how are these limits enforced? Are students encouraged or even compelled to go outside to play after a certain time has been spent playing video games inside? Similar questions could be asked regarding students' consumption of television programs.

Access

In addition to knowledge and education about "healthy" and "unhealthy" food choices in the context of childhood obesity, access to healthy foods is a frequently discussed concern – especially in rural areas. Since the last grocery store in Midwest Town closed in the summer of 2018, there is no grocery store in the entire school district, making the district a food desert and increasing the challenge for district families to access healthy and nutritious foods. The closest grocery stores are located between eight and 30 miles away in the small urban centers to the east and west of Midwest Town.

Would Better Access Really make People Choose "Healthy"?

However, until very recently, such foods *were* available in Midwest Town and those students at Midwest Elementary – my study participants as well as other students I have seen at the school – who are overweight or obese did not become overweight or obese in the few weeks between when the last grocery store closed down and the time this research began in late August 2018. Availability of fresh fruits, vegetables, and other healthy food options are a necessary prerequisite to healthy eating but availability in itself does not yet create or guarantee that healthy choices *can be* and are *being* made. It is possible, and a few students have cautiously hinted at this possibility, that families do not have enough money to purchase fruits and vegetables. In addition, many kids have long lists of fruits and vegetables they do not like and will not eat, including generally popular fruits such as apples or bananas. The question underlying these preliminary findings is not whether access to fresh and healthy foods is a problem in rural areas – it certainly is. Instead, the question is whether improved access itself would solve the problem of people not consuming enough "healthy" and/or consuming too many "unhealthy" foods. A child who does not like apples, broccoli, or peas is unlikely to change this preference when access to and availability of these items change. Similarly, if – and this is a complex question that requires additional data – time constraints, convenience, or food as a medium for parental reward/punishment are primary or even simply more pressing considerations for families, would better access really change these practices and preferences in a meaningful way?

Is Access a Matter of Time as Much or More Than Location?

Another facet of access that will need to be addressed through additional data is to what extent and exactly for whom access is a pressing concern and whether geographic location is the biggest barrier to access or if it is something else. Many parents of my study participants work in one of the two urban centers and therefore, at least in theory, have access to the grocery stores available in these locations. However, Midwest Elementary does not offer organized after school-care, which means that it is possible parents would have geographical *access* to grocery stores but may well not have enough *time* to shop in these locations because they need to rush back to Midwest Town to pick up their children from school or be home when the bus arrives. More information is needed to explore this question further, but it is a question well worthy of additional pursuit. Should additional research reveal that *time* is one or possibly the biggest barrier to access for families in this district, potential interventions hoping to improve healthy eating would need to consider and address this aspect.

DISCUSSION: OPEN QUESTIONS AND NEXT STEPS

This chapter presented preliminary findings of a pilot study designed to explore rural children's perspectives on health, well-being, and nutrition. In part because the analysis is ongoing, and data collection is guided by theoretical sampling, some of the questions this study hopes to address have yet to be answered and others have surfaced as important questions to be addressed that were not part of the original research design. Questions that remain to be answered in subsequent cycles of data collection and analysis include those regarding children's own views and definitions of health and well-being and what meanings they ascribe to these concepts, their ideas of "healthy" versus "unhealthy" eating or activity patterns, and the ways in which children's views of health and well-being relate to each other and to their perceptions of an individual's personality, physical appearance, activity levels, and nutritional practices. The initial codes that are included in this chapter offer insights regarding those factors that influence children to engage in certain behaviors in the context of health, well-being, and nutrition, and refrain from others; the relationship between children's own nutritional practices and their ideas of a "healthy" diet; free-time activities; and other factors that affect children's ideas and practices around health and well-being.

At the current stage of analysis, it seems that the children in my study possess a good working knowledge regarding the basic difference between "healthy" and "unhealthy" foods as well as the importance of a well-balanced diet and the need to consume certain foods and drinks only in moderation. However, as much as study participants seem to *possess* this knowledge, preliminary results indicate that this knowledge neither necessarily nor reliably translates into practice: The same students who describe cookies, candy bars, chips, or other high-sugar/high-fat/high-sodium foods as "unhealthy" regularly consume such foods for lunch or report consuming such foods outside of school. In particularly regarding situations in which food choices are made at the family level or with significant influence from adult family members – including what is packed as a lunch, what is permitted for snack consumption, or what meals are consumed outside of school – preliminary results suggest that time constraints and convenience often play an important role in choosing "unhealthy" or *less* healthy options. Participants describe insufficient time to cook or prepare "healthy" meals or that fast food options are selected because they are quicker and more convenient than cooking at home. Even when meals are prepared at home, choices do not always reflect what is generally recommended as "healthy" or well-balanced. Even though children are at the heart of this study, these preliminary findings underline the need to include parents or other adult caregivers in the research. What choices are made (or not made) at the family level and what rationales exist for these choices? How are choices negotiated in the family – between adult members as well as between adults and children? What rules exist in the family regarding types and amounts of food consumed or children's autonomy to make their own food choices? How do these rules differ between different households children live in at different times of the week or month and to what extent do these difference shape children's food practices?

Preliminary results also indicate that the question of physical activity inside and outside of school is more complex than to simply call for or create additional opportunities for children to participate in such activities. On the one hand, students report strong health incentives as a result of being involved in such activities – wanting to perform well incentivizes healthy food choices – on the other hand, students report that time constraints resulting from such activities can lead to time and convenience as the primary factors influencing meal choices. These different facets of being involved in extra-curricular activities highlight the need to collect additional data about the actual *practices* children and families make in the context of food and physical activity: What do children and their families actually eat in which situations and for what reasons? In addition, these findings pose the question whether "unhealthy" food choices are different, better, or preferable if and when they are made by individuals who are physically active. While a child who consumes a fast food meal following high-intensity physical activity may not need to be concerned about her or his weight, the nutritional value of many fast and convenient food options is often limited or inferior to those of more balanced meals. Do we focus only on those children whose dietary choices have made them overweight or obese and exclude those whose diet may not cause them to have weight problems but may well lack important macro- and micronutrients? Does "skinny" mean "healthy" and do we group all students who "kinda look unhealthy" in the same group regardless of individual situation and context?

Related to physical activity is the time children spend playing video games or watching TV. Preliminary results suggest that children consistently associate such activities with "unhealthy" individuals, and yet several participants report that they or their siblings expend much time on these activities, sometimes even at the explicit exclusion of playing outside. Similar to family food rules, additional information is needed regarding rules that govern free time in different families: Who decides what children do in their free time or how much time they are allowed to spend doing certain things? What rationales do parents or caregivers have for their choices? This topic also highlights the need to add families' perspectives to this child-focused study.

Finally, there is the problem of access – a well-known, prevalent, and well-discussed problem in the context of nutritional health, especially in rural areas. While access in this community is definitely a concern, preliminary findings suggest that location is only one dimension of access and that *time* is another dimension worthy of exploration and potentially even more important as a barrier to access – at least for this particular community. In addition, findings suggest that consideration of access needs to be placed in the context of families' food rationales: if there is no time (or if families *perceive* such a lack of time) to cook, improved access may do very little to increase consumption of healthy foods. Similarly, if children reject certain foods (healthy foods are often very high on the list of foods children do not like and my participants regularly confirm this), then families may not *choose* to consume or prepare such products even if they are easily accessible. Finally, access is also always a matter of affordability. Fruits, vegetables, and other "healthy" foods are often very expensive and while the three communities from which Midwest Elementary draws its students have below average poverty rates and median household incomes that are just below or even slightly above the national average, the school's rate of low-income students is much higher than the district and state average, indicating that poverty might be a problem more concentrated in the school than in the community at large.

The next phase of data collection for this study (December 2018–February 2019) will address as many of these open questions as possible, especially those that involve family or caregiver perspectives. The relationships and rapport I have built both with students and with the school community should minimize barriers and allow me to collect at least some families' perspectives through focus groups or individual interviews. In addition, follow-up sessions for the group exercises administered should provide additional insight into those questions that still remain to be addressed. Other aspects that are emerging as relevant – especially those regarding what children and families actually *do* in the context of health and well-being – are beyond the scope of this pilot study. These questions will be addressed in a more in-depth, comprehensive study that is planned as a follow-up to this study for the second half of 2019. That study will be informed and guided directly by findings and hypotheses generated from this study. In the meantime, preliminary results will be incorporated into the ongoing collaboration with our medical school's clinical department and we begin working toward more informed interventions addressing children's nutritional health and well-being in 2019.

REFERENCES

American Nutrition Association. (2015). USDA defines food deserts. *Nutrition Digest*, *38*, 24. Retrieved from http://americannutritionassociation.org/newsletter/usda-defines-food-deserts

Baker, J. L., Olsen, L. W., & Sørensen, T. I. A. (2007). Childhood body-mass index and the risk of coronary heart disease in adulthood. *The New England Journal of Medicine*, *357*, 2329–2337. doi:10.1056/NEJMoa072515

Bernard, H. R. (2002). *Research methods in anthropology: Qualitative and quantitative methods/H. Russell Bernard* (3rd ed.). Walnut Creek, CA: AltaMira Press.

Brady, G., Lowe, P., & Olin Lauritzen, S. (2015). Connecting a sociology of childhood perspective with the study of child health, illness and wellbeing: Introduction. *Sociology of Health & Illness*, *37*, 173–183. doi:10.1111/1467-9566.12260

Centers for Disease Control. (2016). *Causes and consequences of childhood obesity*. Retrieved from https://www.cdc.gov/obesity/childhood/causes.html

Charmaz, K. (2006). *Constructing grounded theory: A practical guide through qualitative analysis*. London: Sage. Retrieved from http://www.loc.gov/catdir/enhancements/fy0657/2005928035-d.html

Charmaz, K. (2014). *Constructing grounded theory* (2nd ed.) (Introducing qualitative methods). London: Sage.

Christensen, P. M., & James, A. (Eds.). (2008). *Research with children: Perspectives and practices/edited by Allison James and Pia Christensen* (2nd ed.). London: Routledge.

Clarke, A. E. (2005). *Situational analysis: Grounded theory after the postmodern turn*. Thousand Oaks, CA: Sage. Retrieved from http://www.loc.gov/catdir/enhancements/fy0657/2004022902-d.html

Corsaro, W. A. (1997). *The sociology of childhood. Sociology for a new century*. Thousand Oaks, CA: Pine Forge Press.

Corsaro, W. A., & Fingerson, L. (2006). Development and socialization in childhood. In J. Delamater (Ed.), *Handbooks of sociology and social research. Handbook of social psychology* (pp. 125–155). Boston, MA: Springer Science + Business Media, LLC. Retrieved from https://doi.org/10.1007/0-387-36921-X_6

Daly, C. M., Foote, S. J., & Wadsworth, D. D. (2017). Physical activity, sedentary behavior, fruit and vegetable consumption and access: What influences obesity in rural children? *Journal of Community Health*, *42*, 968–973. doi:10.1007/s10900-017-0343-6

Dunne, C. (2011). The place of the literature review in grounded theory research. *International Journal of Social Research Methodology*, *14*, 111–124. doi:10.1080/13645579.2010.494930

Freedman, D. S., Khan, L. K., Dietz, W. H., Srinivasan, S. R., & Berenson, G. S. (2001). Relationship of childhood obesity to coronary heart disease risk factors in adulthood: the Bogalusa Heart Study. *Pediatrics*, *108*, 712–718.

Glaser, B. G., & Strauss, A. L. (1967). *The discovery of grounded theory: Strategies for qualitative research*. New York, NY: Aldine de Gruyter.

Goldkuhl, G., & Cronholm, S. (2010). Adding theoretical grounding to grounded theory: Toward multi-grounded theory. *International Journal of Qualitative Methods*, *9*, 187–205. doi:10.1177/160940691000900205

Greene, S., & Hogan, D. (2005). *Researching children's experiences: Methods and approaches/edited by Sheila Greene and Diane Hogan*. London: Sage.

Hales, C. M., Carroll, M. D., Fryar, C. D., & Ogden, C. L. (2017). Prevalence of obesity among adults and youth: United States, 2015–2016. *NCHS Data Brief*, No. 288, October 2017.

Henwood, K., & Pidgeon, N. (2003, 2009). Grounded theory in psychological research. In P. M. Camic, J. E. Rhodes, & L. Yardley (Eds.), *Qualitative research in psychology: Expanding perspectives in methodology and design* (pp. 131–155). Washington, DC: American Psychological Association. Retrieved from https://doi.org/10.1037/10595-008

Hopf, C. (2008). Qualitative interviews: Ein Überblick. In U. Flick, E. V. Kardorff, & I. Steinke (Eds.), *Rororo Rowohlts Enzyklopädie: Vol. 55628. Qualitative Forschung: Ein Handbuch* (6th ed., pp. 349–360). Reinbek bei Hamburg: Rowohlt-Taschenbuch-Verl.

Illinois State Board of Education. (2018). *Illinois report card: Low income students*. Retrieved from https://www.illinoisreportcard.com/State.aspx?source=studentcharacteristics&source2=lowincome&Stateid=IL

James, A., & Prout, A. (Eds.). (1997). *Constructing and reconstructing childhood: Contemporary issues in the sociological study of childhood*. London: Falmer Press.

Johnson, J. A., & Johnson, A. M. (2015). Urban-rural differences in childhood and adolescent obesity in the United States: A systematic review and meta-analysis. *Childhood Obesity (Print)*, *11*, 233–241. doi:10.1089/chi.2014.0085

Krebs, N. F., Himes, J. H., Jacobson, D., Nicklas, T. A., Guilday, P., & Styne, D. (2007). Assessment of child and adolescent overweight and obesity. *Pediatrics*, *120* (Suppl 4), S193–S228. doi:10.1542/peds.2007-2329D

Lempert, L. B. (2012). Asking questions of the data: Memo writing in the grounded theory tradition. In A. Bryant & K. Charmaz (Eds.), *The Sage handbook of grounded theory* (pp. 245–264). London: Sage. Retrieved from https://doi.org/10.4135/9781848607941.n12

Lobstein, T., Baur, L., & Uauy, R. (2004). Obesity in children and young people: A crisis in public health. *Obesity Reviews An Official Journal of the International Association for the Study of Obesity*, *5*, (Suppl 1), 4–104. doi:10.1111/j.1467-789X.2004.00133.x

Mandell, N. (1988). The least-adult role in studying children. *Journal of Contemporary Ethnography*, *16*, 433–467. doi:10.1177/0891241688164002

Michell, L. (1997). Pressure groups: Young people's accounts of peer pressure to smoke. *Social Sciences in Health*, *3*, 3–17.

Must, A., & Strauss, R. S. (1999). Risks and consequences of childhood and adolescent obesity. *International Journal of Obesity*, *23*, S2–S11. doi:10.1038/sj.ijo.0800852

Pavis, S., Cunningham-Burley, S., & Amos, A. (1996). Young people and smoking: Exploring meaning and social context. *Social Sciences in Health*, *2*, 228–243.

Pavis, S., Cunningham-Burley, S., & Amos, A. (1997). Alcohol consumption and young people: Exploring meaning and social context. *Health Education Research*, *12*, 311–322. doi:10.1093/her/12.3.311

Prout, A. (2002). Researching children as social actors: an introduction to the children 5-16 programme. *Children & Society*, *16*, 67–76. doi:10.1002/chi.710

Prout, A., & James, A. (1997). A new paradigm for the sociology of childhood: Provenance, promise, and problems. In A. James & A. Prout (Eds.), *Constructing and reconstructing childhood: Contemporary issues in the sociological study of childhood*. London: Falmer Press.

Rey-López, J. P., de Rezende, L. F., Pastor-Valero, M., & Tess, B. H. (2014). The prevalence of metabolically healthy obesity: A systematic review and critical evaluation of the definitions used. *Obesity Reviews: An Official Journal of the International Association for the Study of Obesity*, *15*, 781–790. doi:10.1111/obr.12198

Scheer, A. (2017). Maneuvering the Stormy Waters of ethnography in an inner-city school: Reflections from the field. In I. E. Castro, M. Swauger, & B. Harger (Eds.), *Sociological studies of children and youth: Volume 22. Researching children and youth: Methodological issues, strategies, and innovations* (Vol. 22, pp. 59–80). Bingley: Emerald. Retrieved from https://doi.org/10.1108/S1537-466120180000022004

Scott, J. (2008). Children as respondents: The challenge for quantitative methods. In P. M. Christensen & A. James (Eds.), *Research with children: Perspectives and practices/edited by Allison James and Pia Christensen* (2nd ed., pp. 87–108). London: Routledge.

Singh, A. S., Mulder, C., Twisk, J. W. R., van Mechelen, W., & Chinapaw, M. J. M. (2008). Tracking of childhood overweight into adulthood: A systematic review of the literature. *Obesity Reviews: An Official Journal of the International Association for the Study of Obesity*, *9*, 474–488. doi:10.1111/j.1467-789X.2008.00475.x

Stead, M., McDermott, L., MacKintosh, A. M., & Adamson, A. (2011). Why healthy eating is bad for young people's health: Identity, belonging and food. *Social Science & Medicine*, *72*, 1131–1139. doi:10.1016/j.socscimed.2010.12.029

Thornberg, R. (2008). 'It's not fair!'-Voicing pupils' criticisms of school rules. *Children & Society*, *22*, 418–428. doi:10.1111/j.1099-0860.2007.00121.x

Thornberg, R. (2012). Informed grounded theory. *Scandinavian Journal of Educational Research*, *56*, 243–259. doi:10.1080/00313831.2011.581686

Thornberg, R., Halldin, K., Bolmsjö, N., & Petersson, A. (2013). Victimising of school bullying: A grounded theory. *Research Papers in Education*, *28*, 309–329. doi:10.1080/02671522.2011.641999

Tummers, L., & Karsten, N. (2012). Reflecting on the role of literature in qualitative public administration research. *Administration & Society*, *44*, 64–86. doi:10.1177/0095399711414121

Walls, P., Parahoo, K., & Fleming, P. (2010). The role and place of knowledge and literature in grounded theory. *Nurse Researcher*, *17*, 8–17. doi:10.7748/nr2010.07.17.4.8.c7920

PART IV
GENDER CONCERNS

PUBLIC PERCEPTION ON GENDER ISSUES AND WOMEN'S HEALTHCARE CONCERNS RELATED TO LEPROSY: IMPLICATIONS FOR LEPROSY CONTROL PROGRAM IN SOUTHEAST NIGERIA

Ignatius Uche Nwankwo

ABSTRACT

Purpose – *This research chapter focuses on gender issues and women's health concerns relevant to leprosy disease and their implications for leprosy control program in Southeast Nigeria. Four research questions guided the study, two of which were to ascertain the ways in which gender affect both awareness of leprosy and community support and post-treatment reintegration of persons affected by leprosy (PAL) into their communities.*

Methodology/Approach – *A sample size of 1,116 adults drawn through cluster and random sampling methods were the study participants from whom quantitative data were collected via questionnaire. Qualitative data were generated through focus group discussion (FGD) among PAL, and in-depth interview (IDI) of both leprosy control staff, and other stakeholders purposively drawn from the area. The Statistical Package for the Social Sciences (SPSS) software was employed to process data, while frequency tables, bar charts, and chi-square were used to present, analyze, and test the hypothesis.*

Underserved and Socially Disadvantaged Groups and Linkages with Health and Health Care Differentials
Research in the Sociology of Health Care, Volume 37, 165–187

ISSN: 0275-4959/doi:10.1108/S0275-495920190000037013

Findings – *The study found that level of awareness about leprosy (which has several local names in the area) was relatively high (89.6%). However, significant differences exist in levels of awareness on leprosy between males and females. Also, men were perceived as less likely to comply with treatment instructions due to their gender roles of family economic upkeep. Males affected by leprosy were also found to encounter severest forms of social discrimination and post-treatment reintegration challenges.*

Research Limitations/Implications – *The study scope was limited to the examination of public perception of gender issues and women's healthcare concerns related to leprosy and their implications for leprosy control program in Southeast Nigeria. Only PAL registered with Nigeria's Leprosy Control Programme participated with other non-patient respondents. The study focused on social aspects of leprosy (other than its biophysical component).*

The implication of the research outcome includes need for deliberate strategy by leprosy control team to improve the level of awareness/knowledge as well as treatment compliance across gender. Similarly, differential mode of social reaction (to male and female gender) affected by leprosy should be addressed. Above all, aggressive public enlightenment through public, private, and local media and prohibition of sociocultural practices that promote spread of leprosy were stressed as measures to enhance leprosy control in the area.

Originality/Value of Paper – *The study fills the knowledge gap with respect to gender issues and women's healthcare concerns related to leprosy and their implications for leprosy control program in Southeast Nigeria. Findings from the concluded research set it apart and differed with earlier and similar studies elsewhere. For instance, men affected by leprosy in the area encounter severest forms of negative social reaction; are less compliant to treatment plans and less aware of leprosy when compared with females. All these affirm the position of the chapter that gender issues relevant to leprosy differ according to cultural setting, time, and place of inquiry and do not align to any universal scheme.*

Keywords: Gender; leprosy; leprosy control; social isolation; women health concerns; segregation

INTRODUCTION

Leprosy is one of the oldest diseases of mankind with devastating social and physical consequences. It has very unique social dimension that often culminates in total destabilization of the social life of its victims and their caregivers. Persons affected by leprosy (PAL) and their caregivers are often ostracized in many societies. Although Meima, Richardus, and Habbema (2004) had observed that leprosy cases detected globally each year have declined considerably since 1985, the disease remains a public health problem especially in developing countries like Nigeria. Lockwood (2000) also observed that the disease is one of the key causes of permanent disability worldwide. According to Porter (2004), the World Health Assembly (WHA) at its 44th meeting adopted 2005 for global attainment of leprosy elimination goal after which eradication of the disease by 2015 will be the next priority. Nigeria has attained the leprosy elimination goal which implies a reduction in the incidence of the disease to less than one case per 10,000 populations. However, the goal of eradication of the disease still eludes the country and the global community.

THE PROBLEMS

According to Nigeria's Federal Ministry of Health (FMOH, 1997), over 80% of all leprosy cases were concentrated in only six countries of the world: India, Brazil, Bangladesh, Indonesia, Myanmar, and Nigeria, which are listed herein in the order of magnitude of reported leprosy cases in their areas. On her part, the World Health Organization (WHO, 2008) ranked Nigeria at the fifth position among nations with high leprosy burden in the world, and in Africa, as second only to Republic of Congo.

A historical review of Nigeria's registered prevalence of leprosy over the years shows that as at 2002, Nigeria had 5,890 registered cases of leprosy (FMOH, 2004). It declined to 5,381 at the beginning of 2008 (WHO, 2008) and dropped further to 3,913 cases at the end of 2010 (Adagba, 2011).

However, with specific reference to the southeast zone of Nigeria, after an initial drop from 504 registered cases in 2005, to 362 cases in 2006; there was annual increases in both new case detection (NCD) and registered prevalence of leprosy in the zone for three subsequent years of 2007, 2008, and 2009 (see Fig. 1). The trend raised questions about the effectiveness of control measures and whether leprosy should be reconsidered as one of the re-emerging diseases in the zone.

Furthermore, the seemingly low number of cases registered annually both at the national and southeast levels may not reflect the true situation on the ground due to incidences of hidden or unreported cases in the country. This fact was further buttressed by Ekiti (2010) who reported that in the year 2008, only 14% of estimated new leprosy cases in Nigeria were actually detected, registered, and commenced on treatment.

Nigeria's leprosy burden is also worrisome because in addition to unregistered cases, there are also many discharged cases that though declared clinically cured, yet they still suffer severe physical and social consequences of the disease (Ezekpeazu, 2000). Such consequences may include rejection by their families, significant others, community, and labor market.

The need to address her leprosy problems culminated in Nigeria's establishment of a National Tuberculosis and Leprosy Control Programme (NTBLCP) in 1988. The program was, however, formally launched by President Ibrahim Babangida in 1991. Ogbeiwi (2005) summed up the aims of the National Leprosy Control Programme as follows:

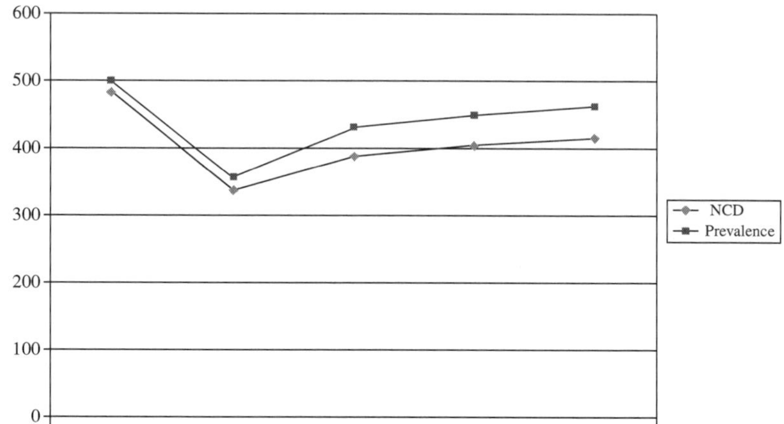

	2005	2006	2007	2008	2009
NCD	488	342	391	406	414
Prevalence	504	360	433	450	461

Fig. 1. Leprosy New Case Detection (NCD) and Prevalence (2005–2009) for Southeast Zone of Nigeria. *Source:* World Health Organization (Southeast Zonal Office, Enugu Nigeria, 2010).

- to reduce leprosy prevalence to a level where it is no longer a public health problem;
- to detect leprosy patients in early stages of the disease and provide comprehensive care to them;
- to provide multi-drug therapy (MDT) for all patients as provided by World Health Organization (WHO);
- to prevent disabilities associated with leprosy; and
- to reduce social and psychological stigma associated with the disease.

Unfortunately, as Nwankwo (2015) observed, the existence of leprosy control strucure over the years in Nigeria has failed to produce significant change in physical characteristics, disability types, and magnitude of social problems associated with the disease in the country. Community participation which is a crucial element in leprosy control has remained weak. Indeed, community response toward those suffering from leprosy is often characterized by avoidance, insult, and rejection of victims. Even discharged leprosy ex-patients are not spared of these actions that also constitute violation of their human rights.

Equally problematic is the fact that PAL still live like outcasts in separate colonies and settlements made of dilapidated structures surrounded by bushes, in more or less inhuman conditions. This is typical to Lockwood's (2000) description of social distance toward PAL which he lamented to be common to many cultures.

In the study area, persistence of colonies also reveals the fact that home-based or ambulatory care arrangement, where most patients ought to access treatment from their homes, with exception of those in critical conditions who may require hospitalization, has not fully materialized. The advantage of home-based care in reducing segregation and facilitating community-based rehabilitation (CBR) cannot be overemphasized. Examples of leprosy colonies or settlements still operating in Southeast Nigeria include those at Okija and Otolo Nnewi/Amichi communities in Anambra state, Mile Four Abakaliki and Uburu communities at Ebonyi state, and at Uzuakoli in Abia state among others.

Furthermore, Smith (2000) notes that Social and Economic Rehabilitation (SER) is usually a major priority in leprosy control projects. However, Ogbeiwi (2005) argued that the SER component of Nigeria's National Leprosy Control Programme does not reflect the priority it deserves.

Also important is the fact that gender dimension and social stratification implications of leprosy, which is the major thrust of this work constitutes crucial subjects that must bother leprosy control program. The gender dimension of leprosy as documented by Kaur and Rameshi (1994); Grand (1997), Rao, Garole, and Walawalker (1996) reflects a pattern that women encounter the severest forms of social, economic, and psychological consequences compared to their male counterparts upon diagnosis of leprosy.

Women do not also occupy important positions in self-help groups formed by patients in their colonies. This is especially so in a highly patriarchal society like the Southeast Nigeria where subservient position and economic dependence of women on men are culturally defined. Nwankwo (2015) observed that in many leprosy colonies in Nigeria, women affected by leprosy get smaller portions of land for cultivation compared to the males. This suggests that equity between male and female gender in accessing rights and privileges accruable from leprosy control program has remained defective.

It is against the backdrop of afore-mentioned problems that the research was undertaken to investigate gender issues implicated in leprosy control program of the states of Southeast Nigeria.

BRIEF REVIEW OF LITERATURE ON GENDER ISSUES RELATED TO LEPROSY AND ITS CONTROL ACROSS SOME SOCIETIES

Both sexes are affected by leprosy, but in most parts of the world, there are more males than females, roughly in the ratio of 2:1 (FMOH, 1997). Some earlier studies in other parts of the world found that women experience greater social, economic, psychological, and physical consequences of the disease when compared to their male counterparts (Grand, 1997; Kaur & Ramesh, 1994; Rao et al., 1996).

Valencia (1989) observes that diagnosis of leprosy results in premature social death of patients whose roles in the family and society are consequently constrained and restricted. In this impasse, Kaur and Ramesh (1994) consider women as more socially vulnerable, given circumstances of low social status and subservient roles they usually play especially in patriarchal societies.

Nwankwo (2006) observed that in patriarchal societies of Africa, beliefs and practices, symbols, public policies, and socioeconomic and political systems are situated within patriarchal definition. According to her, this has far-reaching implications for the socioeconomic status of women, their awareness, and involvement in health decisions that affect them including those related to leprosy control. They also influence their perception in terms of availability, cost, and convenience of leprosy control services. All these, she noted, in the final analysis, affect the outcome of such services.

Grand (1997), in his study at India, also found that women were more affected by leprosy in the following areas:

- Women were more isolated from all activities than men.
- Rejection by spouses, children, and relatives were strong.
- They were completely denied their domestic roles which generate a self-image of being a less valued member of the family.
- Leprosy compounds gender inequality problems between men and females in many regards.

The above submissions amplify Egbue's (2010) position that gender represents a significant form of social stratification across social groups. According to her, men's enduring dominance over women at the household level as well as at the macro-level income earning sphere has resulted in unequal positions in terms of power, prestige, and wealth. She further argues that women generally have less material resources and lower status sustained by various forms of subordination and injustice. These observations are strongly applicable to the field of leprosy as Grand's (1997) study in India has shown.

With respect to the types of leprosy common to each gender, Bryceson and Pfaltzgraff (1990) reported that in Africa, men are more prone to lepromatous leprosy. This could be attributable to the fact that men in Africa engage in greater toils for family upkeep and consequently develop weakened immunity on account of stress. Bryceson and Pfalzgraff (1990) also reported that men in Africa are more prompt in seeking treatment and more compliant to treatment instructions. The explanation given for their action was that the devastating form of lepromatous leprosy leaves those affected with no choice than to comply religiously with instructions of treatment institutions for possible relief. Women, however, tend to be less compliant than men to treatment plans.

An equally important gender issue in leprosy is the observation by Leprosy Mission International (1999) that women involved in leprosy control activities get better results than their male counterparts. They asserted that the use of young graduate girls as Leprosy Control Assistants in Bangladesh and other Asian countries proved the point.

Khulmann (2009) warns that gender inequality has moved away from being "women's problem" to being a "societal concern." The WHO (2002), for instance, advised its member states to implement gender mainstreaming in all its programs. WHO acknowledged that gender mainstreaming in healthcare systems is assigned a double perspective: as an approach to reduce social inequalities in access to health and at the same time improve the quality and efficiency of healthcare. It also provides new opportunities to address women's healthcare needs in all areas including leprosy. Khulmann (2009) asserts that gender mainstreaming opens up new possibilities to address diversity and differences in groups of women and men, thus emphasizing and making it possible to analyze gender relations in all contexts, including leprosy.

Aside from gender divides in access to opportunities and challenges generated by leprosy, Ogoegbulem (2000) reported that male and female patients especially at the colonies often cultivate deep, intimate relationships. Such relationships usually fill emotional gaps created by withdrawal of ties by family and friends from the wider society. According to him, marriages and children are known to have resulted from such relationships over the years.

The culture of social stratification defined along gender lines also has implications for leprosy and its control program in many societies. Several authors have documented that gender dimension of leprosy is such that women encounter severest forms of social, economic, and psychological consequences compared to their male counterparts upon diagnosis of leprosy (see Grand, 1997; Kaur & Rameshi, 1994; Rao et al., 1996).

Social ranking, honor, and prestige generally tilt to the disadvantage of females affected by leprosy in their colonies. This is especially so in a highly patriarchal society like the Southeastern part of Nigeria where subservient position and economic dependence of women on men are culturally defined. Sofola (1999) observed that in many leprosy colonies in Nigeria, women affected by leprosy get smaller portions of land for cultivation compared to the males. This situation suggests that equality of the sexes in accessing rights and privileges accruable from leprosy control program has remained defective in Nigeria.

There are also cases of gender biases that color social relationships and other mechanisms that cushion effects of isolation on leprosy patients. Although CBR is a principal strategy for cushioning the effects of isolation on PAL (see Macaden, 1996; Nash, 2001), other scholars like Ogoegbulem (2000) have documented other forms of social relationships and strategies by which patients themselves attempt to address the problem of isolation and to recreate. Such new approaches are, however, not devoid of elements of male dominance.

For instance, Ogoegbulem (2000) specifically reported that in parts of Nigeria, PAL organize themselves into primary self-help groups with specific rules, goals, and benefits. He noted that there is a strong feeling of oneness and solidarity in such groups, but frowned that women do not also occupy important positions in such self-help groups which are generally headed by males. According to him, women occupy subservient positions. However, members peacefully share donations from the public, distribute farmlands at Leprosaria among themselves, and harvest and sell proceeds of economic trees in the area without much rancor. He further noted that communal life especially at leprosaria and marriages among inmates give some measure of relief to PAL and help them to forget the fact of their social distance from the rest of society.

Adagba (2011) dated the formation of Association of PAL in Kaduna, Northern Nigeria to about 32 years ago. He noted that similar bodies exist at other parts of Nigeria and that male patients are usually the leaders.

At the global level, Lockwood (2000) reported that associations of PAL are being formed. He affirms that such associations have helped to focus more attention to leprosy-related issues like isolation and the use of suitable terms to address patients. They have also been very visible in pursuit of rights of PAL.

On his part, Chukwu (2004) observes that leprosy control programs now engage treatment "helpers", "facilitators," "supporters," or "proxy supervisors." According to him, these concepts refer to individuals in the community who are favorably disposed and willing to assist PAL in their treatment process. He argues that by their level of closeness to patients, such persons cushion their isolation and form supportive bonds of relationships that are socially rewarding. In his opinion, such relationships often grow and surpass primordial ties in the life of a patient. However, Chukwu (2004) maintained that males have dominated such supportive roles across societies.

The researcher notes that equity is a key factor that will optimize successes in the health sector. The present research is an attempt to interrogate gender issues and in particular, women health concerns in the area of leprosy control. Such issues include gender differentials in access to leprosy control services as well as social reactions to leprosy as applicable to southeast area of Nigeria .There is also need to examine gender differentials in reach or uptake of health education and social re-orientation focused on leprosy disease and to ascertain whether leprosy treatment process is truly devoid of discriminatory gender biased policies in the area.

RESEARCH QUESTIONS

The following research questions guided the study:

- How does awareness of leprosy differ among male and female gender in Southeast Nigeria?
- What is the perceived pattern of gender differentials in affliction or exposure to leprosy disease in Southeast Nigeria?
- What is the perceived pattern of gender differentials related to treatment compliance among PAL in Southeast Nigeria?
- In what ways do genders affect community support and reintegration into the community of PAL after treatment in Southeast Nigeria?

HYPOTHESIS

Male respondents are more likely to accept religious and cultural belief systems of their community on leprosy than female respondents.

THEORETICAL FRAMEWORK

The labeling theory postulated by Lemert (1951) is considered most relevant in explaining gender issues associated with leprosy in the study area. Labeling theory was also adopted as theoretical platform because its basic postulations explicitly relate to the process of social definition and stigma surrounding leprosy. These are central issues to leprosy problem in society. Labeling theory is particularly useful in the analysis of the qualitative data because of its emphasis on social constructionism.

Negative cultural imaging of leprosy and the manner in which societies through the instrument of language defined leprosy as curse from gods, or as disease of the unclean, have adverse consequences for its control. People are reluctant to be associated with the disease whether as patients or health workers because of the stigma attached to it. It is therefore not surprising that despite its long history and availability of free and effective drugs (FMOH, 2004), leprosy remains a public health problem in our environment.

Adverse religious perspectives on leprosy have also done much to intensify leprosy stigma and worsen the problems arising from leprosy in our society. Awofeso (2005) notes that biblical references like Leviticus 13:45, Numbers 5:2, and 2 Kings 26:21 create an impression that leprosy is a dreaded disease associated with sinners. He observes also that Buddhist teaching on Karma make it acceptable for believers to frame leprosy sufferers as sinners in their past incarnation. These conceptions compounded by low level of education constitute major obstacles to leprosy control.

Labeling also offers adequate explanation to why PAL try to cover up their disease and fail to avail themselves of early treatment. The situation results in severe deformities and complications. The theory also accounts for the lack of enthusiasm of health workers to leprosy work and for low level of integration of patients into their community.

MATERIALS AND METHODS

The study adopted cross-sectional survey method. It was located in the Southeast zone of Nigeria. The zone was purposively selected because of the need to understand gender and women's health concerns related to leprosy in the area. However, the researcher's attention was first drawn to the area by the fact of steady increases (rather than decrease) in number of leprosy cases registered annually in the area during 2006–2009.

Southeast Nigeria is made up of five states out of which Anambra and Ebonyi States were randomly selected for study. The indigenous ethnic group in the two states (and indeed the entire southeast of Nigeria) are the Igbo group of whom Ifemesia (1979) stated that their territory covers an area of over 15,800 square miles. Nwala (1985) circumscribed the area between 6° and 8½° East longitude and 4½° and 7½° North latitude. He noted that Igbo land is very densely populated.

Anambra and Ebonyi states are rich in natural resources and arable soil. Land cultivation, trading, arts and crafts, animal husbandry, and civil service positions are major economic activities in the two states. However, people of Anambra state are more involved in entrepreneurship and commerce whereas Ebonyi state is notable for her agricultural prowess (Onokala, 2002; Uzozie, 2002).

There is elected civilian government in Anambra and Ebonyi states, in addition to many intricate sociopolitical structures and pressure groups that characterize Igbo traditional societies such as gerontocracy, village assembly, titled men, and women groups. These elements are still relevant to grass root administration in both states. Similarly, Christianity has greater follower ship in the area but exists side by side with traditional religion which still has many adherents.

The total population for the two states was 6,354,775 made up of 3,182,140 males and 3,172,791 females (National Population Commission, 2006). However, the study population consisted of persons aged 18 years and older (adults) who are considered capable of articulating issues related to the subject under investigation.

A sample size of 1,116 members of the public constituting 0.32% of the study population was used to generate quantitative data via the questionnaire. These study participants were drawn from both states on the basis of equality of states in a federation (i.e., 558 respondents from each state). The sample size took cognizance of rural–urban bias at the ratio of 2:1. The sample size was informed by its adequacy to accommodate applicable statistical tests.

The cluster and multistage sampling approach was adopted to enlist study participants. The two states were broken into component local governments areas (LGAs). These were thereafter grouped on the basis of urban and rural characteristics. Then through simple random sampling technique, one urban and two rural LGAs were selected per state. A total of three LGAs were thus selected per state from where one community/village and 62 compounds bearing odd numbers were drawn.

A uniform set of close ended questionnaire with two sections (duly pretested outside the study areas) was other administered by the researcher and five field assistants. Vernacular or English language was used (depending on preference or level of literacy of respondent). The administration was on three adult members/ occupants in those randomly selected 62 houses/compounds per village. Same-sex administration of questionnaire was carried out to prevent any cultural barriers and permit free discussion/responses to questionnaire items. No gender was discriminated in the process. Compounds that lacked three adult members were skipped but those who had one or two adults were complemented from subsequent compounds. The process was continued until the required numbers were achieved. The list of LGAs, communities and villages or streets used in the study is shown in Table 1.

Two qualitative instruments focus group discussion (FGD) schedule and in-depth interview (IDI) guide complemented quantitative tool. Respondents for the qualitative instruments were 64 in number. They included 52 PAL (26 from

Table 1. List of LGAs, Communities and Villages Used in the Study.

States	LGAs	Communities	Villages/Streets	Compounds Visited	No of Respondents
Anambra	Nnewi North (Urban)	Otolo	Orizu Road	62	186
	Idemili South (Rural)	Alor	Ifite village	62	186
	Awka North (Rural)	Achalla	Umudiana village	62	186
Ebonyi	Abakaliki (Urban)	Abakaliki	Ibibio Street	62	186
	Ohaozara (Rural)	Okposi	Okposi-ukwu	62	186
	Ohaukwu (Rural)	Efiom	Akparata village	62	186
Total	Six LGAs	Six communities	Six villages/streets	372	1,116

each state). They participated in four sessions of FGD segmented on the basis of sex. Twelve participants were interviewed. They include six LGA leprosy supervisors (three from Anambra and three from Ebonyi on the basis of one supervisor per selected LGA in each state), four officers from Leprosy Control Units of Ministry of Health in the two states (two from each state), and one official each from Donor Agency supporting leprosy control and World Health Organization. All respondents to the qualitative instruments were purposively selected.

The IDIs were conducted by the researcher and two of the assistants at the offices of the stated officials. Tape recorder and field notebook were used to record responses from interviewees. The interview schedule which addressed the objectives of the study guided the interview. English language was used for the interviews due to respondents' preference and literacy level.

The FGD sessions were conducted at the premises of Mile Four Hospital Abakaliki and Fr Damian Tuberculosis and Leprosy Referral Hospital Nnewi, both of which were accepted and convenient to the patients. Each session was held on leprosy clinic day which is usually a market free day in the area of study. The moderator of the FGD was of the same sex as the FGD group and worked with the co-operation of leprosy control staff on duty. There were also two assistants for each FGD session. The language of administration was vernacular (Igbo). A tape recorder and a field notebook were used to record proceedings. One assistant took notes in the course of each session while the other served as tape recorder operator. Each FGD session, for males or females, had 6–12 PAL as participants

Participants in both FGD and IDI did not respond to the questionnaire but were restricted to distinct unstructured schedules, one used strictly for FGD and the other for IDI.

Quantitative data gathered in the course of research were analyzed with the help of the Statistical Package for the Social Sciences (SPSS) software. Descriptive statistics like frequency distribution tables, mean, median, percentages, and bar charts were used to interpret data collected from field study. The chi-square correlation analysis was employed to test research hypotheses.

However, qualitative data generated through FGDs and IDIs were transcribed, cleaned, and later organized under different aspects/themes of the discussion. They were used to explain quantitative data where applicable. In particular, phrases or statements with contextual or special connotations were noted and pulled out as illustrative quote to complement statistical data.

RESEARCH FINDINGS

After carefully coding and cleaning/ editing validly completed and returned questionnaires, a total of 1,104 were used for analysis out of 1,116 administered on study subjects. Of the number, 549 questionnaires were those administered in Anambra state while 555 were administered at Ebonyi state.

Also included in the analysis were qualitative data collected through four FGD sessions (two in each state) with PAL segmented along gender (i.e., male and female groups of leprosy patients). Similarly, qualitative data collected through IDIs with Leprosy Supervisors at Local Government Areas (LGAs), Leprosy Control Staff at Ministry of Health Headquarters in both States, and officials of the Donor Agency and World Health Organization were also included in analysis. The qualitative data were principally used to support and elucidate the quantitative data.

The presentation of the results and their analysis followed a definite sequence to make for easy comprehension. The sequence which is related to research questions/study objectives has four thematic issues.

Sociodemographic Characteristics of Respondents

The sociodemographic profile of respondents relating to age, sex, marital status, religious affiliation, highest educational attainment, occupation, etc., is presented in Table 2.

Table 2 shows the distribution of respondents by sex, age, marital status, religious affiliation, highest formal educational attainment, and occupation, nature of income, income per quarter, family type, family size, and place of residence. The table shows that females constituted 54.3% of the total respondents, while the males constituted 45.7%. Many of the respondents (29.5%) fall within the age bracket of 38–47 years. The least number of respondents (4.3%) came from the age group of 45 years and older. However, the *modal and median* ages were *41 and 45 years*, respectively. Also, the *mean age* of respondents was *40.33 years* with a *standard deviation of 13.45*.

With regard to the marital status of the respondents, 45.2% were married while 32.9% are single. The widowed, separated, and divorced respondents were very few (11.7%, 5.6%, and 4.6%, respectively). The large number of married respondents illuminates the high premium placed on marriage and family institution in the area. Similarly, divorce is low probably because the value system

Table 2. Distribution of Respondents by Sociodemographic Characteristics.

Sociodemographic Characteristics (Items 1–11)	Frequency $N = 1104$	Percentage
Sex		
Male	505	45.7
Female	599	54.3
Age group		
18–27	246	22.3
28–37	206	18.7
38–47	326	29.5
48–57	201	18.2
58–67	78	7.1
68 and above	47	4.3
Marital status		
Married	499	45.2
Single	363	32.9
Divorced	51	4.6
Separated	62	5.6
Widowed	129	11.7
Religious affiliation		
Christianity	890	80.6
Islam	21	1.9
Traditional religion	189	17.1
Others	4	0.4
Highest formal educational attainment		
No formal education	145	13.1
Primary school certificate	142	12.9
Secondary school certificate	414	37.5
Vocational/technical school certificate	168	15.2
Tertiary	235	21.3
Occupation		
Civil/public servant	239	21.6
Trader/business man	243	22.0
Farmer	260	23.6
Student	119	10.8
Apprentice	85	7.7
Artisan	80	7.2
Unemployed	74	6.7
Others	4	0.4
Nature of income per month		
Regular	239	21.6
Periodic	634	57.4
No income	231	20.9

Table 2. *(Continued)*

Sociodemographic Characteristics (Items 1–11)	Frequency $N = 1104$	Percentage
Income per quarter of a year (every three months period)		
None	232	21
Below N30,000	147	13.3
N31,000–N50,000	141	12.8
N51,000–N70,000	123	11.1
N71,000–N90,000	149	13.5
N91,000–N110,000	124	11.2
N111,000–N130,000	93	8.4
Above N131,000	95	8.6
Family type		
Monogamous	560	50.7
Polygamous	540	49.3
Family size		
Small (1–3 persons)	232	21
Medium (4–5 persons)	384	38.8
Large (above five persons)	488	44.2
Place of residence		
Urban area	369	33.4
Rural area	730	66.1
Don't know	5	0.5

abhors it. Being married and having stable marriage are accorded high esteem and social honor among Igbo people.

With respect to religious affiliation, the table clearly shows that more than three-quarter of the respondents (80.6%) were Christians. A few of the respondents belong to other religious groups including Islam (1.9%), traditional religion (17.1%), and other unspecified groups (0.4%).

In terms of highest formal educational attainment, those who possess secondary school certificate constituted 37.5% of the respondents. Other categories of educational attainment/ certification were tertiary (21.3%), vocational/technical school (15.2%), and primary school certificate holders (12.9%). With only 13.1% of the respondents without any form of formal education, the literacy level in the area is relatively high. However, more respondents from Anambra state (27.7%) had tertiary education than those from Ebonyi state where only 15% had tertiary education.

The respondents were almost equally divided across three major occupations. These are farmers (23.6%), traders (22%), and civil/public servants (21.6%). Students, apprentices, artisans, and the unemployed were few. They constituted 10.8%, 7.7%, 7.2%, and 6.7%, respectively. The occupational distribution of the respondents highlighted above mirrors the popular description of Ebonyi state as food basket (major agricultural zone) of the nation and Anambra state as center for commerce and other entrepreneurial activities. The predominance of farmers and traders in the area of study is therefore not a major surprise. However, the nature of income reveals that most of the respondents (57.4%) earn periodic income; 21.6% earn regular income on monthly basis, while 20.9% earn no income at all.

In terms of actual income earned per quarter (every three months), many of the respondents (21%) earn no income. These include students, apprentices, some artisans, and the unemployed. More than two-thirds of these respondents that earn no income are from Anambra state. Furthermore, 13.5% of the respondents earn below N30,000 per quarter, and only 8.6% earn above N131,000 per quarter. This shows that income status of individuals within the area of study is generally low. The *mean income* per quarter of the respondents is about *N59, 033* with a *standard deviation* of *N45, 933*. The *median income* stood at about *N55, 378*.

Most respondents (44.2%) have large family size containing more than five persons who eat from the same pot. This is likely to compound socioeconomic problems arising from poor income. Only 21% of the respondents have small family size where 1–3 persons form a household that eat from the same pot.

The respondents were almost equally distributed across family types to which they belonged. Those from monogamous family arrangement constituted 50.7%, while the remaining 49.3% were from polygamous family units. This indicates that the two family types are culturally acceptable and enjoy similar measure of importance in the area of study.

The respondents in the study were from urban and rural localities. About two-third (66.1%) were from rural communities while the remaining one-third (33.4%) were from urban towns

Analysis of Substantive Research Issues.

RQ1. How does awareness of leprosy differ among male and female gender in Southeast Nigeria?

Table 3 shows that more than three-quarter (89.6%) of the respondents were aware of leprosy as health problem. However, 3.2% were not aware, while 7.2% claimed they were uncertain. Similarly, more than three-quarter of FGD participants said they were aware of leprosy. They maintained that they had seen cases in the past and heard about the disease through friends and radio, before they were later diagnosed of it (Table 4). A male FGD participant at Mile Four Hospital summarized his awareness of leprosy in these words:

> I know about leprosy before I was diagnosed. It is called "ekpenta" in my community. I have also seen some of the victims in the past but I don't know how and why the disease came to me. None of my close relations have it.

Table 3. Distribution of Male and Female Respondents by Their Awareness of Leprosy.

Response	Frequency			Percentage
	Male	Female	Total	
Yes	440	549	989	89.6
No	17	18	35	3.2
Don't know	48	32	80	7.2
Total	*505*	*599*	*1,104*	*100*

Table 4. Distribution of Respondents by some Sociodemographic Variables, Awareness about Leprosy (% in Parenthesis).

Sociodemographic Variable	Awareness of Leprosy			Total	Statistics
	Yes	No	Don't Know		
Gender					
Male	440 (87.1)	17 (3.4)	48 (9.5)	505 (100)	$\chi^2 = 7.291$, $df = 2$, $p = 0.026$
Female	549 (91.7)	18 (3.0)	32 (5.3)	599 (100)	
Total	*989 (89.5)*	*35 (3.2)*	*80 (7.3)*	*1,104 (100)*	

Table 5. Distribution of Respondents by Their Opinion about Which Gender Encounters Higher Incidence/Exposure to Leprosy in Their Area?

Response	Frequency	Percentage
Male	339	30.7
Female	641	58.1
Don't know	124	11.2
Total	*1,104*	*100*

RQ2. What is the perceived pattern of gender differentials in affliction/exposure or incidence of leprosy in Southeast Nigeria?

Table 5 shows that about 58% of respondents were of the opinion that incidence of leprosy occur more among the female gender.

RQ3. What is the perceived pattern of gender differentials in treatment compliance among persons affected by leprosy in Southeast Nigeria?

On the issue of clinic attendance, Table 6 shows that many respondents (52.4%) were of the view that gender role of men as breadwinners could

Table 6. Distribution of Respondents by Their Opinion on Gender Role That Most Likely Affect Clinic Attendance of Persons Affected by Leprosy in the Control Program.

Response	Frequency	Percentage
Men as breadwinners	670	52.4
Patriarchal social engagements	262	23.7
Domestic chores of women	79	7.2
Don't know	93	8.4
Total	*1,104*	*100*

negatively affect their clinic attendance. This implies that men were perceived to default from anti-leprosy treatment more than females due to their busy socio-economic schedules/roles.

The above findings contradict the submissions of Kaur and Ramesh (1994), Grand (1997), and Rao, Garole and Walawalker (1996) who in their separate studies held that women suffer the severest forms of social and economic deprivation on account of leprosy. Most IDI respondents in the two states also attested that males encounter greatest discrimination on account of leprosy at the communities they serve. However, one IDI respondent from a donor agency supporting leprosy control differed from others. He contended that "success of integration of persons affected by leprosy into their community depends on degree of disability and has little or nothing to do with gender."

> *RQ4.* In what ways does gender affect community support and reintegration into the community of persons affected by leprosy after treatment in Southeast Nigeria?

In attempt to find answers to *RQ4*, the researcher first interrogated the level of isolation generally encountered by PAL in the study area. It was found that the level of isolation of PAL is high. About 57.4% of the respondents acknowledged that they personally isolate or stay away from PAL (see Fig. 2).

The problem of community rejection/isolation of PAL appears to be more severe in Anambra state where 64.3% of respondents identified it as a problem. At Ebonyi state, only 23.6% of the respondents considered it a problem.

Commenting on sociocultural factors and problems affecting leprosy control, an interviewee from WHO Southeast Office at Enugu noted that "what society call leprosy is 'deformity'. If deformity is avoided, social isolation and erroneous belief systems will cease." Another interviewee from Anambra State reported that at Amansea community, an isolated PAL felt so angry and frustrated about his situation that he went about contaminating cassava soaked at the stream for fermentation by villagers with his leprosy sore. Some male FGD participants at

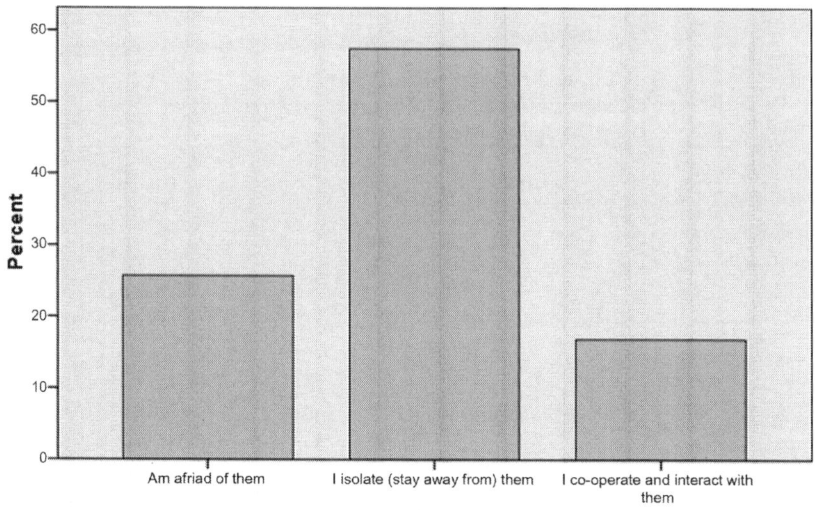

Fig. 2. Respondents' Description of Their Relationship with Persons Affected by Leprosy.

Fr Damian Tuberculosis and Leprosy Hospital, Nnewi/Amichi, expressed their problems and agonies these ways:

- "The community asked me to move away from their midst until I am fully cured. But I have completed treatment, yet they cannot accept me back because of my shortened toes and fingers. I am all alone now. I depend on charity."
- "Once a leprosy patient has sores or wounds, the family and community avoid the person completely."
- "Health workers do not attend clinic again. No doctor comes here. It is up to five months since they last attended. They are afraid of getting leprosy from us."

The above facts suggest that "disposition to leprosy" defined as willingness to maintain forms of association with PAL was generally poor among residents of the study location. This could be related to high level of stigma which accompany leprosy and discrimination/social isolation which its victims encounter.

GENDER-BASED DIFFERENCES IN COMMUNITY SUPPORT AND POST-TREATMENT INTEGRATION

Findings regarding the relationship between gender, community support and post-treatment reintegration of PAL into their community are shown in Table 7.

Table 7 shows that slightly below two-thirds of the respondents (58.1%) stated that females were re-accepted and re-integrated faster than their male counterparts. The major reason advanced for this differential treatment was the belief that men afflicted with leprosy were considered to be in dispute with the

Table 7. Distribution of Respondents by Their Opinion about Which Gender Receives Greater Community Support and Is Re-accepted and Re-integrated Faster into the Community after Anti-leprosy Treatment.

Response	Frequency	Percentage
Male	339	30.7
Female	641	58.1
Don't know	124	11.2
Total	*1,104*	*100*

Table 8. Distribution of Respondents according to Their Gender and Their Acceptance of Belief Systems on Leprosy (% in Parenthesis).

Gender	Acceptance of Communal Belief System on Leprosy as Correct			
	Yes	No	Don't Know	Total
Male	350 (52)	135 (35.7)	20 (37.7)	505 (45.7)
Female	323 (48)	243 (64.3)	33 (62.3)	599 (54.3)
Total	*673 (100)*	*378 (100)*	*53 (100)*	*1,104 (100)*

Note: $\chi^2 = 27.323$, $df = 2$, $p = 0.000$.

ancestors and gods of their land and cannot therefore commune with the people even after treatment.

TEST OF HYPOTHESIS

Only one hypothesis was stated for the study as follows:

"Male respondents are more likely to accept religious and cultural belief systems of their community on leprosy than female respondents." To test this hypothesis, a cross-tabulation between gender and acceptance of belief systems on leprosy was carried out (Table 8).

The computed value of χ^2 is 27.323. The tabulated value of chi-square at 0.05 level of significance with a degree of freedom (*df*) of 2 is 5.991. Having observed that the calculated value of χ^2 is greater than the table value, the researcher consequently accepted the alternative hypothesis. This implies that there is a significant relationship between gender and acceptance of community belief system on leprosy in Southeast Nigeria.

DISCUSSION AND IMPLICATIONS

The study uncovered several interesting differences between the sexes at both patient and community levels. The female gender was found to be more aware of leprosy than their male counterparts. Awareness level as a function of gender indicates that well over four-fifths of the males (87.1%) and slightly above nine-tenth of the female respondents (91.7%) are aware of leprosy. There was therefore a significant difference ($p < 0.05$) in the level of awareness about leprosy between male and female gender ($\chi^2 = 7.291$, $df = 2$, $p = 0.026$). Higher levels of awareness among the female gender could be explained by the absence of restrictive traditions against women such as "purdah" which is practiced by the Moslems. This enabled women in Southeast Nigeria to encounter almost similar social environment with similar opportunities for information acquisition and socialization with the men folk. Regular visits to health institutions for maternal and child healthcare services, however, provide women with additional avenue for acquisition of health information including those related to leprosy. Such visits also provide opportunity for leprosy screening/diagnosis or voluntary reporting of suspicious signs. Thus, women's health concerns in the context of awareness of leprosy swings to the advantage of women. Men lack such privileges; hence, very few of them may be detected by self- /voluntary reporting.

In view of gender differences in levels of awareness and the prevalent low level of knowledge about leprosy, government and private media houses in the two states should be involved in a comprehensive health education and public enlightenment package. The program should commit additional effort to reach the male gender in order to bridge the awareness gap between female and male gender. Also, it will be preferable to use traditional media and local dialect to disseminate correct information about leprosy and interventions in place for its control. This will ensure that both genders understand such enlightenment messages on leprosy.

Differences in sociocultural and economic roles of men and women were identified as key factors that contribute to different levels of exposure to leprosy (prevalence) between males and females in the area. Our data also point to the direction those differences in sociocultural and economic roles which are defined along gender and also account for failures in treatment compliance. In this regard, majority of respondents contended that more men have leprosy disease in the study location than females. They also saw the role of men as breadwinners in their families as capable of exposing them to leprosy and negatively affecting their compliance to treatment. This finding agrees with the position of Bryceson and Pfaltzgraff (1990) who reported that in Africa, men are more prone to lepromatous leprosy. This could be attributable to the fact that men in Africa engage in greater toils for family upkeep and consequently develop weakened immunity on account of stress and over work. The control program should thus incorporate economic support strategies, especially for men to cushion their challenges. Again, women health concerns are positively affected.

However, the submission by Bryceson and Pfalzgraff (1990) to the effect that men in Africa are prompt in seeking anti-leprosy treatment and more compliant to treatment instructions was not supported by data from the current study. This requires further interrogation by scholars. Our data tilt toward the position that women tend to be more compliant than men to anti-leprosy treatment plans. The implication of this is that the control program must take additional measures, specifically targeted at men to stop them from defaulting from treatment. A robust case holding and defaulter tracing plan must be in place.

Due to much superstitions and the association of leprosy to sins against the gods or the breach of local taboos, community support to patients was rated low. Interestingly, our data show that the female gender encounters minimal problems of community support and post-treatment integration into their community when compared to their male counterparts. This is surprising given male dominance and patriarchal structure that characterize most of Southeast Nigeria (Anambra and Ebonyi States inclusive). The finding also contradicts earlier position by Kaur and Ramesh (1994), Grand (1997), Rao, Garole and Walawalker (1996), and Grand (1997) who in their separate studies held that male patients encountered less severe social and economic discrimination during and after treatment in the cultural areas they studied.

The major explanation to the above result could be found within the context of high social ranking enjoyed by males in the social strata of Igbo society. With such ranking, it was considered abominable for males to be afflicted by leprosy (which is attributed to sin and anger of the gods). In view of the above, males afflicted by leprosy encountered extreme difficulties of reintegration into their society because their capacity to obtain pardon or to repair relationship with the gods (after fall from an exalted position of honor) remained doubtful. To counter this biased interpretation of leprosy which sympathize more with women and to cultivate favorable social reaction to both genders, leprosy control program in the area must scale up advocacy and support of traditional and religious institutions as well as public enlightenment. When this is done, both community leaders and the people shall be at the forefront of the crusade to change local perceptions about leprosy. Above all, the involvement of community leaders will improve the level of community involvement, ownership, and participation in the program. With the support and participation of the community, sociocultural practices and beliefs (especially those anchored on gender biases) that negatively affect leprosy control could be abolished /prohibited. Also, the role of social groups like age-grades, women groups, human right groups, clubs, and faith-based associations if harnessed will positively affect decisions toward gender balance in disbursing accruable benefits from leprosy control program.

In addition, leprosy control project must exploit on the job training options to enhance capacity of health workers to understand sociocultural factors and belief systems related to leprosy. Such trainings equip health workers with the rudiments of behavior change techniques. Furthermore, it is imperative that social scientists who are likely to better understand and plan interventions against gender and other sociocultural dimensions of leprosy should be part of leprosy control teams. This is in the spirit of multi- and interdisciplinary cooperation and teamwork which leprosy control requires for better results.

REFERENCES

Adagba, K. (2011). Interview granted to Nigerian television authority (NTA) to mark 50 years of tackling leprosy problem in Nigeria. *NTA Weekend File*, February 5.

Awofeso, N. (2005). Concept and impact of stigma on discrimination against leprosy sufferers – Minimizing the harm. *Leprosy Review*, *76*(1), 101–102.

Bryceson, A., & Pfaltzgraff, R. E. (1990). *Leprosy*. London: Longman Group.

Chukwu, J. N. (2004, April 5–7). *Towards a leprosy free society: The role of tuberculosis and leprosy supervisors (TBLS)*. Address presented at the Quarterly Meeting of Anambra State Tuberculosis and Leprosy Supervisors, Local Government Hall, Amawbia, Nigeria.

Egbue, N. G. (2010). Gender division of domestic roles: Implications for social equality in Nigeria. *The Nigerian Journal of Sociology and Anthropology*, *8*, 13–29.

Ekiti, P. (2010). *Address to mark 2010 World Leprosy Day on theme – justice: Fighting a just course*. Nigeria: World Health Organization.

Ezekpeazu, J. I. (2000, February 9–11). *Leprosy: Causative organism, mode of spread, signs and symptoms, diagnosis, differential diagnosis, classification and treatment*. Paper presented at World Leprosy Day Conference, Madonna University, Okija, Nigeria.

Federal Ministry of Health, Department of Primary HealthCare. (1997). *National tuberculosis and leprosy control programme (NTBLCP), workers' manual* (2nd Ed.).

Federal Ministry of Health, Department of Public Health. (2004). *National tuberculosis and leprosy control programme (NTBLCP) workers' manual* (4th Ed.). Abuja, Nigeria: Federal Ministry of Health, Department of Public Health.

Grand, A. L. (1997). Women and leprosy: A review. *Leprosy Review*, *22*, 40–49.

Ifemesia, C. (1979). *Traditional humane living among the Igbo: An historical perspective*. Enugu: Fourth Dimension.

Kaur, H., & Ramesh, V. (1994). Social problems of women leprosy patients: A study at two urban leprosy centres in Delhi. *Leprosy Review*, *65*, 361–375.

Khulmann, E. (2009). From women's health to gender mainstreaming and back again: Linking feminist agencies and new governance in healthcare. *Current Sociology*, *57*(2), 135–154.

Lemert, E. M. (1951). *Social pathology*. New York, NY: McGraw-Hill.

Leprosy Mission International. (1999). Women in leprosy control. *Partners Magazine for Paramedical Workers*, *2*(36), 9.

Lockwood, D. (2000). Consequences of leprosy and socio-economic rehabilitation. *Leprosy Review*, *71*(4), 417–419.

Macaden, V. P. (1996). An introduction to community based rehabilitation in leprosy. *Partners Magazine for Paramedical Workers*, *1*(30), 3–5.

Meima, A., Richardus, J. H., & Habbema, J. D. F.(2004). Trends in leprosy case – Detection worldwide since 1985. *Leprosy Review*, *75*(1), 19–31.

Nash, J. (2001). *What is rehabilitation*? *Partners Magazine for Paramedical Workers in Leprosy*, *1*(38), 3–7.

National Population Commission. (2006). *Breakdown of 2006 census population according to states*. Awka: National Population Commission (NPC).

Nwala, T. U. (1985). *Igbo philosophy*. Lagos: Literame.

Nwankwo, I. U. (2015). Public assessment of social and economic rehabilitation component of leprosy control programme of Anambra and Ebonyi States of Southeast Nigeria, world family medicine. *Incorporating the Middle East Journal of Family Medicine*, *13*(3), 20–33.

Nwankwo, S. N. (2006). *Compliance status of multiple drug therapy (MDT) by leprosy patients in Imo State from 2000–2004*. Unpublished Postgraduate Diploma thesis, Imo State University, Owerri, Nigeria.

Ogbeiwi, O. I. (2005). Progress towards the elimination of leprosy in Nigeria: A review of the role of policy implementation and operational factors. *Leprosy Review*, *76*(1), 65–76.

Ogoegbulem, S. A. (2000, February 9–11). *Forging new partnerships for effective leprosy control*. Paper presented at a Three Day National Workshop to Commemorate World Leprosy Day, Madonna University, Okija, Nigeria.

Onokala, P. C. (2002). Trade and transport. In G. E. K. Ofomata (Ed.), *A survey of the Igbo nation*. Onitsha: Africana First.

Porter, J. D. H. (2004). Supporting the individual with leprosy: The need for a post elimination strategy. *Leprosy Review*, *75*(1), 2–5.

Rao, S., Garole, V., & Walawalker, S. (1996). Gender differentials in the social impact of leprosy. *Leprosy Review*, *67*, 190–199.

Smith, C. (2000). Leprosy after the year 2000. *Partners Magazine for Paramedical Workers*, *1*(37), 3–6.

Sofola, O. (1999). Leprosy elimination campaigns: The Nigerian experience. *Leprosy Review*, *70*, 465–471.

Uzozie, L. C. (2002). Igbo concepts and beliefs about land. Its classification and tenurial system. In G. E. K. Ofomata (Ed.), *A survey of the Igbo Nation*. Onitsha: Africana First.

Valencia, L. B. (1989). Social science research on social dimensions of leprosy: Where are we going from here? *International Journal of Leprosy*, *57*, 847–863.

World Health Organization. (2002). *Integrating gender perspectives in the work of WHO*. Geneva: World Health Organization.

World Health Organization. (2008). *Weekly epidemiological record* (Vol. 33, pp. 293–300). Retrieved on December 15, 2008. Accessed on http://www.who.int/wer

THALASSEMIC WOMEN'S BIOGRAPHICAL TRAJECTORY: RETRACING GENDER INEQUALITIES IN HEALTH POLICIES

Valentina Raffa

ABSTRACT

Purpose – *Scientific reductionism has made sure that the biological phenomena were abstracted from the social and cultural contexts in which they occur. As a result, institutions of medicine and patient care processes have not taken into account the social and cultural determinants of the illness, therefore concealing a Western and masculine norm. Only recently, gender studies have managed to claim importance of the gender in the process of medical practices capable of dealing with diverse health cultures.*

This chapter proposes further reflections on gender inequalities in health policy for the care and management of thalassemia, taking into account of the differences in health needs, and gendered experience and meanings of illness. It will analyze the medicalization of the female body in the thalassemia experience.

Methodology/Approach – *Qualitative data for this study came from the biographical narratives of 10 thalassemic women in the care of the Polyclinic of Messina (Italy).*

Findings – *The analysis will highlight an inequality between men and women not only in the degree and modes of medicalization of the bodies but also in*

Underserved and Socially Disadvantaged Groups and Linkages with Health and Health Care Differentials
Research in the Sociology of Health Care, Volume 37, 189–201

ISSN: 0275-4959/doi:10.1108/S0275-495920190000037014

the incorporation of an imagination that encages the woman in the necessary role of wife and mother, making the illness an experience particularly dolorous.

Research Limitations/Implications – *These findings can help shape health policies in the cure of thalassemia, which take into account gender differences as an indispensable element in the compliance with the therapeutic process.*

Originality/Value of Paper – *They report on the urgency to deconstruct the social imagination according to which a woman is a "real" woman only if she is also a mother.*

Keywords: Thalassemia; gender; medicalization; health policies; biographical narratives; inequalities

INTRODUCTION

Biomedicine has historically been established and consolidated as a science built on a masculine neutral gender and on two basic assumptions – the Cartesian mind/body dichotomy and a nature/culture divide – which have dominated as unquestionable and universally valid norms for all cultures (Gordon, 1998).

Such scientific reductionism, therefore, ensured that biological phenomena were cut off from their social, economic, historic, and cultural contexts and made independent from patient subjectivity and personal experience. The consequence was the creation of institutions of medicine and processes of treatment which have long failed to take into account the social and cultural determinants of illness, concealing dominant Western and male-related norms.

The process of revealing the social and cultural dimension of illnesses was first tackled by medical anthropology and in particular by the School of Harvard (Good, 2006; Kleinman, 1998, 2006), demonstrating how medical systems are the set of representations, knowledge, and practices which in any particular social and cultural context, allow us to face, prevent, or interpret the illness (Kleinman, 1978). Within these systems, there are care specialists who are repository of knowledge of the body drawing on specific symbolic-cultural sphere.

According to this approach, biomedicine is an ethnomedical system (Good, 2006), expression, and historic product of Western culture, and the way in which Western doctors deal with patients, illnesses, bodies, is the result of the process through which the illness is shaped as social and personal reality, responding to the ethnomedical system of reference (Good, 2006).

Studying disease as social and cultural experience implies that we must focus on the central role of the body. For this reason, Good (2006) and Kleinman (1988) propose the use of storytelling as a primary therapeutic instrument for the reconstruction of the personal world destroyed by the illness. According to anthropology, it allows us to retrace the origins of suffering (Good, 2006), to resist medicalization practices (Cardano & Lepori, 2012), to exchange experiences with people who share similar conditions, and to be relieved from loneliness and labeling.

According to Kleinman (Kleinman, 2006, pp. 199–234), illness storytelling is the first step toward healing, intended as that process through which people not only benefit from medical treatment but become aware of the cultural dimensions of the experience of illness, to which they attribute precise meanings.

The contribution of medical anthropology and health sociology (Cipolla & Maturo, 2009; Cipriani, 2010; Maturo, 2007), therefore, was to consider cultural and social determinants as fundamental in the interpretation of the illness, in treatment practices, and in designing health policies. Ethnopsychiatry follows a similar trajectory, starting with the works by Franz Fanon (1952, 1961), enlightening keys and precious instruments to analyze this issue.

However, only recently have gender studies managed to claim how essential the gender category is in developing medical practices dealing with differing health cultures.

Facchini and Ruspini have written (2001, p. 9):

> the dimension of health is a key element in analysing individual courses of life, in determining citizenship rights and therefore in understanding the system of both social and gender inequalities. (Facchini & Ruspini, 2001, p. 9)

In spite of advances in medicine and the increase in life expectancy in Western countries, gender and class differences continue to exacerbate, and biological factors are unable to explain, the complexity of this system of inequalities (Lombardi, 2005). Research on the relationship between women, health and medicine have, however, revealed a gradual process of medicalization of women's bodies especially regarding reproduction, highlighting the construction and social control of the female body (Lombardi, 2005; Meo, 2012).

Departing from such studies, gender medicine in the 80s, a branch of biomedical sciences whose aim is recognizing and analyzing the differences between men and women in terms of health and practices of treatment, was born. Only recently, however, gender medicine has established itself as a legitimate approach and a necessary instrument for the treatment of women, since immense differences exist between men and women, even in the daily experience of disease, as the evidence from medical literature produced in the last years (Baggio, 2015) increasingly shows.

Adopting a gender approach to analyze health inequalities also means pondering the social consequences of this inequality.

Therefore, this contribution reflects on gender inequalities in health policies targeting the treatment and management of thalassemia and considers differences in health needs, as well as the way in which men and women experience illness and attribute meaning to it.

The medicalization process of female bodies in the experience of thalassemia will be analyzed, and here, the topics of body, sexuality, reproduction, and maternity are central. The analysis will reveal an inequality between men and women, not only in the level and in the ways their bodies are medicalized, through the embodiment of an imaginary necessarily encasing women in the role of wife and mother, making the disease a particularly painful experience, often obstructing the achievement of these objectives.

METHODS

The method used consists in the analysis of biographical interviews of 20 patients (10 men and 10 women. The number of interviews resulted sufficient for saturation of data), out of a total of 47, treated at the center of microcythemia of the General Hospital of Messina, from which interesting illness narratives emerge. The respondents were identified thanks to the help of the medical director and, in some cases, upon indication of people who had already replied to questions. They are patients between the ages of 26 and 57, of differing social and cultural status, of which only five are married and 12 are employed, mainly as public employees.

Interviews were built around four moments considered representative of a person's biography: childhood, adolescence, adulthood, and the future. All respondents were asked to tell their story starting from the most important memories relating to family, school, friendship, love, employment, and of course, their illness experience. Interviews, recorded and entirely transcribed, have been analyzed in their content, highlighting their most interesting points, the common narrative patterns observed in the text corpus, the shared narratives used to portray their experience and their elements of diversity. Life trajectories have been interpreted paying particular attention to what Bruner (1992) defines as turning points, which, within the narrative constructions, help narrators to gain self-awareness, triggering a reinterpretation of their life.

Thalassemia is a hereditary blood disorder entailing the presence of a lower quantity of hemoglobin and red blood cells in the body. The most serious form is thalassemia major, known as Cooley's syndrome; in this case, the person inherited the disease from both thalassemic heterozygotic parents. It is first observed in childhood and is characterized by paleness, yellowish skin, little appetite, and difficulty in growing up, contrasting with an enlargement of the skull, in particular of cheekbones. The person with thalassemia major suffers from minor or severe deformations of the bones, owing to the fact that the bone marrow expands in an effort to produce more red blood cells. Further, the stomach is enlarged and prominent, due to the enlargement of spleen and liver, while the eyes appear slanted and the nose with hollowed base and enlarged wings. Until about 40 years ago, thalassemia made huge impacts on somatic characteristics of people who suffered from it. People who are 40 today therefore bear on their bodies the signs of the disease. The youngest, instead, show absence or a more or less complete reduction in the clinical signs of thalassemia major, as they have been provided with more correct and chelating treatments that allowed them not to have an excessive load of iron in their body. This brings about a difference in the way the illness is experienced by older and younger people.

The impact of thalassemia on reproduction is significant both among men and women, but mainly affects women who, for biologic reasons, are more likely to have fertility problems or in bringing a pregnancy to term. In fact, one of the consequences of thalassemia is often primary or secondary amenorrhea; in such cases, patients who want to have children must undergo treatments with ovulation injections and, in case they get pregnant, must comply with a series of precautionary measures. Male patients who suffer from azoospermia generally respond effectively to a combination of hormone treatments administered for a period of about ninety days (see: http://www.fertilitycenter.it/gravidanza/talassemie-e-gravidanza).

In general, as far as the treatment is concerned, patients with thalassemia major must periodically undergo blood transfusions and follow iron-chelation treatments which reduce the iron accumulating in the body. The main instrument is a pump infusion set that today, differently from the past, is light and portable.

DISCUSSION OF THE RESULTS

The analysis of the collected biographical interviews reported a significant difference between men and women living with thalassemia, strongly developing around the topic of parenthood. The biographical trajectories of the women interviewed show that for many of them maternity, achieved or not, represented a turning point engraved in individual memory, a moment that changed forever the course of their lives. It is shown by the recurrent use of time expressions indicating rupture to the narrate which focuses on the specific moment in time: "since then," "suddenly," "finally," and "only today."

For the 10 women interviewed, except for the youngest for whom the age might still be a limitation to a desire for maternity, being a mother seems to take on a crucial role in the definition of identity. Data show that only two of the women managed to make this wish and life project come true. For the others, thalassemia represented an insurmountable obstacle, often together with the lack of a stable partner.

The issue of maternity is vital to studying gender differences in health policies targeting to thalassemia treatment and management, as it involves the topics of body, sexuality, stigma, and also because reproduction is the privileged field in which the process of medicalization of women's bodies and its social control is developed, according to much of the existing literature (Conrad, 1992; Lombardi, 2005; Connell, 2011; Meo, 2012).

If analyzing the interviewed men's tales, paternity, although central in their biographies, does not seem to be so crucial, for women who did not manage to become mothers, this meant a state of suffering which continues and is a factor in further stigmatization: as a thalassemic woman and as a *non*-mother woman (Goffman, 1983; Raffa, 2016).

The collected stories are alike for their common dynamics; they are all about a moment in history in which pregnancy represented a taboo for thalassemic women even in the medical field. Maternity seemed incompatible with thalassemia; therefore, women often renounced it *ex ante*. For example, M. G. tells:

> [...] Then we got married. Well then from 18 to 19 years old I had some problems, my period stopped from iron accumulation. So one more problem, then well, they gave me the replacement treatment but I wondered: what if I want to have a child? I knew that it was a question mark, at the time there were just two girls in Messina who managed to have children. The topic of pregnancy was a taboo. Step by step we young people together with doctors went to conferences to try to understand. A friend of mine, as she had the same problem as I did, told me she had known a gynecologist dealing with thalassaemic girls and since then I started the battle to have a child. I went to Palermo, I talked to this gynecologist, a person very skilled but very rude [...] not rude, very blunt, he spoke his mind, he didn't have certain attitudes [...] at the beginning when he saw some tests that I had brought he told me "well, it's a bit difficult, but let's try." First weeping. (M. G., 38 years old, divorced, unemployed)

Those women who made their mothering dream come true followed a common path: the difficulty in getting pregnant obliged them to go to specialized doctors to undergo specific treatments and in some cases assisted fertilization. Their body, therefore, has doubly become an arena for the exercise of biopower (Foucault, 1978): on the one hand, undergoing necessary and invasive treatments for thalassemia tending to destroy the world of daily life; on the other hand, obtrusive techniques which, taking direct action in the field of life, controlling their bodies and producing a certain set of social regulation (Meo, 2012).

Some narratives confirm that the interviewed women embody an imaginary that sees them irretrievably as wives and mothers, sole model of normality outside which it does not seem to be possible to find a social role. Again, M. G.'s narrative proves particularly significant:

> [...] In those years maybe you start to understand more things, you try to plan your life, I started to get more informed about the disease, I started to pay more attention in taking Desferal in order to get pregnant, I did everything. Later, growing up, I was told I had hepatitis, and at the beginning, when I was told, I didn't understand, I didn't realize; then I started to get information and I started to be scared about the consequence of this hepatitis. In short, the more I knew, the worse I felt. [...]. The doctor told me to wait a bit, he said let's try, I had this desire to complete the marriage. My husband had the same desire and I wanted to reply to his mother, as the first thing she had said was "she can't have children and she will die soon." I wanted to reply to let her understand that I was nothing less than others. With the treatment I immediately got pregnant, a pregnancy almost completed, she was a baby girl and one night I don't know what happened. The following morning I didn't feel her, but there was nothing to do when I went to the hospital. Eight months and a half, not three days [...]. They had me deliver spontaneously. After 11 hours of labor I delivered spontaneously, later I had to have urgent surgery because the placenta didn't detach. I left, and more checkups because I didn't have my period, not even with the treatment, actually they had performed curettage badly on me and there were some adhesions in the uterus and I had to set it free because I didn't have my period. It should have been a day-hospital experience, but at the General Hospital I had my uterus drilled, three months after delivering. (M. G., 38 years old, divorced, unemployed)

As we can see, the issue for M. G. is not just linked to her maternal desire, but, as she herself says, to the wish to feel accepted and acknowledged by the husband and his family in the social roles of wife and mother that the stigma linked to thalassemia risked blurring. In order to understand such a mechanism, shared by most of the females interviewed, it can be useful to adopt the analysis offered by Bourdieu about what he defines "symbolic violence." M. G. would be the product and at the same time the producer of a system of power that wants her ruled and a victim of "that violence that is exercised on social agents with their complicity" (Bourdieu, 1992), of which ruling male is its paradigmatic form (Meo, 2012, p. 68).

The topic of unachieved maternity comes back in other women's narratives who blame the illness for not being able to carry out their life projects. For example, L. says: "if only at this age I had twenty year old sons like my friends, instead I couldn't," or G.:

> thalassemia has limited me very much. Today I'm happy, but my sorrow is that I didn't have any children and that other women had them [though they too were] ill.

G. also had to face her husband's illness:

> the only wish that I have left is to have a baby, we decided this because he would take two diseases and it does not make any sense just for the selfishness of having a child. I wasn't very happy in making this decision, but for my husband it was even worse. It means that it had to be like that, not everything is as you want it to be.

As demonstrated in these narratives, for these women, the illness represents a particularly painful experience because it prevented them from fully complying with socially acceptable norms of healthy womanhood, fulfilled in the role of wife, and above all of mother.

This social imagery has therefore produced a specific type of female subjectivity (Berger & Luckmann, 1966). As feminist theories pointed out (Balbo, 1978, 2008; Barazzetti, 2007; Butler, 1996a,1996b; Cammarota, 1984, 2005; Lombardi, 2005; Piccone & Saraceno, 1996), women's bodies are placed within a gendered *habitus* linked to the reproductive field and different from the male one, connected to production field (Illich, 1894). This aspect emerges, for example, in E.'s narrative:

> In any case, I used to play with dolls, with the kitchen […] and above all I wanted to be a mummy, I wanted to act like a mummy. I wanted the doll, who, if I went to another room, would call me mummy and that was impossible. And my mother always tells me that I have always had this torment because as soon as I perceived, as soon as I was the age to understand that there was a problem in my life, my obsession was to be able to become a mother. I have a memory, while she was taking me to middle school, I remember asking her: "mummy do you think that I will ever be able to have children?" And I remember my mother's reply: "darling, I can't know that now, in life you can never know, why shouldn't you have them, mummy can't give you an answer, because I can't foresee the future!" but this has always been my worry, my real obsession. (E., 42 years old, divorced, unemployed)

E. and C. too, the two women out of 10 who managed to have children, had to undergo hard procedures of assisted fertilization. Their bodies were invasively checked to monitor the fetus's status and to inspect that it was healthy. These elements of the narration lead us to a further consideration.

The reproductive arena is the space where the maintenance of social forms must take place, but at the same time, it hides the risk that the social order is overturned (Connell, 2011; Meo, 2012, p. 73). Techniques of assisted reproduction become an instrument to control births, giving these women their "normality" back and reproducing a normalized social order (Pizzini, 2009). In other words, it could be said that they are medical-scientific techniques through which the power of control on the species is exercised. Of course, in the case of thalassemic women because of the infertility caused by the disease, and for which there is also the expected problem of genetic transmission of the disease to children, this issue takes on multifaceted aspects and implications.

Among the 10 men whose story of life has been collected, four have become fathers. As for the others, the two youngest put paternity among their future projects, while the other four have no children and do not deal with the topic. D., for example, says:

> […] My wife does, but I don't feel this need to have a child, I understand that my wife is five years older, she is a woman […] I always see thalassemia as an obstacle distracting me and then there is always the fear of not being up to it. Also, because I had some checkups to see if we can, I don't have to undergo who knows what treatments […]. (D., 38 years old, married, employed)

Comparing female and male narratives, a considerable gender difference is evident. A first difference, as we have noted, is of biological origin. In this sense, it can be interesting to look at the way one of the interviewed men represents this difference:

> For a thalassemic woman having children is challenging. You perfectly know that out of a sample of 20 healthy women there can be one who is unlucky, poor thing, and maybe she has ovaries (that are not working); out of 10 thalassemic women five can have children and five can't, maybe I'm being generous. So you see that it's quite frustrating, choosing not to have children is one thing, not being able to have them is frustrating. So yes, it's different, according to me of course, then it can be that I'm spouting bullshit. This is the perception that I have. If I am not wrong, there is somebody who has even lost a child […]. (T., 39 years old, married, employed)

Other factors can also impact the production of a determined female and male subjectivity, factors not necessarily related to illness and body, but rather to cultural and social domains. For example, more freedom of movement for men and therefore more opportunities for meeting potential mates, as opposed to the greater restriction imposed on women by their families. It is not a coincidence that male narratives regarding the topic of sexuality are characterized by more personal experiences, with respect to those of women interviewed.

In this regard, it must be underscored that the incidence that some aspects of southern Italian culture have historically had in constructing ideal womanhood, where they are consigned to the private domestic sphere while men dominate public space. For example, G. (55 years old, unemployed, married) says she was the only one of four daughters given more freedom of movement, but only together with a church group:

> maybe because I have been at home longer. They let me go out with the parish group (I started going out when I was over 18 years old), and I started feeling more accepted and sometimes I felt excluded maybe for the illness. That is, I thought that all the times they called me, they did it because I was ill.

It is interesting to point out that not always is so-called patriarchal culture the result of men's decisions, in G.'s family (40 years old, unemployed, married), for example, it was the mother, particularly "anxious and possessive," who had introjected it:

> I left home with my father and my brother's help and I flew away. My mother was absolutely against it, she wanted me to stay at home with her and she hasn't talked to me for a while. When I left, for me it was great, it was my space and I did what I wanted.

Generally, for many of the women interviewed, that condition was deciphered in terms of dependence on parents or partner or incapacity to look at themselves as subjects capable of agency. However, some instead have willfully fought to conquer their own independence and not adhere to the image of weak and vulnerable womanhood – due to either gender or illness, as L.'s story shows (46 years old, employed, unmarried):

> I wanted to work, I didn't want to be pensioned like everybody else. I wanted to be a psychologist. Even a minor job, but I wanted to be independent, I wanted to get a driver's license, to travel, to have a family, a few children [...] I have always been in love with children. I could have been a policewoman but thalassemia has always stopped me. I wanted to have a job allowing me to travel but with thalassemia I couldn't [...] Even the family, I had problems, for example, not being able to have children as other women [...] I could have had 20 year old children as my friends, and instead I couldn't [...] I felt like an adult when I got my driver's license, I could do what I wanted without bothering anyone. I had a second-hand car, I took the car and I traveled alone.

In this case, it seems that the higher the level of education, the greater the sense of independence, ability, and self-determination, as it does for healthy women (Cammarota, 2005).

Judging from the interviews, fear of transmitting the illness to the child, is probably higher in men than is any desire for paternity.

Their stories too recall memories of checkups to monitor fertility and the possible risk of having a thalassemic child, as well as the re-emergent representation of the female body as a medicalized reproductive body, as in G.'s narrative:

> I had my wife tested and I knew my child could not be born with thalassemia, but I had huge anxiety, more than any other father, that my child could have any pathologies, because it's painful and I think that, in any case, I'm telling you foolishly that I would have a hard time caring for a child with a pathology today, since mine already requires a huge effort, even psychological. You have commitments, deadlines, so caring for your child as well would mean starting all over again, and without end, because I myself have never finished. It would be hard! Fortunately, there is no problem. (G., 43 years old, married, freelance)

It must be pointed out that in many cases the pain expressed by women is connected not so much to a missed pregnancy, but to the fact that the illness affects the possibility of procreation. It is the idea of not being able to be potential mothers because of thalassemia that provokes such a sense of frustration and suffering. From research carried out in 2005 in Messina on a group of young healthy women (Cammarota, 2005), it is revealed that maternity is central in self-fulfillment plans; however, it is not everyone's wish, nor an essential element in building their identity as women. If, therefore, healthy women can voluntarily decide to be or not to be mothers (without this affecting their being women), thalassemic women do not have the same self-determining possibility.

Generally, through the possibility to imagine themselves as women, regardless of being mothers or wives is higher in women with a higher level of education (Cammarota, 2005).However, in the case we have analyzed, the level of education is not a determining factor: even women with a higher level of education connect their womanhood to the possibility of reproduction and missing this opportunity represents a weakening of their identity.

A study carried out in 2007 in Sardinia (Italy) (Smorti & Sanna, 2007), out of a sample of 230 subjects with thalassemia major (110 men and 120 women), shows strong resistance in accepting the illness, a negative perception of the future, and a low ability to use coping strategies based on solution of the problem and on research of social support to cope with stressful events. Analyzing qualitative interviews carried out in Messina, a partial confirmation of these data can be highlighted. As far as women are concerned, they show a higher predisposition, with respect to men, in accepting thalassemia and a good use of coping strategies. However, some psychological problems which are typical of adolescence but exacerbated in adulthood and characteristic above all in women, persist. Self-image is influenced both by social factors, due to objective limitations the illness imposes, and due to physical factors, due to the clinical complications the illness entails. Social integration is moreover limited by constant and prolonged therapeutical practices and by the perception of being unable to form a family (Ratip & Modell, 1996). Therefore, for example, A. (43 years old, unemployed, unmarried) says:

> From the age of 18, my body and I have started to change. I changed my way of dressing, I saw my friends who got engaged, whereas I didn't. Actually, men made fun of me. I wasn't comfortable with myself because everybody made fun of me. Because I was ugly, they gave me nicknames. I didn't have close friends to trust, only friends to go out with sometimes. I don't have a memory of a close friendship. I didn't have much to tell, I didn't have a love life, I got engaged very late.

Or again G. (55 years old, unemployed, married):

> I didn't talk about thalassemia when I was little; it was evident because I was paler, my teeth stuck out and it was more evident. My childhood was not beautiful because I suffered more, both physically, and then I felt uncomfortable because my teeth stuck out, and it bothered me because they made fun of me and I always cried.

Although, from the interviews, it is evident that women tend to have an attitude of greater attention toward health and toward behaviors aiming at protecting it (perseverance in treatments, attention to food habits and lifestyle [...]), they claim they feel fragile and vulnerable more than men do:

> in ten years time I see myself as old. Imagine, if I am 43 years old and I feel so tired, how is this going to be in 10 years time? I hope to have my husband next to me, but I don't know how I will feel physically. (G., 43 years old, unemployed, married)

This trend seems to confirm indications coming from an investigation of the Italian National Institute of Statistics in 2010 on health perception in Italy. It highlights that women live on average longer than men, but if health conditions are considered, only 67.2% of Italian women declares they are fine, against

75.1% of men. According to this research, therefore, women feel more vulnerable to illness.

Recent developments in gender medicine (Biancheri, 2016) have shown that medical diagnostics underestimate or do not consider women's life conditions in determining diagnosis and treatment plans, favoring therefore a series of failures that are seriously prejudicial for women's health and life. In particular, gender medicine has pointed out how a mainly naturalistic approach in observing women creates a hiding effect for other types of illness etiology, in particular veiling interactions and connections between women's health and conditions of oppression (Biancheri, 2016).

Based on such considerations, it could be vital first, to plan or increase in case where they already exist, measures to support and promote health for thalassemic women considering the different levels thalassemia affects, from the organic to the psychological, the social and cultural. Second, it is evident that the need to read gender differences not in terms of inequalities, but as elements necessary to building new values opposed to a male dominant technical-scientific medical approach, around which our main theoretical and methodological frameworks have been consolidated (Biancheri, 2014). Narrative medicine is useful to achieving these goals. It is based on narrative competence: the ability of physicians to listen to the narratives of the patients, honor their meanings, and be moved to act on the patient's behalf. Narrative medicine is a model for medical practices that provide physicians and surgeons the skills and texts to learn how the factors and objects of health and illness are constructed, as well as their consequence and meanings for individual patients and physicians (Charon, 2001). The use of narrative allows physicians to contextualize clinical data, needs, and offers the patient the possibility of not feeling apart and secondary, but at the very heart of care practices. Narrating illness helps the patient to make decisions more consciously, to interact with others, to express emotion and hardship, and to share experiences – all of which can be useful to other patients and/or physicians.

Considering the results of our research, we might consider offering workshops on reflective writing for women in the care of the Microcythemia Centre of the General Hospital of Messina. It would be possible not only to create a stronger and more communicative relationship with physicians and surgeons for a better compliance but also to work on the stigma associated with thalassemia, as well as the social construction of gender, female identity, and mothering.

CONCLUSION

The results of our research demonstrate the existence of a considerable gender difference in the way in which thalassemia affects men and women's bodies that is abundantly illustrated in the "reproductive arena" that socially defined arena where cultural definitions of gender are consolidated (Connell, 2011).

This difference means gender inequality in health policies targeted to treatment and management of thalassemia – starting from differences in health needs and in the way in which women and men live the experience of illness and give meanings to it.

Analyzing biographical trajectories we report that, in the case of almost all the interviewed women, the main core around which the narration of the illness is developed, is maternity, whether achieved or not. It is therefore on the possibility to fulfill the socially-shared role of wife-mother that thalassemia reveals its capacity to have a significantly painful impact on female lives.

If for men, the problem of fertility is far less important, or the desire for paternity not as central, for women the possibility to procreate seems to be decisive in defining self-identity with regard to complying with s socially-shared female image.

The female body, therefore, in this way becomes the defenseless field upon which the dynamics of power play out, transforming it into a medicalized body, through medical-scientific techniques. A body that, on the one hand, fights against thalassemia and, on the other, faces futile medical care in order to exercise its "natural" reproductive function, that is, a culturally determining female "normality."

Thalassemia, therefore, ends up being a particularly painful experience of illness especially for those women who cannot have children.

The topic points to the need to rethink and achieve more "humanized" health policies, which are capable of meeting these women's needs. But long before this, it must work to deconstruct female subjectivity created by social imagery that contributes to a painful sense of social inadequacy and stigma in women that add to the difficulties of daily life of living with the illness.

Lastly, it is still an open debate whether intervention through medical-scientific techniques on the bodies of women as carriers of the disease, aimed at ensuring a "healthy" fetus, can legitimize the dangerous idea that being different from a standard of normality is wrong, putting in crisis the precious principle of diversity.

REFERENCES

Baggio, G. (2015). Dalla medicina di genere alla medicina genere-specifica. *Gendermedjournal, 1*, 3–5.

Balbo, L. (1978). La doppia presenza. *Inchiesta*, marzo-aprile, 3–6.

Balbo, L. (2008). *Il lavoro e la cura*. Torino: Einaudi.

Barazzetti, D. (2007). *C'è posto per me? Lavoro e cura nella società del non lavoro*. Milano: Guerini e Associati.

Berger, P. L., & Luckmann, T. (1966). *The social construction of reality*. New York, NY: Garden City.

Biancheri, R. (2014). Dalla medicina di genere al genere in salute. *Salute e Società, 1*, 17–33.

Biancheri, R. (2016). *Narrare la malattia, costruire la salute*. Convegno nazionale AIS, Pisa, 26 febbraio, Pisa, Edizioni ETS.

Bruner, J. (1992). *La ricerca del significato*. Torino: Bollati Boringhieri.

Bourdieu, P. (1992). *Risposte. Per un'antropologia riflessiva*. Torino: Bollati Boringhieri.

Butler, J. (1996a). *La disfatta del genere*. Roma: Meltemi.

Butler, J. (1996b). *Corpi che contano. I limiti discorsivi del sesso*. Milano: Feltrinelli.

Cammarota, A. (1984). *Donna, identità, lavoro. Il movimento femminista di fronte alla complessità sociale*. Milano: Giuffrè.

Cammarota, A. (2005). *Femminismi da raccontare. Un percorso attraverso le lotte e le speranze delle donne di ieri e di oggi*. Milano: FrancoAngeli.

Cardano, M., & Lepori, G. (2012). *Udire la voce degli dei*. Milano: FrancoAngeli.

Charon, R. (2001). Narrative medicine. A model for empathy, reflection, profession and trust. *JAMA*, *286*(15), 1897–1902.

Cipolla, C., & Maturo, A. (Eds.). (2009). *Con gli occhi del paziente. Una ricerca nazionale sui vissuti di cura dei malati oncologici*. Milano: FrancoAngeli.

Cipriani, R. (Ed.). (2010). Narrative-based medicine: una critica. *Salute e Società* (n. 2). Milano: FrancoAngeli.

Connell, R. W. (2011). *Questioni di genere*. Bologna: Il Mulino.

Conrad, P. (1992). Medicalization and social control. *Annual Review of Sociology*, *18*, 209–232.

Facchini, C., & Ruspini, E. (2001). *Salute e disuguaglianze. Genere, condizioni sociali e corso di vita*. Milano: FrancoAngeli.

Foucault, M. (1978). *La volontà di sapere. Storia della sessualità* (Vol. 1). Milano: Feltrinelli.

Goffman, E. (1983). *Stigma. L'identità negata*. Milano: Giuffrè Editore.

Good, B. J. (2006). *Narrare la malattia. Lo sguardo antropologico sul rapporto medico-paziente*. Torino: Einaudi.

Gordon, D. (1998). Tenacious assumptions in Western medicine. In M. Lock & D. Gordon (Eds.), *Biomedicine examined*. Boston, MA: Kluwer Academic Publishers.

Illich, I. (1894). *Il genere e il sesso. Per una critica storica dell'uguaglianza*. Milano: Mondadori.

Kleinman, A. (1978). Concepts and a model for the comparison of medical systems as cultural systems. *Social Science and Medicine*, *12*, 85–93.

Kleinman, A. (1988). *The illness narrative: Suffering, healing and the human condition*. New York, NY: Basic Books.

Kleinman, A. (1998). *Experience and its moral modes: Culture, human condition and disorder*. Stanford, CA: Stanford University.

Kleinman, A. (2006). Alcuni concetti e un modello per la comparazione dei sistemi medici intesi come sistemi culturali. In I. Quaranta (Ed.), *Antropologia medica* (pp. 5–29). Milano: Raffaello Cortina Editore.

Kleinman, A., & Kleinman, J. (2006). La sofferenza e la sua trasformazione professionale: verso una etnografia dell'esperienza interpersonale. In I. Quaranta (Ed.), *Antropologia medica* (pp. 199–234). Milano: Raffaello Cortina Editore.

Lombardi, L. (2005). *Società, culture e differenze di genere. Percorsi migratori e stati di salute*. Milano: FrancoAngeli.

Maturo, A. (2007). *Sociologia della malattia. Un'introduzione*. Milano: FrancoAngeli.

Meo, M. (2012). *Il corpo politico: biopotere, generazione e produzione di soggettività femminili*. Milano: Mimesis.

Piccone, S., & Saraceno, C. (1996). *La costruzione sociale del femminile e del maschile*. Bologna: Il Mulino.

Pizzini, F. (2009). *Corpo medico e corpo femminile. Parto, riproduzione artificiale, menopausa*. Milano: FrancoAngeli.

Raffa, V. (2016). *Identità croniche? La talassemia tra costruzione sociale ed esperienza biografica*. Milano: FrancoAngeli.

Ratip, S., & Modell, B. (1996). Psychological and sociological aspects of the thalassaemia. *Seminars in Haematology*, *33*(1), 53–65.

Smorti, M., & Sanna, A. (2007). Atteggiamento verso il futuro, verso la salute e locus of control in soggetti affetti da β-talassemia major. *Social Science and Medicine*, *2*, 25–39.

PART V
HEALTH CARE WORKERS

WORK–LIFE BALANCE IN MEDICAL PRACTICE: THE REPRODUCTION OF PATRIARCHY AND THE POLITICS OF GENDER

Jennifer McDonald and Claudia Chaufan

ABSTRACT

Purpose – *To shed light on how gender norms are reproduced in medical training and practice through an exploration of representations of the problem of "work–life balance." Women physicians and women physician-researchers (WPs/WPRs) in Canada and in the United States experience social and health inequities when compared to their men colleagues. Despite current medical school acceptance parity, upon entering the medical workforce, women work harder than men to succeed within the historically male-dominated structures and value system of the medical profession.*

Methodology – *We performed a critical discourse analysis of articles retrieved from academic databases and leading Anglo-American journals that discussed "work–life balance," to investigate how the discourse contributed to, or challenged, the reproduction of gender norms in medicine.*

Findings – *While the medical literature acknowledges that the social and health inequities experienced by WP/WPR result from discriminatory norms and practices, it neglects to challenge built-in gendered inequities in benchmarks for success in the profession. Instead, proposed solutions require that WP/WPR themselves learn to cope and make better lifestyle choices, including downloading domestic responsibilities on socially disadvantaged – racialized and poor – women. Authors' gender appears to make no difference.*

Underserved and Socially Disadvantaged Groups and Linkages with Health and Health Care Differentials
Research in the Sociology of Health Care, Volume 37, 205–223

ISSN: 0275-4959/doi:10.1108/S0275-495920190000037017

Research Limitations – *Our search was limited to the Anglo-American literature, often retrieved articles inaccessible via our university library, excluded informal venues (e.g., blogs), and did not include cases of same-sex couples or interviews of WP/WPR. All these may have challenged components of our argument by revealing more nuanced debates, occurring under different political, cultural, and economic contexts.*

Policy Implications – *While individual choices of WP/WPR are important to the protagonists, to successfully address the very real problem of work–life balance experienced by WP/WPR, patriarchal norms should be challenged, failure to comply with these norms should be rejected as explanations for work–life balance challenges, and norms themselves should become the focus of analysis and intervention.*

Originality/Value – *The medical language used by physicians of both genders normalizes gendered inequities, favoring the success of medical men over women, and reproducing the professional and personal disadvantages experienced by the latter, further burdening socially disadvantaged women.*

Keywords: Work–life balance; women in medicine; gender inequities; critical discourse analysis; critical functionalism; medical social control

INTRODUCTION

Women physicians and women physician-researchers (WPs/WPRs) in Canada and the United States do not experience the same success, inclusion, and health as do their comparable male colleagues (Ash, Carr, Goldstein, & Friedman, 2004; Ferris, Mackinnon, Mizgala, & McNeill, 1996; Reed & Buddeberg-Fischer, 2001; Woodrow, Gilmer-Hill, & Rutka, 2006). At least in the Western world, it is well documented that medicine has been a historically male-dominated profession that largely excluded women from medical practice, and it was not until the 1960s and 1970s that women began entering the profession in greater numbers (Jefferson, Bloor, & Maynard, 2015). As the number of WP/WPR grew, the breadth and depth of knowledge concerning women choosing a medical career increased, hand-in-hand with literature highlighting their problems – of motherhood timing, lower pay for equal work, and the balance between a medical career and domestic life, that is, "work–life" balance (see Clem et al., 2008; Heru, 2005; Miller, 2011). Other identified challenges as well as indicators of poor health for WP/WPR have included barriers to career advances (Ash et al., 2004), insufficient networking or mentorship opportunities (Phillips & Clarke, 2012), and higher rates of burnout and depression (Frank & Dingle, 1999). Scholars attribute these challenges and poor health indicators to gendered norms that selectively disadvantage, stereotype, and stand in the way of WP/WPR's professional progress (Mayer, Files, Ko, & Blair, 2008; Valian, 1999).

Be that as it may, some progress has been achieved, as women are accepted into medical school at increasing rates (Micieli, Trope, & Buys, 2016; Office of

Research & Information Services, 2015). Nevertheless, significant challenges for WP/WPR persist (Mobilos, Chan, & Brown, 2008; Sonnad & Colletti, 2002). For instance, women tend to avoid medical specialties, such as surgery, that appear to pose greater challenges to work–life balance, and in these specialties, women are underrepresented (Gautam, 2001; Marschall & Karimuddin, 2003; Woodrow et al., 2006). The literature documents well, and quantifies, these challenges (see, e.g., Barnett & Gareis, 2002; Merchant, Hameed, & Melck, 2013; Micieli et al., 2016; Shanafelt et al., 2016), thus indicating that they exist. Yet quantitative research, by its very nature, cannot interpret the meaning of these challenges for those experiencing them, nor can it reveal why a phenomenon, in our case differential professional and health outcomes for WP/WPR as compared to men, occur and persist.

A clue can be gleaned when examining how the literature discursively treats "work–life" balance issues when experienced by women (Potee, Gerber, & Ockovics, 1999; Stentz et al., 2016). Generally, women appear to face "tough choices" between the demands of profession and family, while this is hardly the case for men. In fact, in the past the literature described men physicians who placed work before home life as commendable, or working above and beyond the call of duty, yet never as experiencing "work–life balance" conflicts (Dunn, Arnetz, Christensen, & Homer, 2007; Uhlenberg & Cooney, 1990). While in our day the demands of medical practice are rarely presented in this explicitly gendered way, our investigation suggests that gendered norms continue to be legitimized within the medical literature itself, even as this literature acknowledges and critiques these norms that pose work–life balance issues and disadvantage women. This is because, at least in our knowledge, the literature does not probe how the problem of "work–life balance" is framed, or how the notion of "work–life balance" is discursively treated, such that the literature itself may reproduce rather than challenge patriarchal structures built into the practice of medicine.

We propose that an investigation of the framing and discursive treatment of "work–life balance" in the medical literature is warranted, thus the goal of our article: to examine the debate around "work–life" balance in medicine as this debate appears in the literature produced by the medical profession. We focus on how this debate is framed, compare how it is presented when it concerns women and men, respectively, and attempt to reveal how built-in gendered inequities in medicine concerning values, practices and benchmarks for success reproduce patriarchal structures. We conclude by proposing policies with the potential to address these inequities, improve the well-being of WP/WPR, and contribute to their professional integration in Canada, the United States, and elsewhere.

THEORETICAL AND METHODOLOGICAL CONSIDERATIONS

Our analysis is informed by the Marxian tradition, especially the work of Howard Waitzkin (1989) and Vicente Navarro (1980), which help reveal how medical language reproduces structural inequalities, by naturalizing the social order, ignoring relevant context, and excluding challenges to this order and process of naturalization. We also draw from critical functionalism, specifically from the work of Herbert Gans (1972), who applies a Mertonian, that is, functionalist, analysis to identify processes that contribute to the persistence of norms and practices – in our case patriarchal norms and practices in medicine – despite their "dysfunctionality" to disadvantaged groups – in this case WP/WPR – and despite manifest, official attempts to address the harmful effects of these norms and practices. Finally, we draw from a critical discourse analysis approach to investigate how discourse and social practices dialectically interact to reproduce, or challenge, structures of domination (Fairclough, 2013).

Contemporary critical discourse has been described as a method of analysis that explores how structures of domination often not perceived by protagonists – in our case WP/WPR – are constructed and legitimized through the language used in the discourse of a community, while the language is in turn shaped by those structures (Fairclough, 2013). Such is the discourse of the medical community, as represented by articles identified for our analysis. Critical discourse analysis, originating from large-scale immigration and postwar sociological theory that was concerned with institutional inequalities in education for minority groups has been described by Luke (1997) as a way of examining language as a process that shapes the identities and practices of subjects. Michel Foucault (1980) further elaborated on early critical discourse theory and suggested that language was not merely a means of describing and analyzing society but also a tool to construct, regulate, and control the dissemination of knowledge. In the spirit of these authors, we focused on language that revealed structures of domination as it addressed and explained work–life balance challenges in the medical profession. We further observed how the authors framed, resisted, or otherwise complied with existing hierarchies (van Dijk, 1993).

DATA SELECTION

Using "work–life balance" and "women physicians" as keywords, we searched for articles indexed in Scopus, PubMed, Google Scholar, and leading North American medical journals, such as the *Canadian Medical Association Journal* (CMAJ), the *New England Journal of Medicine* (NEJM), and the *Journal of the American Medical Association* (JAMA). We included original research, commentary, editorials, and opinions written in English by women or men physicians or physician-researchers, produced in Canada or the United States. The rationale for including opinion pieces and editorials rather than only original research was that we were less interested in the accuracy of, or empirical support for, claims, than we were in the discourse produced by and for the medical community as an object of inquiry in itself. We chose "work–life balance" as the focus of our analysis and key search word because it compellingly captures the challenges faced by WP/WPR as they juggle between traditionally assigned domestic roles and the responsibilities of a historically male-dominated profession.

The database and journal searches produced a large number of articles. We included all articles in English that were fully accessible and addressed the topic of work–life balance or a functional equivalent (e.g., articles that discuss family responsibilities in relation to career responsibilities in medicine. See Guille, Frank, Zhao, Kalmbach, Nietert, Mata, & Sen, 2017; Jolly, Griffith, DeCastro, Stewart, Ubel, and Jagsi, 2014), regardless of the medical specialty or inclusion of other issues. We excluded articles in languages other than English or that were not accessible via the York University library system, and a few that did not address in sufficient detail comparisons and interactions between a medical career and domestic life. This search, started in September of 2017 and completed in October of 2017, produced a sample of 50 articles (list available upon request).

To analyze our sample, we identified key themes (Aronson, 1995) pertaining to four categories: (1) how the concept of work–life balance or functional equivalents was defined, (2) problems associated with work–life balance, (3) causes of work–life balance tensions, and (4) recommendations for addressing problems of work–life balance. We decided upon these categories based on our personal experience as a prospective medical student (first author) and a trained, currently non-practicing medical doctor and experienced social researcher (second author). While most of the articles were quantitative and communicated self-reported data, all had introductions, conclusions, and discussion sections that shed light on the object of our investigation. We read the articles in their entirety, compiled and listed themes pertaining to each category according to their prevalence in the literature, selected examples to illustrate, elaborate on, and clarify these themes, and resolved discrepancies by consensus.

FINDINGS

Out of the 50 articles selected, four% ($N = 2$) journal articles were written solely by men authors, 48% ($N = 24$) by women authors and 48% ($N = 24$) by both men and women. All articles with the exception of two were written by at least one author or researcher who had a medical degree, and many were written exclusively by medical doctors. The articles typically began with a brief description of the work–life balance problem and why it was important for physicians. While the narrative produced by authors of both genders suggested that work–life balance was a challenge inherent in the profession of medicine, it subsequently elaborated that the challenge resided in the greater number of hours spent on domestic activities, for example, child-rearing, which undermined the chances of professional development for WP/WPR, whereas for medical men this was not the case – in fact, it was even the opposite. Most of the time, authors did not elaborate further. An example of this narrative follows:

> A majority of women are combining motherhood and career. Compared with their male counterparts, these women have greater domestic responsibilities and lower levels of career involvement. For female physicians, marriage and child-rearing clearly are associated with reduced hours worked and lowered earnings, while for men the effects of marriage and children are just the opposite. (Uhlenberg & Cooney, 1990)

While implicit gender-specific negotiations of home and life were pervasive, many articles, while data heavy, excluded references to a gender context, but instead linked work–life balance issues to specific medical specialties or to the practice of medicine more generally when compared to other occupations (Keeton et al., 2007; Roberts et al., 2014; Shanafelt et al., 2012; Shanafelt et al., 2014; Shanafelt et al., 2015; Shanafelt et al., 2016; Szender et al., 2016). Another interesting, recurrent theme was the acknowledged inequalities in success rates, yet these inequalities were more often attributed to the high tuition fee of medical school and gap in pay among specialties typically chosen by either men or women than to existing patriarchal structures and standards (see Table 1 for key themes that illustrate the categories of inquiry as defined by our study). In the

Table 1. Identified Categories and Themes on Work–life Balance in the Medical Literature.

Issue	Common Themes	Quotations
Defining work–life balance for physicians	• The trade-off/interplay between career and family responsibilities • Tension between family and career generated by competing demands • A way to increase productivity and well-being • Professional and personal choices made by physicians • Achieving fulfillment from work and family • The search for greater gender equality in life and career • WLB is not a set of balancing scales, but a pyramid of values or blend of priorities • "Having it all"	"How highly career-driven contemporary male and female physician-researchers allocate time to professional and domestic responsibilities." (Jolly et al., 2014) "The concept of work–life balance acts as quicksand in our professional and personal lives resulting in slow drowning in frustration, depression, and exhaustion." (Schwingshackl, 2014) "While the daily practice of balance is certainly a valuable aspiration, fulfillment may be, for some physicians, a more encompassing and guiding state to strive for as we seek satisfaction in our personal and professional lives." (Harrison, 2008)
Problems associated with work–life balance for physicians	• Poor mental and physical health including burnout and stress symptoms • Women physicians and researchers leave medicine or there is a reduction in clinical/surgical/academic hours and direct increase in domestic responsibilities for female physicians because of WLB priorities (including general loss of income compared to male colleagues) • Conflict within personal life or marriage • Career trajectory before, during and after maternity/paternity leave	"Depression levels are reported to be markedly higher in physicians than in the general population." (Raja & Stein, 2014) "While the trend toward part-time clinical practice may not harm patient outcomes, it is occurring in the midst of a growing physician shortage in North America." (Jovic et al., 2006) "A common theme for women was perhaps a sense of guilt about their performances as both mothers and family doctors at all stages of their careers." (Parsons et al., 2009)

Table 1. *(Continued)*

Issue	Common Themes	Quotations
	• Women physicians forego demanding specialties because of lack of WLB • Concept of WLB does not actually exist and often worsens rather than improves because of unrealistic expectations • Glass ceiling and gender inequities/ assumptions	"Female physician teachers with children had lower job satisfaction, less institutional support and slower career progress than male physician teachers with children." (Cujec et al., 2000) "Women, far more than men, consider the balancing of family, parental, and occupational roles when making career decisions." (Verlander, 2004)
Causes of work–life balance problems among physicians	• Result of behavioral and individual choices that cause tension such as taking on more domestic/child-rearing responsibilities and maternity leave • "Role strain" on women physicians and being mothers/spouses • Lack of role models and mentors for female physicians • Professional stressors such as time-constraints, lack of resources, decline in compensation, erosion of professional autonomy and decision-making capabilities • Socialized gender differences • Result of a demanding speciality choice or prioritizing career over life • Lack of perceived or actual control of work or domestic environment • Discrimination • Employers only concerned with financial profits/ physician has different priorities than institution • Lack of good support system	"In marriages between two physicians, wives are more likely to make accommodations in their career based on consideration of the effects on spouses and children whereas men were less likely to do so." (Robinson, 2003) "It may be that there are challenges inherent to the practice of clinical academic medicine that are fundamentally at odds with balancing family care responsibilities." (Beckett et al., 2015) "Barriers to work–life balance appear to be deeply rooted within professional culture [...] gendered societal expectations of women's roles, within and outside the workplace, continue to have a substantial impact." (Strong, 2013) "Female physicians perceived significantly less control than male physicians regarding a variety of daily work activities [...] In addition, control of workplace issues was related to risk of burnout for women, but not men." (McMurray, 2000)
Solutions to work–life balance problem for physicians	• Behavioral suggestions like better time management, monitoring stress, networking, prioritization, having a supportive spouse, finding inner-peace • Policy/programming interventions to promote well-being and success within medical organizations • Need more positive mentorship and support	"Nurturing and protecting our personal and professional relationships are keys to avoiding burnout." (Shenoi, 2016) "The opportunity for variable and flexible work scheduling, as well as the support of spouses, life partners, or other family members, were cited as key facilitating factors." (Phillips et al., 2016)

Table 1. *(Continued)*

Issue	Common Themes	Quotations
	• More research is needed/no solution • More on-site day-care, flexible scheduling, job sharing, and replacement staff for maternity leave • Integrate work and what we consider to be life • Specialty choice in medicine should be conducive to physician's anticipated future lifestyle • Embrace medical culture of spending more time at work because that is what a physician's life entails • Need new work–family paradigms • Address structural and systemic inequalities that specifically affect women physicians	"Strategies to improve the work experience of middle career physicians are needed to maintain productivity, minimize turnover, and improve patient care." (Dyrbye et al., 2013) "Women physicians should press for institutional changes that could reduce stress on and discrimination against women." (Robinson, 2003) "We must have realistic expectations of what one can accomplish [...] we need to foster the right kind of mentoring [...] we need to develop collaborative links between women to support and learn from each other through coaching and networking." (Figueroa, 2016) "Every medical school and residency program should have a written policy regarding parental leave." (Potee et al., 1999)

following sections, we expand on the themes present in the literature and elaborate on their equity implications for WP/WPR.

Defining Work–life Balance: The "Competing" Demands of Work and Life

One dominant theme in the definition of work–life balance was that a medical profession, on the one hand, and life (i.e., domestic life). on the other hand, are two separate and contrasting, often incompatible, realms, and as such, require that *both* men and women balance competing demands. However, the literature pointed out that WP/WPR make choices that increase the likelihood of their experiencing work–life balance problems more than their men colleagues (Kuehn, 2012; Phillips, Hustedde, Bjorkman, Prasad, Sola, Wendling, Bjorkman, & Paladine, 2016; Tarquinio, 2016). This was apparent in the language used by the authors in our article selection, particularly when discussing specialty choices of WP/WPR. An example follows:

> The flexibility offered in family practice is one of the reasons more women physicians than men physicians enter the discipline [...] and many women choose specialties based not only on their passion for that field, but because of the lifestyle it offers. (Mobilos et al., 2008)

This ostensibly factual statement implies that some specialties, say surgery, are not "flexible," because they do not offer the "lifestyle" that would enable a medical *woman* to achieve the desired work–life balance. Of note, specialty considerations are seemingly not worth mentioning when it comes to medical *men*. The literature also occasionally mentioned the need to pursue greater gender equity in the practice of medicine to address the disproportionate burden of work–life balance for women (Carnes, Morrissey, & Geller, 2008), yet the overall balancing act between work and the domestic sphere was often described as a women's issue (see Gautam, 2001; Harrison, 2008; Mobilos et al., 2008; Parsons, Duke, Snow, & Edwards, 2009). Many authors appeared confident that women would be able to navigate work and life (Wang, 2015), but perhaps not to the same extent as men physicians, due to additional "unique" stressors such as child-rearing (Phillips et al., 2016; Sandler, Tackett, Longo, & Yoo, 2016), harassment in the workplace (Gautam, 2001), and marriage or partnership to a surgeon (Dyrbye, Shanafelt, Balch, Satele, & Freischlag, 2010; Perlman, Ross, & Lypson, 2015). Others appeared less confident, suggesting that WP/WPR could not "have it all" without modifying their lifestyles, such as their choice of partner (Perlman, Ross, & Lypson, 2015). Finally, 56% ($N = 28$) of the articles proposed or implied that work–life balance for WP/WPR was either very difficult to achieve or not attainable, and that at best WP/WPR would be "able to combine career and family with *some* degree of success" (Sasser, 2004, emphasis added). Now, "with *some degree of* success" is not the same as "successfully," yet this one example illustrates the elusive nature of work–life balance – for women.

Overall, the literature portrayed the seemingly inevitable and intractable struggle of work–life balance both as inherent in the medical profession yet almost exclusively pertaining to women. And it fell on WP/WPR to decide how much time to devote to a career or a life at home, and to prioritize between the two. Not a single article questioned whether, much less how, men physicians should balance the practice of medicine with the responsibility to raise a family.

Problems Related to Work–life Balance: Prioritizing Family over a Medical Career

Based on the findings, the literature subtly assumed that WPs will, and indeed do, spend more time in the domestic sphere than male physicians. A particular set of problems arises when WP/WPR has another physician as a partner (Dyrbye et al., 2013; Raja & Stein, 2014) and their medical specialty (theirs, not their partner's) is surgery:

> Surgeons whose domestic partner [DP] is another physician appear to experience greater challenges balancing personal and professional life than surgeons whose DP is a working nonphysician or whose DP stays at home. (Dyrbye et al., 2010)

As the quote indicates, the work–life balance conflict was associated with WP/WPR having greater domestic responsibilities despite working full-time in a demanding medical setting. Unsurprisingly, higher rates of depression, stress, and burnout ensue from role strain and competing commitments. Authors noted the disproportionate amount of time spent by WP/WPR in domestic roles, regardless of the (in)flexibility of the medical institution, or of where WP/WPR are positioned in their career, and attributed this to gender bias:

> Promotions and tenure are biased in favour of men due to the male-oriented career framework in medicine [...] with no flexibility in timing of promotion or tenure for physicians with heightened family responsibilities. (Verlander, 2004)

Authors also often cited that WP/WPR tended to be overlooked for career advancement because they were seen as less ambitious or able to balance work and family life as are men or because of the "mommy track" (Strong et al., 2013). Findings in one article suggested that gender bias against WP/WPR affects their ability to fully participate in, and produce, medical research, and that this bias makes them less likely than their male colleagues of similar backgrounds, professional roles, and achievements to receive a full professorship (Carnes, Morrissey, & Geller, 2008; Verlander, 2004). This bias also appears to explain the lower income and greater number of hours at work spent by WP/WPR:

> Women physicians with children may not be able to return to their previous earnings trajectory even if they return to their previous work schedules. (Sasser, 2004)

Yet another problem related to work–life balance identified in our sample was that even considering maternity leave or the fact that women spend a greater number of hours as a primary caregiver of children, many WP/WPR work as long hours as do their men colleagues (Jinapriya, Cockerill, & Trope, 2003). This fact notwithstanding, as hiring committees evaluate candidates, they tend to judge women as less able to juggle career and family life, and present candidates with scenarios and questions that they would not present to men candidates (Carnes, Morrissey, & Geller, 2008). This is because, as one author put it bluntly, "women bear the brunt of child-rearing responsibilities" (Cujec et al., 2000, p. 637).

This bias also applies to medical students or physicians-in-training. Because women are assumed to be less committed to a career once it conflicts with family, female medical students are often maligned as, for instance, potential surgeons or career-focused specialists, and these attitudes contribute to their choices of medical specialization (Beckett et al., 2015; Carnes, Morrissey, & Geller, 2008). The literature also indicates that WP/WPR tend to feel that they must work harder than males to demonstrate their ability and commitment to the profession when their values are called into question, and they are automatically relegated to "mother" rather than physician by their colleagues and superiors (Phillips & Clarke, 2012).

Causes of Work–life Balance Tensions: Inherent Gender Roles and Behaviors

In most articles causes of work–life tensions leading to worse health, poor career outcomes, or non-desired choices of "flexible" specialties included biases against WP/WPR, normative gender roles, and a greater amount of time involved in domestic chores and child care, despite equivalent clinical hours worked (Jolly et al., 2014). Discrimination was a frequent cause of tension, drawing WP/WPR away from otherwise desirable specialties, such as surgery. One particular study of medical students described explicit disdain by medical educators and practicing physicians for women surgeons-to-be because of an assumption of inferior skills and issues of motherhood (Phillips & Clarke, 2012).

A frequent, often implicit, cause of work–life balance tension was the (wrong) timing for parenthood. Thus a recurring theme in the literature was that it would be easier if WP/WPR chose specific times during their training and career to become parents (Potee, Gerber, & Ickovics, 1999). These recommendations were usually presented as an observation, couched in neutral and matter-of-fact language, for instance, the ostensibly straightforward statement that "[t] he optimal timing for parenthood appears to be after the completion of medical training" (Cujec et al., 2000). Neither this nor any article in our sample ever wondered whether optimizing the timing for parenthood was an issue for medical men.

Recommendations to Address Work–life Balance Tensions: "Let Us Teach Them How to Cope"

As to how to deal with work–life balance, a running theme in our sample was the observation that the ability to "think carefully before acting" leads to lesser stress and burnout, thus the recommendation, for WP/WPR, albeit not for their men colleagues, to think carefully before responding to a discriminating, male-dominated work environment, by "monitor[ing] their stress level and address [ing]it productively." (Gautam, 2001). While we wholeheartedly agree with this sound advice for individual cases, the proposed solution to work–life balance tension does not address the source of discrimination. Instead, it offers a seemingly reasonable advice on how to react to it politely and without essentially challenging the norms. Training to develop coping skills, as well as "educating" women, were also suggested as ways to deal with the challenges of work–life balance (Gautam, 2001; Robinson, 2003), as well as the advice to prioritize – example, making intimate relationships a priority – accessing appropriate child care, and hiring outside help for the home in order to help shoulder domestic responsibility (Armstrong, Alvero, Dunlow, Nace, Baker, & Stewart, 2009; Mattessich, Shea, & Whitaker-Worth, 2017; Robinson, 2003; Verlander, 2004). These recommendations were undoubtedly sound (i.e., one enabling child care or the hiring of outside help) yet were all but absent with reference to men physicians, and in themselves did not present a challenge to gendered norms. Moreover, they implicitly assumed a class affiliation that would enable WP/WPR to outsource domestic labor to other women – generally working poor women of color – a strategy that may support the health and well-being of *some* women, but clearly not of women broadly. Indeed, the very proposal of such a strategy speaks to the implicit acceptance of not only of the gendered but also of the class, and likely the racial, hierarchies that the medical profession operates within.

Interestingly, some authors praised WP/WPR who challenge traditional domestic roles and who "appear to be getting better at relinquishing household and childcare tasks to spouses and others" (Robinson, 2003). Again, while it is encouraging that some women challenge traditional roles and managed to relegate traditional women tasks to others, this framing blames the victim, as those women who *fail* to challenge these roles and *fail* to delegate domestic tasks are implicitly blamed for experiencing work–life tensions, while the structural victimizers get a pass. While *individual* challenges in a male-dominated medical world are to be encouraged and may benefit *particular* women, they will not change the structural basis of gender inequities in medical practice.

Yet other articles vaguely suggested that structures and institutions unfavorable to women ought to be challenged, yet stopped short of recommending major changes, calling instead for modest policy changes such as greater support for breastfeeding practices in medical establishments for WP/WPR (Parsons et al., 2009; Sarma et al., 2017).

> [W]orkplaces should strive to create supportive environments for breastfeeding women, and enough flexibility to sustain this practice. (Sarma et al., 2017)

We wholeheartedly support breastfeeding if that is what a woman chooses to do and encourage its support, not only for WP/WPR but for all women in the workforce. That being said, supporting breastfeeding without calling attention to the need to also transform the hierarchical, male-dominated structures and norms pervading the medical profession risks making these structures and norms even more invisible. A notable instance of their invisibility was the case of authors suggesting behavioral adjustments – developing better time management skills, finding supportive spouses, and seeking suitable mentors to work–life problems – that would help WP/WPR to achieve greater work–life balance (Armstrong et al., 2009; Dyrbye et al., 2013; Keeton et al., 2007; Phillips et al., 2016; Strong et al., 2013).

These calls were persuasive as they were framed as collaborative and were paired with suggestions that WP/WPR could build networks of support for women peers (Gautam, 2001; McMurray et al., 2000; Robinson, 2003; Shenoi, 2016; Tarquinio, 2016). Nevertheless, they neglected to indicate, or better still, challenge, why better time management, supportive spouses, or suitable mentors were not required to succeed as a medical *man*. Moreover, these suggestions, while reasonable, are not easy to follow. As indicated by the literature, there are already too few WP/WPR role models and mentors, certainly fewer than men, and the ones who succeed to do so by standards of a male-dominated profession (Mattessich, et al., 2017). Finally, role models and mentors in and of themselves cannot challenge or change the patriarchal normative structure of medicine, and in fact may paradoxically help reproduce them if they "mentor" women to succeed by meeting patriarchal standards.

DISCUSSION

Our findings indicate that WP/WPR work harder to meet clinical benchmarks and societal standards designed for them by men physicians and often reproduced and legitimized by WP/WPR themselves, however, unintentionally. The medical literature largely acknowledges and even critiques the hardships experienced by WP/WPR – including the multiple-role demands affecting their physical and emotional well-being and creating "work–life" balance tensions. Nevertheless, it directly or indirectly downloads the responsibility on women for these hardships, often framing the effects of gendered norms as caused by gender-specific lifestyle and behavioral decisions, using instances of these decisions to illustrate how the choices of WP/WPR lead to career successes or failures. In so doing the literature neglects to challenge, and even legitimizes the male-dominated construction of medical practice. Burnout, depression, tensions with work–life balance, and overall dissatisfaction with life and career are often presented as outcomes of individual choices and circumstances, followed by behavioral suggestions and individual solutions to combat the said challenges. In the meantime, the normative, patriarchal structures built into the practice of medicine remain invisible. The social order, produced by men physicians and maintained by WP/WPR, is legitimized when the latter tacitly consent to male-constructed norms of behavior.

Persuasive notions of empowerment and personal choice facilitate gender inequity by further separating work and domestic responsibilities (Gascoigne, Parry, & Buchanan, 2015), a separation that mostly benefits men physicians. The emphasis is placed on the individual rather than on medical institutions, the profession of medicine, or the state, thus exacerbating the very real conflict between the demands of a medical career and the domestic sphere. Recommendations for amelioration appear to ultimately contribute to the reproduction of patriarchy in medicine. This is because, while well-meaning, the recommendations do not challenge the patriarchal paradigm in the medical profession, a paradigm that in itself is at odds with achieving "work–life" balance, for women *and* men. Calls to address the problem are frequent, yet do not appear to challenge how medical institutions operate, nor do they demand a reconsideration of the social values that are the real sources of conflict. As noted by Waitzkin close to three decades ago (1989), when medical language used is devoid of a critical appraisal of social norms, institutional dynamics and power structures, it becomes a contributor to the reproduction of the status quo. In our case, language contributes to the persistence of patriarchal domination in medical practice.

The phenomenon whereby oppressed social groups contribute to their own domination has been observed in other areas of social life involving matters of health. For instance, research indicates that individuals from populations experiencing high rates of diabetes tended to blame themselves for their "high-risk" status and to propose behavioral solutions (Chaufan, Constantino, & Davis, 2013) and diabetic patients tend to blame themselves for poor treatment outcomes (Chaufan, Fielding, Chesla, & Fernandez, 2015). Similarly, in our current investigation of work–life balance challenges in medical practice, WP/WPR themselves perform the ideological work of patriarchy. Research also indicates the limits of medical discourse to "diagnose" problems beyond the boundaries of medical interventions: in a study of low-income patients with diabetes in an urban teaching hospital, attending physicians who had been trained in the social determinants of health acknowledged that poor treatment outcomes resulted from patients' disadvantaged position yet were unable to articulate solutions beyond the boundaries of the health system (Chaufan, Hong, & Fernandez, 2017).

The language used in academic medical literature by women authors fails to advance the status of women in medicine and often puts the onus of responsibility for dealing with "appropriate" lifestyle choices on WP/WPR themselves. This language largely neglects, when not altogether ignores, a deeper critique of the social and institutional context of the profession of medicine, a profession in which the standards of successful performance are themselves gendered, and therefore *cannot but contribute* to the disadvantaged status of WP/WPR. One such instance calls for institutional support for *maternal* policies yet not *paternal* policies (Mattessich, Shea, & Whitaker-Worth, 2017), a support that further enforces the gender stereotype that not only it is largely women who effectively are responsible for child-rearing and homemaking, but that this is how it *should* be, while the main role of their male counterparts is, and should be, that of breadwinner. Against this background, calls for better, that is, "adaptive," behavioral, and lifestyle choices for WP/WPR overshadow deeper discussions of persisting patriarchal norms, policies, and practices.

Building upon our findings, we propose that the relative privilege that comes with practicing medicine, and likely the class and ethnic background of those women most likely to enter the medical profession, discourages WP/WPR from critiquing the system, leads them to adjust to societal expectations, encourages behavioral explanations for their successes and failures in the medical sphere – a subtle form of self-blame – and has implications, however, inadvertently, for the welfare of more disadvantaged women. Maintaining the status quo and unintentionally supporting a patriarchal system makes it more difficult for future WPs to succeed. Even when women succeed, their success plays into a male-dominated model of "successful physician," as it implicitly mandates that success for WP/WPR requires that they reach the career echelons and benchmarks reached by men. Whether success entails a high-ranking surgical position at a hospital for a single WP/WPR, or the ability to balance a professorship, clinical work and a family, women have learned to maneuvre through a male-created and male-dominated system, and the lesson learned understandably weakens any motivation they may have to critique the system.

Challenges to these standards exist yet are scarce and occur not within but outside the medical literature – in the social sciences. While not in the context of work–life balance, thus not part of our sample, authors in these disciplines recognize the inequities experienced by WP/WPR, yet do not recommend ways to cope or to help them meet *existing* benchmarks. Rather, they *critique* these benchmarks – the structure of medical leadership, organization chairs, and hierarchy in medical academia – and recommend changes toward more collegial orientations in organizational structure and less hierarchical, more collaborative and transparent decision-making (Conrad et al., 2010). The inability of medical discourse to articulate challenges to disease producing, oppressive social structures is not unusual, as illustrated in a critical discourse analysis on the invisibility of poverty as a cause of diabetes, which found the scant challenges to these structures in the boundaries of the medical literature – medical sociology and public health journals (Chaufan & Weitz, 2009).

Our study has limitations. For instance, our scoping databases and leading journals at times produced articles that were not accessible via York University's library. Articles that were not included may have offered information that challenged key findings and components of our argument. Further, our focus was primarily literature produced by medical professionals themselves within the boundaries of peer-reviewed journals – findings might have been different had we included blogs, podcasts, and other forms of media, also produced by medical professionals, yet with potential to harbor more nuanced debates. Additionally, we did not interview WP/WPR to explore in depth their views on patriarchal norms and medicine. Importantly, we did not seek to explore WP/WPR in same-sex relations, what their work–life issues would be, and how they would be handled. We note, however, that the literature rarely mentions such cases, a silence that may be itself revealing issues relevant to work–life balance. In addition, from a global perspective, the literature we investigated represented a narrow segment of WP/WPR. Work–life balance issues in the practice of medicine may reveal significant differences and challenges in other parts of the world, under different political, cultural, and economic contexts.

That being said, we believe that our findings reveal important features of the gendered nature of the medical profession and medical practice, and importantly, *how this nature and practice may be reinforced by women themselves*, even as these features impinge on their own health and well-being. We also believe that our findings can offer fruitful venues for further investigation of structural barriers to women's health and well-being in other settings, contexts, and professions. In the United Kingdom for instance, female students in engineering and technology were found to uphold contradictory views about women in these professions, often believing that women are less suited to succeed yet believing as well that they themselves were equally well prepared as men are to meet benchmarks of success (Powell, Dainty, & Bagilhole, 2012).

PRACTICE, POLICY IMPLICATIONS, AND RECOMMENDATIONS

Ensuring social and health equity among genders in the practice of medicine requires that historically patriarchal practices and attitudes be challenged. A sheer increase of the *number* of WP/WPR in and of itself is unlikely to produce the needed paradigm shift and breakdown of patriarchal standards, especially if women are socialized to perform the ideological work of reproducing these standards. A movement led by women from within the medical community and genuinely supported by their men colleagues is necessary, but unlikely to emerge if both are engaged in the reproduction of gendered inequities, even if this happens at the micro-level of language – never mind policy and practice.

Challenging gendered norms and structures will allow WP/WPR to succeed in the same time frame as their male colleagues, equitably and with realistic expectations. Establishing programs that critique and erode social norms and tradition (Woodrow et al., 2006) are positive steps, but further attention and action are needed. The idea that choices made by WP/WPR may lead to success or failure, while seemingly reasonable, and probably true at the individual level, should be rejected. It is not individual choices, but rather the patriarchal structures of medicine, that shape how men and women practice the profession, and that are responsible for the negative effects experienced by WP/WPR. Even the success of *some* women could paradoxically work against the success of *all* women, if success compels women to follow on the footsteps of men and comply with gendered standards. The continuation of this pattern of disadvantage will harm WP/WPR, as well as their families and patients.

REFERENCES

Armstrong, A., Alvero, R., Dunlow, S., Nace, M., Baker, V., & Stewart, E. (2009). Balancing the professional and personal. *Fertility and Sterility*, *91*(1), 18–21.

Aronson, J. (1995). A pragmatic view of thematic analysis. *The Qualitative Report*, *2*(1), 1–3.

Ash, A., Carr, P., Goldstein, R., & Friedman, R. (2004). Compensation and advancement of women in academic medicine: Is there equity? *Annals of Internal Medicine*, *141*(3), 205–212.

Barnett, R., & Gareis, K. (2002). Full-time and reduced-hours work schedules and marital quality: A study of female physicians with young children. *Work and Occupations*, *29*(3), 364–379.

Beckett, L., Nettiksimmons, J., Howell, L., & Villablanca, A. (2015). Do family responsibilities and a clinical versus research faculty position affect satisfaction with career and work-life balance for medical school faculty? *Journal of Women's Health*, *24*(6), 480–489.

Carnes, M., Morrissey, C., & Geller, S. (2008). Women's health and women's leadership in academic medicine: Hitting the same glass ceiling? *Journal of Women's Health*, *17*(9), 1453–1462.

Chaufan, C., Constantino, S., & Davis, M. (2013). 'You must not confuse poverty with laziness': A case study on the power of discourse to reproduce diabetes inequalities. *International Journal of Health Services*, *43*(1), 143–166.

Chaufan, C., Fielding, H., Chesla, C. A., & Fernandez, A. (2015). "It's not the doctor – it's me": How self blame obscures language and other structural barriers to diabetes care among low-income Latinos with limited English proficiency. *Research in the Sociology of Health Care*, *33*, 187–208.

Chaufan, C., Hong, M.-K., & Fernandez, A. (2017). "Lost in translation": How clinicians make sense of structural barriers to diabetes care among US Latinos with limited English proficiency. *Research in the Sociology of Health Care*, *35*, 127–144.

Chaufan, C., & Weitz, R. (2009). The elephant in the room: The invisibility of poverty in research on type 2 diabetes. *Humanity & Society*, *33*, 74–98.

Clem, K., Promes, S., Glickman, S., Shah, A., Finkel, M., Pietrobon, R., & Cairns, C. (2008). Factors enhancing career satisfaction among female emergency physicians. *Annals of Emergency Medicine*, *51*(6), 723–728.e8.

Conrad, P., Carr, P., Knight, S., Renfrew, M., Dunn, M., & Pololi, L. (2010). Hierarchy as a barrier to advancement for women in academic medicine. *Journal of Women's Health*, *19*(4), 799–805.

Cujec, B., Oancia, T., Bohm, C., & Johnson, D. (2000). Career and parenting satisfaction among medical students, residents and physician teachers at a Canadian medical school. *Canadian Medical Association Journal*, *162*(5), 637–640.

Dunn, P., Arnetz, B., Christensen, J., & Homer, L. (2007). Meeting the imperative to improve physician well-being: Assessment of an innovative program. *Journal of General Internal Medicine*, *22*(11), 1544–1552.

Dyrbye, L., Shanafelt, T., Balch, C., Satele, D., & Freischlag, J. (2010). Physicians married or partnered to physicians: A comparative study in the American college of surgeons. *Journal of the American College of Surgeons*, *211*(5), 663–671.

Dyrbye, L., Sotile, W., Boone, S., West, C., Tan, L., Satele, D., … Shanafelt, T. (2013). A survey of U.S. physicians and their partners regarding the impact of work-home conflict. *Journal of General Internal Medicine*, *29*(1), 155–161.

Dyrbye, L., Varkey, P., Boone, S., Satele, D., Sloan, J., & Shanafelt, T. (2013). Physician satisfaction and burnout at different career stages. *Mayo Clinic Proceedings*, *88*(12), 1358–1367.

Fairclough, N. (2013). *Critical discourse analysis: The critical study of language*. London: Routledge.

Ferris, L., Mackinnon, S., Mizgala, C., & McNeill, I. (1996). Do Canadian female surgeons feel discriminated against as women? *Canadian Medical Association Journal*, *154*(1), 21–27.

Figueroa, M. (2016). Work-life balance does not mean an equal balance. *Frontiers in Pediatrics*, *4*(18), 1–2.

Foucault, M. (1980). *Power/knowledge: Selected interviews and other writings, 1972–1977*. New York, NY: Pantheon Books.

Frank, E., & Dingle, A. (1999). Self-reported depression and suicide attempts among U.S. women physicians. *The American Journal of Psychiatry*, *156*(2), 1887–1894.

Gans, H. J. (1972). The positive functions of poverty. *The American Journal of Sociology*, *78*(2), 275–289.

Gascoigne, C., Parry, E., & Buchanan, D. (2015). Extreme work, gendered work? How extreme jobs and the discourse of 'personal choice' perpetuate gender inequality. *Organization*, *22*(4), 457–475.

Gautam, M. (2001). Women in medicine: Stresses and solutions. *Western Journal of Medicine*, *174*, 37–41.

Guille, C., Frank, E., Zhao, Z., Kalmbach, D., Nietert, P., Mata, D., & Sen, S. (2017). Work-family conflict and the sex difference in depression among training physicians. *Journal of the American Medical Association: Internal Medicine*, *177*(12), 1766–1772.

Harrison, R. (2008). Evolving trends in balancing work and family for future academic physicians: A role for personal stories. *Medical Teacher*, *30*, 316–318.

Heru, A. (2005). Pink-collar medicine: Women and the future of medicine. *Gender Issues*, *22*(1), 20–34.

Jefferson, L., Bloor, K., & Maynard, A. (2015). Women in medicine: Historical perspectives and recent trends. *British Medical Bulletin*, *114*, 5–15.

Jinapriya, D., Cockerill, R., & Trope, G. (2003). Career satisfaction and surgical practice patterns among female ophthalmologists. *Canadian Journal of Ophthalmology*, *38*(5), 373–378.

Jolly, S., Griffith, K., DeCastro, R., Stewart, A., Ubel, A., & Jagsi, R. (2014). Gender differences in time spent on parenting and domestic responsibilities by high-achieving young physician-researchers. *Annals of Internal Medicine*, *160*(5), 344–353.

Jovic, E., Wallace, J., & Lemaire, J. (2006). The generation and gender shifts in medicine: An exploratory survey of internal medicine physicians. *BMC Health Services Research*, *6*(55), 1–10.

Keeton, K., Fenner, D., Johnson, T., & Hayward, R. (2007). Predictors of physician career satisfaction, work-life balance, and burnout. *Obstetrics and Gynecology*, *109*(4), 949–955.

Kuehn, B. (2012). More women choose careers in surgery: Bias, work-life issues remain challenges. *Journal of the American Medical Association*, *307*(18), 1899–1901.

Luke, A. (1997). Theory and practice in critical discourse analysis. In L. Saha (Ed.), *International encyclopaedia of the sociology of education* (pp. 50–56). Oxford: Pergamon.

Marschall, J., & Karimuddin, A. (2003). Decline in popularity of general surgery as a career choice in North America: Review of postgraduate residency training selection in Canada, 1996–2001. *World Journal of Surgery*, *27*, 249–252.

Mattessich, S., Shea, K., & Whitaker-Worth, D. (2017). Parenting and female dermatologists' perceptions of work-life balance. *International Journal of Women's Dermatology*, *3*, 127–130.

Merchant, S., Hameed, S., & Melck, A. (2013). Pregnancy among residents enrolled in general surgery: A nationwide survey of attitudes and experiences. *The American Journal of Surgery, 206*(4), 605–610.

McMurray, J., Linzer, M., Konrad, T., Douglas, J., Shugerman, R., & Nelson, K. (2000). The work lives of women physicians: Results from the physician work life study. *Journal of General Internal Medicine, 15*, 372–380.

Micieli, J., Trope, G., & Buys, Y. (2016). Gender gap and declining surgical activity among new graduates: Cataract surgery in Ontario. *Canadian Journal of Ophthalmology, 51*(3), 154–169.

Miller, A. (2011). The effects of motherhood timing on career path. *Journal of Population Economics, 24*(3), 1071–1100.

Mobilos, S., Chan, M., & Brown, J. (2008). Women in medicine: The challenge of finding balance. *Canadian Family Physician, 54*, 1285–1286.e5.

Navarro, V. (1980). Work, ideology, and science: The case of medicine. *International Journal of Health Services, 10*(4), 523–550.

Office of Research and Information Services. (2015). *Canadian medical education statistics 2015* (Vol. 37, pp. 9–32). Ottawa: The Association of Faculties of Medicine of Canada.

Parsons, W., Duke, P., Snow, P., & Edwards, A. (2009). Physicians as parents: Parenting experiences of physicians in Newfoundland and Labrador. *Canadian Family Physician, 55*, 808–809.e4.

Perlman, R., Ross, P., & Lypson, M. (2015). Having it all: Medicine and a family. *Mayo Clinic Proceedings, 90*(6), 713–715.

Phillips, S., & Clarke, M. (2012). More than an education: The hidden curriculum, professional attitudes and career choice. *Medical Education, 45*, 887–893.

Phillips, J., Hustedde, C., Bjorkman, S., Prasad, R., Sola, O., Wendling, A., … Paladine, H. (2016). Rural women family physicians: Strategies for successful work-life balance. *Annals of Family Medicine, 14*(3), 244–251.

Potee, R., Gerber, A., & Ockovics, J. (1999). Medicine and motherhood: Shifting trends among female physicians from 1922 to 1999. *Academic Medicine, 74*(8), 911–919.

Powell, A., Dainty, A., & Bagilhole, B. (2012). Gender stereotypes among women engineering and technology students in the UK: Lessons from career choice narratives. *European Journal of Engineering Education, 37*(6), 541–556.

Raja, S., & Stein, S. (2014). Work-life balance: History, costs, and budgeting for balance. *Clinics in Colon and Rectal Surgery, 27*(2), 71–74.

Reed, V., & Buddeberg-Fischer, B. (2001). Career obstacles for women in medicine: An overview. *Medical Education, 35*, 139–147.

Roberts, D., Shanafelt, T., Dyrbye, L., & West, C. (2014). A national comparison of burnout and work-life balance among internal medicine hospitalists and outpatient general internists. *Journal of Hospital Medicine, 9*(3), 176–181.

Robinson, G. (2003). Stresses on women physicians: Consequences and coping techniques. *Depression and Anxiety, 17*, 180–189.

Sandler, B., Tackett, J., Longo, W., & Yoo, P. (2016). Pregnancy and parenthood among surgery residents: Results of the first nationwide survey of general surgery residency program directors. *Journal of the American College of Surgeons, 222*(6), 1091–1098.

Schwingshackl, A. (2014). The fallacy of chasing after work-life balance. *Frontiers in Pediatrics, 2*(26), 1–3.

Shanafelt, T., Boone, S., Tan, L., Dyrbye, L., Sotile, W., Satele, D., … Oreskovich, M. (2012). Burnout and satisfaction with work-life balance among US physicians relative to the general US population. *Archives of Internal Medicine, 172*(18), 1377–1385.

Shanafelt, T., Raymond, M., Kosty, M., Satele, D., Horn, L., Pippen, J., … Gradishar, W. (2014). Satisfaction with work-life balance and the career and retirement plans of US oncologists. *Journal of Clinical Oncology, 32*(11), 1127–1136.

Shanafelt, T., Hasan, O., Dyrbye, L., Sinsky, C., Satele, D., Sloan, J., & West, C. (2015). Changes in burnout and satisfaction with work-life balance in physicians and general US working population between 2011 and 2014. *Mayo Clinic Proceedings, 90*(12), 1600–1613.

Shanafelt, T., Hasan, O., Hayes, S., Sinsky, C., Satele, D., Sloan, J., … Dyrbye, L. (2016). Parental satisfaction of U.S. physicians: Associated factors and comparison with the general U.S. working population. *BMC Medical Education*, *16*(228), 1–10.

Shenoi, A. (2016). Unbalanced but satisfied? *Frontiers in Pediatrics*, *3*(120), 1–3.

Sonnad, S., & Colletti, L. (2002). Issues in the recruitment and success of women in academic surgery. *Surgery*, *132*, 415–419.

Stentz, N., Griffith, K., Perkins, E., DeCastro Jones, R., & Jagsi, R. (2016). Fertility and childbearing among American female physicians. *Journal of Women's Health*, *25*(10), 1059–1065.

Strong, E., DeCastro, R., Sambuco, D., Stewart, A., Ubel, P., Griffith, K., & Jagsi, R. (2013). Work-life balance in academic medicine: Narratives of physician-researchers and their mentors. *Journal of General Internal Medicine*, *28*(12), 1596–1603.

Szender, J., Grzankowski, K., Eng, K., Odunsi, K., & Frederick, P. (2016). Evaluation of satisfaction with work-life balance among U.S. gynecologic oncology fellows: A cross–sectional study. *Gynecologic Oncology Reports*, *16*, 17–20.

Tarquinio, K. (2016). Work-life balance? It is not about balance, but priorities. *Frontiers in Pediatrics*, *4*(6), 1–3.

Uhlenberg, P., & Cooney, T. (1990). Male and female physicians: Family and career comparisons. *Social Science and Medicine*, *30*(3), 373–378.

Valian, V. (1999). *Why so slow? The advancement of women*. Cambridge, MA: MIT Press.

van Dijk, T. (1993). Principles of critical discourse analysis. *Discourse and Society*, *4*(2), 249–283.

Verlander, G. (2004). Female physicians: Balancing career and family. *Academic Psychiatry*, *28*(4), 331–336.

Waitzkin, H. (1989). A critical theory of medical discourse: Ideology, social control, and the processing of social context in medical encounters. *Journal of Health and Social Behavior*, *30*(2), 220–239.

Wang, T. (2015). Work-life balance: Hopeless endeavour or rather, a true privilege? *Frontiers in Pedatrics*, *3*(99), 1–3.

Woodrow, S., Gilmer-Hill, H., & Rutka, J. (2006). The neurosurgical workforce in North America: A critical review of gender issues. *Neurosurgery*, *59*, 749–758.

VULNERABLE CAREGIVERS: A COMPARISON OF DIRECT CARE WORKERS' HEALTH RISKS IN SKILLED NURSING FACILITIES AND PRIVATE HOMES

Kim Price-Glynn and Carter Rakovski

ABSTRACT

Purpose – *This chapter explores variation in direct care workers' health risks within institutional and home-based settings, according to the demographic composition of workers and the gendered, raced, and citizenship-based expressions of their work roles.*

Methodology/Approach – *This quantitative intersectional study draws on two nationwide datasets from the US National Center for Long-term Care Statistics, a division of the Centers for Disease Control and Prevention, the National Nursing Assistant Study (NNAS), and National Home Health Aide Survey (NHHAS).*

Findings – *Workplace context was the strongest predictor of workers' health risks and working conditions. Physical injuries affected more than half of facility-based workers annually compared to less than 10% of home-based workers. Facility-based workers are more likely to report insufficient time for tasks, lower job satisfaction, and less respect and appreciation from patients. Home-based workers may be more likely to experience emotional distress, be offered fewer benefits, but experience fewer injuries, due to the better relative health of their patients and having more time for client care. Women reported*

Underserved and Socially Disadvantaged Groups and Linkages with Health and Health Care Differentials
Research in the Sociology of Health Care, Volume 37, 225–238

ISSN: 0275-4959/doi:10.1108/S0275-495920190000037018

more injuries and more time pressure than men across racial and citizenship groups within the same work setting.

Research Limitations/Implications – *There are limitations to the NHHAS and NNAS public-release data file data. We are unable to fully capture citizenship, some racial/ethnic categories, workers over age 65, supervisory workers, facilities with fewer than three residents, and facilities not certified with Medicare or Medicaid. The exclusion of these questions, workers, and contexts is a weakness of the present study.*

Originality/Value of Paper – *Analyses draw on data from the first nationally representative sample surveys of home health aides and nursing assistants in the United States. Direct care workers are an important population to capture through intersectional research since care work is done predominantly by multiracial women and immigrants. This research also underscores the importance of workplace contexts in shaping the labor performed and the workers' experiences.*

Keywords: Care work; nursing assistant; home health aid; workplace risks; intersectionality

INTRODUCTION

Caring labor is essential throughout the life course. For the aged and those with short and long-term disabilities, care work takes place through home health agencies and care institutions, like hospitals and nursing homes. Though care work varies considerably by location and organization, workers typically describe their jobs as both rewarding and challenging. Care work rewards stem from the intrinsic significance of caring for others (Stacey, 2005). Care work challenges stem from the often hurried pace of physically and emotionally demanding work performed for low wages (Duffy, 2005, 2007; Stacey, 2005).

In the United States, people are living longer, expanding the need for caregiving. For many scholars studying care work, US care needs at the end and beginnings of the life course constitute a national (and increasingly global) crisis in care. Particularly for currently aging baby-boomers, projections are that US direct care worker (DCW) jobs will grow "faster than the average for all occupations" over the next decade (BLS, 2018). DCW jobs are unlikely to be lost to relocation or automation. These jobs require a human touch.

In *Making Gray Gold* (1995), Timothy Diamond's moving study of institutionalized elder care, his vocational school administrator began class by saying, "welcome to the firing line of health care" (p. 13). While he was referencing the *front lines* of health care delivery, this military metaphor also captures how care workers occupy a dangerous position near an adversary. The question is who or what fosters this adversarial condition – is it the workplace administrators, workplace setting, clients, or broader cultural norms?

This chapter explores the variation in DCW health risks by setting, according to the sex and race composition of workers and the gendered and raced expressions of their work roles, as well as their citizenship status. In addition to demographic considerations, DCWs face many workplace hazards in terms of the labor performed as well as the workplace context. Work risks include: care related injuries, physical and emotional trauma, and contact with environmental toxins and diseases from clients. Workers' differing risks for negative physical and emotional health outcomes are setting dependent and vary depending on whether they are performed in skilled nursing facilities or in private homes (Price-Glynn & Rakovski, 2015). By exploring the risks associated with DCW jobs we hope to address how these workers' vulnerabilities can be addressed and mitigated.

Our analyses draw on data from the US National Center for Long Term Care Statistics, a division of the Centers for Disease Control and Prevention, National Nursing Assistant Study (NNAS) (Bercovitz et al., 2011; Squillace et al., 2009) and National Home Health Aide Survey (NHHAS). The NNAS provides nationally representative data that includes the nature and risks associated with DCWs in skilled nursing facilities, as well as the demographics of the nearly 3,000 workers surveyed. The NHHAS examines home-based DCWs using 582 agencies across the United States.

LITERATURE REVIEW

Caring labor performed by DCWs entails both nurturant and non-nurturant reproductive labor (Duffy, 2005). Nurturant caregiving relationships are face-to-face and often emotionally and physically intimate (Duffy, 2005; England, 2005; Himmelweit, 1999). DCWs help clients with nurturant activities of daily living (ADL), such as dressing, bathing, eating, transferring, and toileting. Non-nurturant, reproductive labor is also required, including house cleaning, grocery shopping, and food preparation, particularly for private home workers.

Care work, generally, has been culturally defined as women's work, though it can be performed by anyone. Despite being skilled work that is not easily outsourced to other places or to technology, DCW jobs are not well compensated and workers face a number of challenges. A vast majority of DCWs are women (about 90% in the United States). The extreme gender segregation of the work contributes to the perception that it is unskilled, performed naturally, and intrinsically rewarding, rather than for money (Hays, 1996; Palmer & Eveline, 2012).

Like other workplaces, research has documented the ways in which DCW workplaces reproduce social hierarchies found in the broader culture (Price-Glynn & Rakovski, 2012). DCWs are diverse in terms of their race, nationality, and citizenship (Rakovski & Price-Glynn, 2010). Nursing facilities foster inter-occupational racial and gender stratification, with African American nurses performing disproportionate amounts of "dirty work" compared to their White colleagues (Duffy, 2007). Male African American nurses are stereotyped by their race and gender and perceived by others as less well suited for patient care and have reported difficulty in gaining seniority (Harvey Wingfield, 2009). White men nurses, by contrast, advance more quickly to more prestigious and better-paid nursing positions (Price-Glynn & Rakovski, 2012; Wingfield, 2009). Immigrant DCWs, many of whom come from marginalized countries in the global south, vary considerably in terms of their circumstances and access to economic and cultural resources (Arends-Kuenning, 2006; Portes, 1993). Previous research drawing on the NNAS found that immigrant DCWs were more likely working in urban, large-scale facilities, and reported significantly less respect from residents and families, but not supervisors (Sloane, Williams, & Zimmerman, 2010). Given variations by gender, race, nationality, and citizenship, analyses that examine multiple facets of identity simultaneously are likely to more accurately capture DCW employment.

Risks associated with caring labor stem from the kinds of labor performed as well as the context and circumstances therein. Some of the risks faced by DCWs are inherent to emotional labor, such as alienation and bodywork (England & Dyck, 2011; Hochschild, 1979; Kang, 2010). Clients may also present risks to workers including: musculoskeletal pain and injuries from lifting patients; exposure to drugs and chemicals; contact with infectious diseases; emotional stress from traumatic situations and client deaths; as well as physical and verbal assaults from clients (Miranda, Punnett, Gore, & Boyer, 2011; Sophie, Belza, & Young, 2003). Some circumstances workers faced are conditional and not inherent to the work: inadequate staffing, worker turnover, low wages/benefits, long hours, unpaid work, night shifts, and discrimination by administrators and clients (Brannon, Zinn, Mor, & Davis, 2002; Castle, Endberg, Anderson, & Men, 2007; Diamond, 1992; Dodson & Zincavage, 2007; Foner, 1994; Gass, 2004; Harrington et al., 2000).

Context shapes the organization of care work. There is a higher chance of physical injury in skilled nursing facilities than in private homes (Price-Glynn & Rakovski, 2015). Institutions have a faster pace of work, higher institutional demands, longer hours, and sicker clients. There may be an increased risk for mental strain, such as secondary traumatic stress, in private homes than in hospitals. Risks for direct care workers based in private homes are not as well documented as those in skilled nursing facilities, but are likely different due to the unpredictable private home context, differences in the tasks preformed, and better relative health of home-based patients (Price-Glynn & Rakovski, 2015). Home-based workers are at risk of exploitation through invisibility and distancing that justifies low pay and preserves the dignity and perceived independence of clients (Hondagneu-Sotelo, 2007; Rivas, 2003; Solari, 2006; Stacey, 2005). DCWs working independently in client's homes may experience isolation that comes from working alone (Froymovich, 2007). Home-based work may also include cooking, cleaning, and grocery shopping – the catch-all combination of caring labor provides few boundaries around caregivers' work (Stacey, 2005). Moreover, workers are encouraged by supervisors to use family metaphors when thinking about clients to foster more intimacy and connectedness in their caregiving, blurring the boundaries between care work as paid employment or as something more freely exchanged, as in families (Berdes & Eckert, 2007). The family metaphor is deliberately used as a strategy by employers to extract more emotional and physical labor from DCWs without increasing monetary compensation or worker benefits (Berdes & Eckert, 2007). Despite the family rhetoric, the exchange of care mostly flows only one way.

METHOD

Analyses draw on data from the first nationally representative sample surveys of home health aides and nursing assistants in the US, the NHHAS and the NNAS (Bercovitz et al., 2011; Squillace et al., 2009). The Centers for Disease Control and Prevention's National Center for Health Statistics in conjunction with the Department of Health and Human Services' Office of the Assistant Secretary for Planning and Evaluation (ASPE) sponsored the surveys to evaluate issues related to worker satisfaction and retention. The NNAS, a two-stage probability sample survey, was a supplement to the 2004 National Nursing Home Survey (NNHS). NHHAS was modeled after the NNAS to be its equivalent with home health aides in 2007. The first stage was the sampling of facilities (NNAS, $n =$ 790) and agencies (NHHAS, $n = 955$), and the second stage was the sampling of workers (NNAS, $n = 2{,}909$; NHHAS, $n = 2{,}707$). Aides who worked in agencies that participated in the facility surveys and who provided ADL assistance (i.e., direct patient care) were sampled and interviewed using computer-assisted telephone interviewing in either English or Spanish.

Drawing on Leslie McCall's work, we use existing analytical categories to examine relationships and inequalities within and between social groups (McCall, 2005). Despite the strengths of the sampling methods and data collection procedures, the NHHAS does not include some variables in the public-release data file. For example, citizenship status was not released and its exclusion is a weakness of the present study. Few intersectional identities can be studied using the NHHAS. In both surveys, race included three categories: White, Black, and other. Asian is also included in the NNAS. In the NHHAS Asian was not an option in the survey questions on race. Latinx was asked as a separate ethnic category. Age was limited at the upper end (65 years and older).

Our analysis is limited to NNAS non-supervisory workers with available current job data and NHHAS home-based workers. Aides working at agencies not included in the NHHCS or NNHS are not eligible for inclusion. The NNAS did not reach aides who worked in facilities with fewer than three residents, or those not certified with Medicare or Medicaid. Further details of the sampling and data collection can be found at https://www.cdc.gov/nchs/nnhs/nnas.htm.

Individual characteristics, such as demographics, income, and education, and organization characteristics, such as facility type and location, were tabulated for facility-based workers (NNAS) and home-based workers (NHHAS). Working conditions, satisfaction with work, and benefits were tabulated for workers by setting, based on individual survey items.

Reproductive labor measures draw on sets of survey items. Time for tasks was measured by the following questions: "During a typical work week, how much time do you have to give individual attention to residents with ADL assistance?" and "During a typical work week, how much time do you have to complete other duties not directly related to residents?" Organizational support for care work was measured by questions such as, "Are you assigned to care for the same residents on most days that you work?" and "In general, does supervisor encourage you to discuss the care and well-being of residents with their families?" Survey questions also included measures of workers-client relationships. The percentage of workers who were supported in their caring labor was calculated for each setting. To determine whether categorical variables, such as job satisfaction, were significantly different for the two groups of workers, chi-square tests were used.

FINDINGS

Worker Characteristics

Worker characteristics are compiled in Table 1. Facility-based workers (n = 2,909) were from the NNAS, whereas home-based workers (n = 2,077) were from the NHHAS. The overwhelming majority of direct care workers across both samples were women, with slightly more women employed in homes (94.4%) than in institutions (92.3%). Given the greater compensation (pay and benefits) in institutional settings, it is not surprising that men comprise a greater number (7.7%) of those workers. Workers across settings were diverse with slightly over half identifying as White. Home-based workers were older (mean age = 46) and more likely to be citizens (94.2%) than facility-based workers (mean age = 38; 90.7% of citizens). A little over half of all workers across both settings received public assistance, currently or in the past. Home-based workers worked fewer hours per week, had the fewest benefits, but reported higher household incomes than facility-based workers. Total household income differences may be partly due to inflation (the NNAS was conducted in 2004 and NHHAS in 2007); however, they also suggest that home-based workers have access to other household financial support. Home-based workers were also more likely to be employed by for-profit agencies in urban areas.

Working Conditions

The care work context is important. Table 2 details working conditions across both settings. Both groups of workers overwhelmingly expressed satisfaction with their work (88% of home-based and 81.6% of facility-based workers). On-the-job injuries were reported far more in facilities (56.2%) than in homes (8.6%). These percentages indicate one or more on-the-job injuries in the past year that were reported to a supervisor, needed medical attention, or caused the worker to miss work. The large gap in injury prevalence may stem from caring for facility-based patients, who have more serious health-related concerns than clients well enough to live at home. By definition, clients receiving facility care need help with at least two of the four ADLs, which means caregivers perform more lifting and transferring. Injuries are most likely to occur when workers are rushed. Under time constraints, caregivers are less likely to use lifting equipment or wait for another worker to become available to help with a lift (Sophie et al., 2003). Over 40% of facility-based workers report that they lack sufficient time to

Table 1. Worker Characteristics by Setting NNAS ($n = 2{,}909$) NHHAS ($n = 2{,}077$).[a]

	Facility-based Workers % or Mean (SE)	Home-based Workers % or Mean (SE)
Individual characteristics		
Women	92.3	94.4
Ethnicity		
Latino/Latina	9.4	8.9
Race		
Black	38.8	37.6
White	53.3	51.7
Other racial group	7.9	10.8
Citizenship		
Not a US citizen[b]	9.3	5.8
Age[c]	38.4 (0.3)	46.3 (0.7)
High school graduate	87.7	87.4
Household characteristics		
Ever received public assistance	56.7	56.4
Total household income (US)		
<$20,000	37.5	23.2
$20,000 to < $30,000	28.1	28.2
$30,000 to < $40,000	14.2	20.8
$40,000 to < $50,000	10.0	11.8
> $50,000	10.2	16.1
NA cares for family/friend with disability or health problem	15.3	20.0
Children living at home	58.7	48.0
Organization type and location		
For-profit facility or agency	58.5	88.9
Chain affiliation	54.1	51.5
Metropolitan location	75.9	82.9

Notes: [a]Data sources are the National Nursing Assistant Survey (NNAS, 2004) and the National Home Health Aide Survey (NHHAS, 2007). Sample sizes for individual characteristics are sometimes smaller. The following responses were treated as missing: don't know, refused, and not ascertained. Percentages are reported for non-missing cases.

[b]Citizenship status was not released in the public-use data for NHHAS. The estimate is from the NHHAS report (Bercovitz et al., 2007).

[c]Age was coded as 65 when age was 65 or greater in the NNAS data. Therefore, mean age reported here is lower than it should be.

Table 2. Working Conditions by Setting: Facility (NNAS, $n = 2{,}909$), Home (NHHAS, $n = 2{,}077$).[a,b]

	Facility-based Workers %	Home-based Workers %
Satisfaction with current job		
Extremely satisfied	30.1	47.6
Somewhat satisfied	51.5	40.4
Somewhat dissatisfied	14.6	9.9
Extremely dissatisfied	3.7	2.1
Injuries on the job		
Injured in the past year	56.2	8.6
Time for tasks		
Not enough time to assist patients[c]	42.6	5.3
Not enough time for other duties[d]	43.8	12.1
Organizational support		
Encouraged to talk with family members about patient's health and well-being	28.8	55.1
Usually care for the same patients	47.1	86.7
Supervisor respects worker as part of health care team[e]	58.0	78.8
Supervisor tells worker doing a good job[e]	52.9	77.6
Supervisor supportive of career progress[e]	48.0	80.2
Relationships with patients		
Patients respect worker as part of health care team[e]	71.7	92.1
Patients tell worker doing a good job[e]	72.2	90.7
Benefits and training		
Health insurance available	89.7	71.4
Training prepared worker well for job	66.2	83.3

Notes: [a]Data are from the Centers for Disease Control (cdc.gov), specifically the National Nursing Assistant Survey (NNAS, 2004) and the National Home Health Aide Survey (NHHAS, 2007). Sample sizes for individual characteristics are sometimes smaller. The following responses were treated as missing: don't know, refused, and not ascertained. Percentages are reported for non-missing cases.

[b]The two samples were tested for statistical differences on each of the reported items using Chi-square tests. All items were significantly different at the $p < 0.001$ level.

[c]Not enough time to assist patients with activities of daily living, such as bathing, eating, dressing, and transferring.

[d]Not enough time for other duties that do not directly involve the patients, such as food preparation, making beds, cleaning, laundry, or record keeping.

[e]Percentages are given for responses that were the most positive (a great deal, always or most of the time, and strongly agree).

assist patients (42.6%) and complete other duties (43.8%). The most commonly cited cause of injuries was "lifting, reposition, bathing, handling patients, and/or bumping or hitting equipment." The most common type of injury was back pain, pulled back muscle, or other muscle strain.

Across all measures, home-based workers reported more workplace support than facility workers. More home-based patients tell DCWs they are doing a good job more than do facility-based clients (92.1% vs 71.7%). A similar pattern emerges for supervisors of home-based compared to facility-based workers (77.6% vs 52.9%). Home-based DCWs also reported that their training prepared them well for their employment.

Injuries

Intersectional injury results by context are found in Table 3. Almost across the board, women are more likely to report injuries than men. In facilities, White women were the most likely to be injured (66.7%) about 10% higher than White men (56.9%). For citizens, women were injured at about a 5% higher rate than men, and this gap widens to nearly 15% for noncitizen women and men (52.0% and 34.3%, respectively) and for Asian women and men (50.8% and 33.3%, respectively). The gender imbalance did not hold for Black, Latinx, and other groups. Men who identified as Other racial group reported the highest injury rate (72%), although this sample size is small ($n = 11$).

Among home-based workers, intersectional analysis showed again that men were injured less frequently than women across groups. Women's injury rates ranged between about 15% and 20%. Black women at 13.1% were on the low end, and women identifying as Other were on the high end at 22.3%. Men's injury rates ranged from about 5 to 15% (6.3% Black and other to 15% White). Workplace setting was more important than sex or race in understanding injury rates. Even the group with the highest injury rate within the home setting could not approach the group with the lowest injury rate in facilities.

Table 3. Percentage of Workers with Injuries in the Past Year by Identity and Setting: Facility (NNAS, n = 2,814), Home (NHHAS, n = 2,077).[a,b]

Setting	White %	Black %	Asian %	Other	Latinx[a] %	Citizen %	Noncitizen %
Facility							
Male	56.9	45.2	33.3	72.7	63.0	55.6	34.3
Female	66.7	46.7	50.8	66.4	59.6	60.4	52.0
Home							
Male	15.5			6.3 [c]	10.0		
Female	20.0	13.1		22.3 [d]	16.9		

Notes: [a]NNAS Sample size for Latinx (n = 2,804).
[b]NNAS Sample size for citizenship (n = 2,811); NHHAS citizenship data not available.
[c]NHHAS Black and Other male participants combined due to small sample size (n = 32).
[d]NHHAS Asian was not an option in the NHHAS survey questions on race or ethnicity.

Time for Tasks

Having enough time to complete tasks is an important indicator of both working conditions and risk of injury. Intersectional analysis of time for tasks is outlined in Table 4. Reports of dissatisfaction with the pace of work were most common among women across almost all categories. White women in facilities had the highest reports of not having enough time for tasks (ADLs 48.9% and other tasks 47.9%). Among home-based workers these pressures were felt most by Black women (15.5%) and Latinas (16.2%) who more often report having not enough time for tasks than other groups of workers.

Like injuries, facility-based workers had dramatically worse outcomes across all groups than home-based workers. There was only one case of overlap between the most pressured home workers (16.2% of Latinas not having enough time for other tasks) and the least pressured facility workers (13.3% of Asian men not having enough time for ADLs). Generally, the workers across settings were not at all close in terms of having enough time for their work. Facility workers also worked longer hours. They were employed on average approximately 38 hours per week, compared with roughly 30 hours per week for home-based workers (Table 2). The harried pace of work and time pressures add to other challenging circumstances of facility-based workers, namely, youth, poverty, increased parenthood responsibilities, and more frequent uncertainty due to non-citizenship status.

CONCLUSION

Results from this analysis suggest that identity characteristics like country of origin matter and underscore the importance of examining identity using a multifaceted approach that considers not just race, ethnicity, and gender but also citizenship, intersectionally. DCWs are an important population to capture through intersectional research since care work is done predominantly by multiracial women and immigrants (Misra, 2003). Intersectional analysis shows patterns for both facility and home-based workers – Whites, women, and citizens are more likely to report injuries than minorities, men, and non-citizens. These findings for DCWs support some of the internal hierarchies at the intersections of gender, race, ethnicity, and nationality found among other care workers (Duffy, 2005; Duffy, 2007; Nakano Glenn, 1992). Previous research has documented discrimination against African American DCWs from clients and families (Dodson & Zincavage, 2007). Nursing facilities foster inter-occupational racial and gender stratification compared to their White colleagues (Duffy, 2007). Institutional discrimination and interpersonal prejudice may keep minorities from systematically reporting injuries as more empowered groups do.

While the majority of direct care workers are women, there may also be gendered differences that are better captured through intersectional analysis. Normatively care work is defined as women's work – labor that is seen as unskilled and performed naturally rather than for money (Hays, 1996; Palmer & Eveline, 2012). Subject to prevailing gender norms that value men's strength and

Table 4. Percentage of Workers with Not Enough Time For Tasks by Identity and Setting: Facility (NNAS, $n = 2{,}814$), Home (NHHAS, $n = 2{,}077$).

	White		Black		Asian		Other		Latinx		Citizen		Noncitizen	
Setting Facility	% ADL	% Other	% ADL	% Other	% ADL	% Other	% ADL	% Other	% ADL	% Other	% ADL	% Other	% ADL	% Other
Male	39.8	39.0	26.7	29.3	13.3	26.7	36.4	36.4	22.2	18.5	34.8	34.8	26.3	34.2
Female	48.9	47.9	36.7	38.6	23.1	27.3	42.7	44.9	39.9	39.5	44.6	45.1	37.3	30.6
Home														
Male	4.3	10.4					9.4	7.1	0.0	0.0				
Female	3.8	10.6	6.0	15.5			4.8	12.9	7.1	16.2				

Note: For home health workers, Latino ($n = 10$), Black and other men combined ($n = 28$); For facility health workers, Asian men ($n = 15$), Other men ($n = 11$).

competence, men may be more likely to minimize ailments and refrain from injury reporting.

Citizenship status and country of origin may be significant to workers' experiences. Non-citizens may feel more vulnerable to deportation and less able to disclose their concerns. That may explain non-citizens lower injury reporting than citizens, despite simultaneously indicating that they do not have enough time for ADLs and other tasks. Qualitative research could uncover whether differences in rates of injuries and job satisfaction could be explained by differences in social comparisons or with perceived alternate work options available to citizens and non-citizens.

The caring context matters. Home settings may provide both benefits and drawbacks to workers who experience more protection from risk of physical injury and simultaneously less protection from racism than institutionally based workers. The independence and autonomy workers may experience caring for relatively healthier clients in private homes may also lead to isolation and invisibility from other workers and supervisors. Decreasing isolation and supporting workers over clients in some critical situations could mitigate the risks of home care work. Conversely, DCWs working in institutions may be at greater relative risk of physical injury due to sicker patients with greater needs, frequent insufficient staffing levels, and a fast pace of work.

REFERENCES

Arends-Kuenning, M. (2006). The balance of care: Trends in employment of immigrant nurses in the US between 1990 and 2000. *Globalizations*, *3*(3), 333–348.

Bercovitz, A., Moss, A., Sengupta, M., Park-Lee, E. Y., Jones, A., Harris-Kojetin, L. D., & Squillace, M. R. (2011). An overview of home health aides, 2007. *National health statistics reports*. US Department of Health and Human Services: Centers for disease control and Prevention National Center for Health Statistics.

Berdes, C., & Eckert, J. M. (2007). The language of caring: Nurse aides' use of family metaphors conveys affective care. *The Gerontologist*, *47*, 340–349.

Brannon, D., Zinn, J., Mor, V., & Davis, J. (2002). An exploration of job, organizational, and environmental factors associated with high and low nursing assistant turnover. *The Gerontologist*, *42*, 159–168.

Bureau of Labor Statistics. (2018). U.S. Department of Labor, *Occupational outlook handbook*. Retrieved from https://www.bls.gov/ooh/healthcare/nursing-assistants.htm. Accessed on June 26, 2018.

Castle, N. G., Endberg, J., Anderson, R., & Men, A. (2007). Job satisfaction of nurse aids in nursing homes: Intent to leave and turnover. *The Gerontologist*, *47*, 193–204.

Diamond, T. (1992). *Making gray gold: Narratives of nursing home care*. Chicago, IL: University of Chicago Press.

Dodson, L., & Zincavage, R. (2007). 'It's like a family': Caring labour, exploitation, and race in nursing homes. *Gender & Society*, *21*, 905–928.

Duffy, M. (2005). Reproducing labor inequalities: Challenges for feminist conceptualizing care at the intersections of gender, race and class. *Gender & Society*, *19*, 66–82.

Duffy, M. (2007). Doing the dirty work: Gender, race and reproductive labor in historical perspective. *Gender & Society*, *21*, 313–336.

England, P. (2005). Emerging theories of carework. *Annual Review of Sociology*, *31*, 381–399.

England, K., & Dyck, I. (2011). Managing the body work of home care. *Sociology of Health and Illness*, *33*, 206–219.

Foner, N. (1994). *The caregiving dilemma: Working in an American nursing home*. Berkeley, CA: University of California Press.

Froymovich, E. (2007). How managers can retain qualified in-home caregivers in a competitive job market. *Home Health Care Management and Practice*, *19*, 169–173.

Gass, T. E. (2004). *Nobody's home: Candid reflections of a nursing home aide*. Ithaca, NY: Cornell University Press.

Harrington, C., Kovner, C., Mezey, M., Kayser-Jones, J., Burger, S., & Mohler, M., (2000). Experts recommend minimum nurse staffing standards for nursing facilities in the United States. *The Gerontologist*, *40*, 5–16.

Hays, S. (1996). *The cultural contradictions of motherhood*. New Haven, CT: Yale University Press.

Himmelweit, S. (1999). Caring labor: Emotional labor in the service economy. *Annals of the American Academy of Political and Social Science*, *561*, 27–38.

Hochschild, A. (1979). *The managed heart: Commercialization of human feeling*. Berkeley, CA: University of California.

Hondagneu-Sotelo, P. (2007). *Domestica: Immigrant workers cleaning and caring in the shadows of affluence*. Berkeley, CA: University of California Press.

Kang, M. (2010). *The managed hand: Race, gender, and the body in beauty service work*. Berkeley, CA: University of California Press.

McCall, L. (2005). The complexity of intersectionality. *Signs: Journal of Women in Society*, *30*, 1771–1800.

Miranda, H., Punnett, L., Gore, R., & Boyer, J. (2011). Violence at the workplace increases risk of musculoskeletal pain among nursing home workers. *Occupational and Environmental Medicine*, *68*, 52–57.

Misra, J. (2003). Caring about care. *Feminist Studies*, *29*, 387–401.

Nakano Glenn, E. (1992). From servitude to service work: Historical continuities in the racial division of paid reproductive labor. *Signs*, *18*, 1–43.

Palmer, E., & Eveline, J. (2012). Sustaining low pay in aged care work. *Gender, Work and Organization*, *19*(3), 254–275.

Portes, A. (1993). Embeddedness and immigration: Notes on the social determinants of economic action. *American Journal of Sociology*, *98*(6), 1320–1350.

Price-Glynn, K., & Rakovski, C. (2012). Who rides the glass escalator? Gender, race and nationality in the national nursing assistant study (NNAS). *Work, Employment & Society*, *26*(5), 699–715.

Price-Glynn, K., & Rakovski, C.. (2015). The best of both worlds? How direct care workers perceive home health agencies and long-term care institutions. In M. Duffy, A. Armenia, & C. Stacey (Eds.), *Caring on the clock: The complexities and contradictions of paid care work, Part II: The contexts of care, Chapter 3* (pp. 31–41). New Brunswick, NJ: Rutgers University Press.

Rakovski, C., & Price-Glynn, K.. (2010). Nursing assistants, caring labor, and intersectionality. *Sociology of Health & Illness*, *32*(3), 400–414.

Rakovski, C., & Price-Glynn, K. (2012). Intersectional identities and worker experiences in home health care: The national home health aide survey. *Research in the Sociology of Health Care, Issues In Health And Health Care Related To Race/Ethnicity, Immigration, SES and Gender*, *30*, 261–280.

Rivas, L. M. (2003). Invisible labours: Caring for the independent person. In B. Ehrenreich & A. R. Hochschild (Eds.), *Global woman: Nannies, maids and sex workers in the new economy* (pp. 70–84). London: Granta Books.

Sloane, P. D., Williams, C. S., & Zimmerman, S. (2010). Immigrant status and intention to leave of nursing assistants in U.S. nursing homes. *Journal of the American Geriatric Society*, *58*, 731–737.

Solari, C. (2006). Professionals and saints: How immigrant careworkers negotiate gender identities at work. *Gender & Society*, *20*(3), 301–331.

Sophie, J., Belza, B., & Young, H. (2003). Health and safety risk at a skilled nursing facility: Nursing assistants' perceptions. *Journal of Gerontological Nursing*, *29*(2), 13–21.

Squillace, M. R., Remsbur, R. E., Harris-Kojetin, L. D., Bercovitz, A., Rosenoff, E., & Han, B. (2009). The national nursing assistant survey: Improving the evidence base for policy initiatives to strengthen the certified nursing assistant workforce. *The Gerontologist*, *49*(2), 185–197.

Stacey, C. L. (2005). Finding dignity in dirty work: The constraints and rewards of low-wage home care labor. *Sociology of Health & Illness*, *27*, 831–854.

Wingfield, A. H. (2009). Racializing the glass escalator: Reconsidering men's experiences with women's work. *Gender & Society*, *23*, 5–26.

THE HEALTH OF MIGRANT WOMEN WORKING AS HOME CARE ASSISTANTS IN ITALY: AN ANALYSIS OF THE MOST HAZARDOUS FACTORS OF HOME CARE WORK

Francesca Alice Vianello

ABSTRACT

Purpose – *The aim of this chapter was to analyze of the most hazardous aspects of home care work in Italy.*

Methodology/Approach – *The chapter is based on a multi-method analysis conducted in Italy, including a survey on a sample of 867 home care assistants, and four focus groups organized with home care assistants.*

Findings – *The data collected show that: (1) there is a strong correlation between the physical and emotional complexity of the work and the workers' malaise; (2) the live-in formula is not clearly linked with high levels of psychophysical malaise, while isolation is associated much more strongly with a high index of malaise; and (3) violence in the workplace is clearly one of the main risks to which home care assistants are exposed.*

Research Limitations/Implications – *The findings may suffer from limitations due to the type of data collected. First, it was a convenience survey, so the results are not generalizable and they may be negatively influenced by bias relating to sample self-selection. Second, the empirical research was not*

Underserved and Socially Disadvantaged Groups and Linkages with Health and Health Care Differentials
Research in the Sociology of Health Care, Volume 37, 239–258

ISSN: 0275-4959/doi:10.1108/S0275-495920190000037019

designed to investigate occupational health alone, so accurate information on symptoms, causes of ill-health, experiences of violence, and the meaning of respondents' malaise and of the episodes of violence were not available. Third, with the help of an epidemiologist, we could have included some diagnostic tests to better ascertain the workers' state of health.

Originality/Value of Paper – *The chapter offers an original contribution to sociological research on the occupational health hazards from a gender-specific perspective. First, it investigates workers' health risks in an understudied and highly feminized and racialized occupational sector. It also analyzes the implications of both the emotional and the body work on the workers' health. It deals with the correlation between cohabitation and health problems. Finally, it looks into the impact of workplace violence on workers' health, which is a strongly gendered issue, and rooted in social processes that stigmatize and racialize migrant women employed as home care assistants.*

Keywords: Occupational health; home care work; migrant women; Italy; body work; emotional work; isolation; violence

INTRODUCTION

In the last 30 years, Europe has seen a process of care commodification, in northern and southern regions alike, that has resulted in increasing numbers of people being employed in the care services sector (Williams, 2012). In Southern Europe in particular, which is characterized by a weak and familistic welfare state, the diffusion of domestic and care services can be interpreted as the way in which families respond to a complex scenario comprising an aging population, more women in employment outside the home, new gender and family models, and a longer working life, alongside the persistence of a family-based long-term care model (Bettio, Simonazzi, & Villa, 2006).

The well-being of a significant proportion of Southern Europe's elderly and people who are not self-sufficient relies on home care assistants, who are usually migrant women. An abundance of literature has been published on such migrant home care workers (Ambrosini, 2013; Lutz, 2008; Triandafyllidou & Marchetti, 2015), but few studies have focused on the consequences of this type of employment on the workers' health (Ahonen et al., 2010; Christensen & Manthorpe, 2016; Sarli, 2014; Taylor & Donnelly, 2006).

There is an urgent need to investigate the occupational health of home care assistants because they are a particularly vulnerable category of workers, often discriminated against and exploited. They consequently risk developing health issues related both to their occupation and to their experience of migration (European Institute for Gender Equality, 2016; Rakovski & Price-Glynn, 2012; Rechel et al., 2011; Schenker, 2008, 2010). Scientific research has abundantly demonstrated that protecting care assistants' well-being is a prerequisite to ensuring that people who are frail, elderly and not self-sufficient receive good-quality care (Aiken, Clarke, & Sloane, 2002; George, Hale, & Angelo, 2017; Poghosyan, Clarke, Finlayson, & Aiken, 2010; Walsh & Shutes, 2013).

This chapter helps to fill this gap by examining the health issues of home care assistants, also taking into consideration that this is one of the most gendered, feminized and ethnicity-associated occupations. The aim of the study described here was to conduct an exploratory analysis on the most hazardous factors of home care work in Italy. It revealed the main causes of ill-health in this category of workers by means of a multi-method analysis carried out in Italy. The innovative sociological contribution of the analysis lies primarily in that it investigated how both the emotional and the body work involved affected the home care assistants' health, as suggested by Wolkowitz (2002). The analysis also looked into the experience of violence in the workplace – a phenomenon little studied in the setting of in-home care work.

HOME CARE ASSISTANTS IN ITALY: THE JOB CONTOURS

Before discussing the characteristics of paid home care work in Italy, we need to briefly mention the main features of domestic and care-providing work in general. Domestic and care-providing jobs entail a set of material and emotional tasks regarding the provision of care for life in the private space of the home (Federici, 2012). It is a very demanding and intensive job, both physically and emotionally, but it is often unpaid or underpaid, underestimated, and socially undervalued because it is considered the "natural" work of women (England, 2005). People employed to do domestic work and provide care are usually women belonging to the lower social classes and the more marginalized social groups, such as migrants or racialized people (Anderson, 2000; Duffy, 2007; Lutz, 2008). The social construction of domestic and care-providing work is the result of the sexual division of labor, a historical process rooted in a patriarchal and capitalistic society that associates women with reproduction, confining them to a subaltern position in relation to men and the male sphere of production (Mies, 1986).

In Italy, home care assistants take care of people who depend on others, the elderly and the disabled, in the latter's own homes. Care assistants usually have no specific qualifications or training. They are generally employed directly by the family under a national collective agreement for care assistants and domestic workers. According to official data, there were 375,560 people employed as home care assistants in Italy in 2015 (INPS, 2015), the majority of them migrant women (Andall, 2000; Marchetti, 2014; Vianello, 2009). However, this type of work is often undertaken informally, without any proper labor contract (or it may be registered as hourly domestic work), so the real number is certainly higher. There are two types of home care assistant: those who live in with the person in their care and those who only provide day care. They are occupied mainly in providing personal care, but they also keep house, doing the cleaning, cooking, shopping, etc. (Alemani et al., 2016; Catanzaro, & Colombo, 2009; Sarti, 2010).

This section focuses on clarifying the specific nature of such home care work. It combines many of the features of domestic work (which involves housekeeping chores, such as cleaning, cooking, washing and ironing, but not providing personal care) with those of healthcare work. The main characteristics considered here concern the "body work" involved, the relational/emotional dimension, and the spatial setting.

Rather like nursing, home care work involves both body work and face-to-face emotional labor (Dyer, McDowell, & Batnitzky, 2008; James, 1992). According to Kang's conceptualization of body work, the home care assistant's job also entails the "provision of body-related services and the management of feelings that accompany it" (Kang, 2003, p. 820). Home care work is associated with a human body that is usually old and frail (Wolkowitz, 2002). It is this body that is the object of the assistant's activities (Gimlin, 2007), which involve being in intimate contact with the person in their care (for feeding, bathing, medicating wounds, dressing, brushing hair, shaving, lifting, and so on). As these actions are physical, their bodies are the primary tools of their work.

Although it is not written in the labor contract, home care workers also have an emotional job to do, however. They have to display specific sets of emotions (both verbally and nonverbally) designed to induce particular feelings and responses from their clients (Hochschild, 1983). A good home care worker is not detached and professional, but caring like a relative ("like a daughter" is how their behavior is usually described), devoted and patient. It is very difficult for home care assistants to manage the delicate balance between emotional distance and empathy (Anderson, 2000).

As for the spatial conditions, home care assistants do their job in their client's home. This is particularly meaningful for live-in care workers because they live in their place of work, which is their client's own private space. Research on the complex relationship between private and public spaces in the case of live-in workers has taken into consideration both domestic and care workers, since the two categories share the same condition of seclusion. The overlap between the employee's working and reproductive space and the employer's domestic space fosters an extension of the former's working day, and a consequent erosion of the time when they should be resting. In fact, it is common for domestic and home care workers to work during their time off or days off (Yeoh & Huang, 1998).

It is important to consider some other differences between domestic and home care workers, too. The first concerns their level of autonomy. Home care workers usually have a greater degree of independence in the way their work is organized because they live alone with their clients, whereas live-in domestic workers are routinely under their employers' control. Going along with Goffman's dramaturgical analysis, domestic workers are continuously on stage (Goffman, 1959). The second distinction regards the dimensions of the home. In Italy, home care assistants often work for middle-, lower middle-, or even working-class families who live in small- to medium-sized apartments, in which case worker and client occupy the same spaces and both have little privacy. Live-in domestic workers, however, are usually employed by upper- or middle-class families living in large houses, where there is a clear spatial separation between the spaces occupied by the domestic worker and their employers, and both enjoy a good deal of privacy (Lan, 2003). A third difference concerns the definition of internal boundaries. When the home becomes a workplace, employers try to establish multi-layered borders to defend their privacy. Recalling the concept of "spatial deference" (Rollins, 1985), Parreñas (2001) argues that these borders are defined by differentiating between employers' and employees' food and dishes, as well as by banning employees from certain areas (such as the living room) at certain times of day. This may be true of domestic workers, but the majority of home care assistants share the same spaces, food, and life rhythms with their employers. That is why the line between the private and public spheres is less distinct for home care workers than for domestic workers.

In conclusion, the job of home care assistant in Italy is very poorly paid, physically and emotionally very demanding, and done by people who have not been trained to do this kind of work. The live-in formula makes it even more demanding because the home care assistants work long hours without any real breaks or rest periods. In addition, because these workers are usually migrant women who live isolated from the community and are unfamiliar with the health services of their adopted country, we can expect the risk of developing health problems to be particularly high among home care assistants.

HOME CARE WORKERS' HEALTH RISKS: LITERATURE REVIEW AND HYPOTHESIS

The available literature on the risks to home care workers includes studies conducted mainly in European countries, with the exception of the report from Ayalon (2012) on Filipino home care workers in Israel, where the private care market has expanded considerably in recent years (Ahonen et al., 2010; Christensen & Manthorpe, 2016; Sarli, 2014; Taylor & Donnelly, 2006). In Europe, the increasing demand for home care has been met by female migrant workers, so most of the published studies have focused on the risks run by migrant workers. They highlight that these workers' status as migrants adds to the risks they run because it makes them more vulnerable, more isolated, easier to blackmail, and more willing to accept intensive working rhythms in order to earn more money to send home.

Christensen and Manthorpe (2009), Sarli (2014) and Ahonen et al. (2010) converge in identifying the main hazards for migrant home care workers as follows: an informal employment relationship; a vague description of their tasks, role, rules, working hours, and workload; cohabitation and isolation; intimacy and deep emotional involvement. Such working conditions engender a malaise that particularly affects the worker's psychological well-being. These studies stress that the various psychological disorders reported by live-in caregivers, such as insomnia and anxiety, are caused by the lack of control over their working time, while depression can develop as a result of their severe isolation and prolonged contact with human pain.

Ahonen et al. (2010), and Taylor and Donnelly (2006) also report physical hazards relating to the conditions of their physical and social environment, such as issues with access to the house where they work, hygiene and infections, aggression and harassment, domestic and farm animals, the safety of equipment used in the home, and exposure to chemicals.

The above-mentioned studies have their shortcomings. First of all, apart from the one by Ayalon (2012), they do not provide an in-depth analysis of the correlation between specific working conditions and workers' health. They also fail to consider the experience of violence in the workplace, and gender-related violence in particular, as one of the most common risks run by home care workers. Some of the studies mention it (Ayalon, 2012; Taylor & Donnelly, 2006), but no research has been done to correlate such violence and the workers' health problems.

In the light of these studies, the present work starts from the premise that both physical and mental disorders should be considered because home care work involves the body as well as the emotions, and because hard physical work affects both body and mind, and vice versa. I hypothesize that a home care assistant's health is at greater risk the more complex the mental and/or physical health issues of the person in their care.

I also hypothesize that the live-in formula is one of the main reasons for the home care assistants' work-related malaise. This assumption is supported by several studies on living in the workplace, such as in factory dormitories, on cruise ships, or in the case of professionals with offices at home. These studies have underscored the implications for workers of the overlap between their working and private lives (Moore, 2006; Smith, 2003; Trees Bolt & Lashley, 2015). The most important (partly physical, but largely psychological) causes of worker malaise are: longer working days, isolation, loneliness due to separation from family, and overlapping social roles.

Finally, in light of studies conducted on domestic workers and nurses on the close correlation between the experience of violence in the workplace and health problems (mainly in the psychological sphere), I hypothesize that violent behavior towards home care workers can cause them severe malaise. The domestic environment and the relational dimension of home care work exposes workers to specific risks of violence. The few studies on this topic focus mainly on live-in domestic workers, and show that living in their employers' homes increases their risk of being harassed due to their economic reliance on the host family, their greater interaction and proximity with family members, and their isolation from other people (DeSouza & Cerqueira, 2009, p. 1266). Because of their social class and racial otherness, domestic workers occupy a low position in the hierarchy of the household, subordinated not only to the male members of the family but also to the women and children, who may exercise different kinds of violence (Huang & Yeoh, 2007; Scrinzi, 2013).

According to Ayalon (2012) and DeSouza and Cerqueira (2009), home care workers' problems with depression are strongly connected to abuse they experience in their working environment, in the form of physical aggression from people with dementia, or unwanted sexual advances. Other studies on workplace violence against nurses have likewise shown the correlation between the experience of violence (harassment, bullying, physical and verbal aggression) and the levels of these workers' psychological distress (Demir & Rodwell, 2012; Magnavita & Heponiemi, 2011; Miranda, Punnett, Gore, & ProCare Research Team, 2014; Zampieron, Galeazzo, Turra, & Buja, 2009).

In short, I analyze the implications for the workers' health of the following aspects of home care work, which the available literature identifies as the most perilous: the compound effects of emotional work and body work; cohabitation; and violence in the workplace.

RESEARCH DESIGN AND METHODS

Data Collection

This chapter draws on broad research conducted on home care workers in Italy. The general goal of the study was to analyze the most important changes in the home care sector in times of economic recession. The research was designed and supervised by a scientific committee comprising scholars and experts in this field (the author, Claudia Alemani, Raffaella Maioni, Sabrina Marchetti, Raffaella Sarti, Clorinda Turri, and Olga Turrini), and it was conducted by Gianfranco Zucca (researcher at the Institute for Education and Training Research – IREF).

A mixed method was used, combining focus groups with a survey. The research was completed between April and July 2013, and involved workers employed as home care assistants. The first stage involved nine focus groups with home care workers. In the second stage, self-completion questionnaire were completed in person by 867 home care assistants.

Focus Groups

The aim of the focus groups was to collect home care workers' opinions on various topics in order to construct a questionnaire covering the most significant characteristics and problems of their job. Using the mixed-method approach, the workers' narrations were also very useful for interpreting the results of the questionnaires. The quantitative results were therefore supported by the analysis of the focus groups expressing how workers perceived and explained the relationship between certain working conditions and their health.

Participants in the focus groups were recruited through local representatives of the ACLI Colf home care and domestic workers' association (the promoter of the study), who assured the socio-demographic heterogeneity of participants. The focus groups were held in various Italian cities situated in different regions to obtain a representative picture of the situation nationwide. Every meeting involved around eight people, for a total of 74 workers. The discussions lasted from about 100 to 120 minutes. The meetings were conducted in Italian and the moderator was the above-mentioned researcher. This choice of language may have hindered the participants' free expression, since most of them were not native Italian speakers, but it was judged necessary because of the participants' multiple nationalities. The focus groups consisted almost entirely of women (73

Table 1. Topics Covered by Focus Groups.

Agrigento	• work contract and immigration documents • professional figures
Cosenza	• sexual harassment in the workplace • labor brokers/brokering • importance of correct information on working conditions
Foggia	• implications of clients' poverty • request for medical assistance
Milan	• relational distance • precarity
Naples	• job loss • labor market changes during the economic recession
Rome	• working conditions, tasks and salaries • recognition of skills • class inequalities between employers and employees
Treviso	• worker-client relationships • problems with work-life balance
Trieste	• physical burden of care work • length of working day
Turin	• extension and diversification of care needs • relationship with clients' families

out of 74 participants) – a gender composition reflecting that of the employment sector considered. Participants were also almost always foreigners (in 87.8% of cases), coming from 14 different countries. The most represented countries of origin, in descending order, were: Romania, Peru, Morocco, Philippines, Moldova, Tunisia, and Ukraine.

Every focus group started from similar inputs, but the discussion developed in different directions. The most significant topics that emerged are listed in Table 1. In this chapter, I consider only the focus groups most relevant to the issue of interest here, that is, those held in Cosenza, Milan, Treviso, and Trieste.

The Survey

The questionnaire was designed on the basis of an analysis of the focus groups' output. The survey contained questions about workers' personal details, working conditions (wages, working hours, employment contract, and workload), their relationship with clients and their families, their education and training, their attitudes to care work, their health and their experience of violence. The questionnaire was written in Italian and, here again, this may have hindered its thorough comprehension by non-Italian workers and affected their ability to answer the questions. To minimize this risk, we paid particular attention to the wording, using simple sentences and everyday language. In addition, although the questionnaires were self-administered, they were distributed by a trained representative of the ACLI Colf association, who offered to assist respondents if necessary.

Although the survey was based on a convenience sampling, as it was impossible to obtain a representative random sample of home care workers, every effort was made to secure a maximally diverse sample. A total of 867 questionnaires were collected in 30 Italian provinces distributed all over the country, through the local ACLI Colf offices. This does not mean that only members of this association were involved: 46.5% of respondents were not members of ACLI Colf (because the organization provides information services for other people too).

As shown in Table 2, the majority (94.2%) of the sample surveyed were adult women, and 36.9% were 45–54 years old. Most respondents were married, but

Table 2. Socio-demographic Characteristics of the Sample (Frequencies: Absolute Number and Percentage).

	N	%
Sex		
Male	50	5.8
Female	809	94.2
Total	859 (missing cases, 8)	100
Age (in years)		
18–34	98	11.5
35–44	220	25.9
45–54	314	36.9
55 <	219	25.7
Total	851 (missing cases, 16)	100
Marital status		
Single	172	20.1
Married	298	34.8
Separated	100	11.7
Divorced	197	23
Widowed	90	10.5
Total	857 (missing cases, 10)	100
Macro-areas of origin		
Eastern Europe	551	66.1
Latin America	117	14
Africa	75	9
Asia	50	6
Italy	41	4.9
Total	834 (missing cases, 33)	100
Average years of formal education	11.45	
Type of job		
Live-in home care worker	519	59.9
Live-out home care worker	332	38.3
Total	851 (missing cases, 16)	100

many were separated or divorced. Almost all of the respondents were migrants, coming mainly from Eastern Europe (66.1%), especially Romania, Moldova and Ukraine; Italians accounted for only 4.9% of the sample. Finally, 59.9% of the respondents were employed as live-in care workers.

These data do not perfectly reflect the national figures for home care workers, because: (1) Italians are a minority in the sector, but account for 17.2% of the total, and (2) around 12% of the total are men.

In analyzing the questionnaire for the present study, I focus only on certain questions specifically relating to the workers' health. Table 3 shows the frequencies of the answers to the question "Since you started working as a home care assistant, have you begun to suffer from [...]." Numerous workers associated their job with the onset of one or more disorders: more than one in two suffered from backache since they started working as home care assistants; around one in three experienced insomnia; and more than one in four suffered from anxiety and/or depression. It is important to note that these conditions were self-diagnosed. The focus groups had been helpful in illustrating the significance home care workers of migrant origin attributed to their health problems.

Table 3. Disorders Perceived by Respondents (Frequencies: Absolute Number and Percentage).

Since you Started Working as a Home Care Assistant, have you begun to Suffer from:		
Backache		
No	381	47.1
Yes	428	52.9
Total	809 (missing cases, 58)	100
Other physical pains		
No	521	67.3
Yes	253	32.7
Total	774 (missing cases, 93)	100
Insomnia		
No	539	68.4
Yes	249	31.6
Total	788 (missing cases, 79)	100
Anxiety and/or depression		
No	565	72.5
Yes	214	27.5
Total	779 (missing cases, 88)	100
Other disorders		
No	517	74.4
Yes	178	25.6
Total	695 (missing cases, 172)	100

Table 4. Psychophysical Malaise Index (Frequencies: Absolute Number and Percentage).

Psychophysical Malaise	*N*	%
Absent	242	27.9
Low	248	28.6
Intermediate	186	21.5
High	191	22.0
Total	867	100.0

Note: Missing, 0.

The results presented here are based on a bivariate analysis of the correlation between the psychophysical malaise index (dependent variable) and several variables concerning the conditions I consider more hazardous. The malaise index (Table 4) was developed by counting the affirmative answers to the above-mentioned question, where: "absent" means that respondents reported no health issues; "low" means they reportedly had one or two problems; "intermediate" means they two or three; and "high" means four or five. From a first analysis of the frequencies, the majority of respondents had no or only low levels of malaise, but the proportion of workers with intermediate or high malaise indexes was far from negligible.

RESULTS

The Compound Effects of Emotional Work and Body Work

Analyzing the focus groups' output suggests that the emotional burden on care workers and its implications for their health override the physical strain of the body work involved, although workers recognize and name body work issues too. Backache was the type of malaise most often reported (see Table 3), but participants in the focus groups mainly insisted on the hazards of the relational and emotional aspects of their job, while they saw the physical strain as easier to cope with, and less important. They dwelt a great deal on explaining the emotional dedication required in their work, stressing the complexity of their relationship with the family as a whole, and with their clients especially, who demand constant attention. In Milan, all the focus group participants agreed on two aspects: (1) that their job has to be done with a heartfelt commitment; and yet (2) it is important for them to keep the right distance between themselves and their clients, otherwise they risk burnout (Maslach, 2003).

> You have to define a boundary. I put all my heart and soul into the previous family, and became very fond of the lady. Her sons left her to me. But in the end I suffered a lot. So I realized it's important to set a limit. I'm here, you're there. Without love, it's impossible to do the job. But it has to be a rational love. (Milan focus group)

> You have to be more than just a worker who works physically; you have to be a psychologist too. You have to understand your role in the household. If you work as a home care assistant,

you have to understand that you are dealing with a person who is ill, and first of all you have to comfort this person. It isn't a simple job. If you keep too much distance, you're just an assistant who helps physically, who offers no affection. On the other hand, if you are too involved, you make yourself ill, because it isn't easy to spend 24 hours a day near people who are ill. You have to find a balance: being a worker, being part of the family, but still being yourself. (Milan focus group)

The work is physically demanding, and complex from a technical and relational standpoint, because of the clients' health issues; and the more complex their condition, the greater the risk of the care workers developing psychophysical disorders. Assisting people with limited mobility, dementia, or severe disease has pronounced implications for the workers' health: they experience the physical strain of moving and handling their clients and the mental strain of having to manage many tasks and cope with great responsibilities. One of the focus group participants, for instance, underscored the physical implications of not having a hoist, while another spoke of the strain of working with someone very ill and completely reliant on the assistant.

If there's no hoist we break our backs, because we have to move our clients without any help. Even if they are thin, it's still hard. Usually, there's no hoist in people's homes, they're not equipped for people who're not self-sufficient. The home care worker breaks her back, her hands. (Trieste focus group)

I assisted a couple of elderly people who took lots of medicines. He, in particular, was very ill. Nurses came every day. I was very scared of making a mistake. I was afraid I might hurt him. I felt responsible for them. It was a very hard job, both physically and psychologically. [...] In the end, I had to leave them, because I couldn't take it anymore, I felt bad. (Treviso focus group)

Based on findings of the focus groups, I have tried to identify the implications of both emotional and body work for home care assistants' well-being by means of questions on clients with motor disabilities (Table 5), and a question on the amount of cooperation received from clients (which alludes to people with

Table 5. Psychophysical Malaise Index for Physical Strain (Absolute Number and Percentage).

Psychophysical Malaise Index	Your Client [...]						Total	
	Is Self-sufficient		Has Some Mobility Problems		Is Unable to Move Unassisted			
	N	%	*N*	%	*N*	%	*N*	%
Absent	74	34.7	94	24.5	64	25.6	232	27.4
Low	65	30.5	111	29.0	65	26.0	241	28.5
Intermediate	39	18.3	97	25.3	46	18.4	182	21.5
High	35	16.4	81	21.1	75	30.0	191	22.6
Total	213	100	383	100	250	100	846	100

Note: Missing, 21.

Table 6. Psychophysical Malaise Index for Relational Strain (Absolute Number and Percentage).

Psychophysical Malaise Index	Convincing Your Client to do Something (e.g., to Eat, Wash, or Wake Up)						Total	
	Takes Little Time		Takes a Long Time		The Client Decides What to Do			
	N	%	*N*	%	*N*	%	*N*	%
Absent	81	28.8	61	21.3	84	30.8	226	26.9
Low	87	31.0	66	23.0	88	32.2	241	28.7
Intermediate	53	18.9	79	27.5	52	19.0	184	21.9
High	60	21.4	81	28.2	49	17.9	190	22.6
Total	281	100.0	287	100.0	273	100.0	841	100.0

Note: Missing, 26.

mental disabilities) (Table 6). Workers who take care of self-sufficient people have fewer health problems, while those assisting people who are partially or totally dependent on others have far more health issues (Table 5). That said, when home care assistants working with people who were not self-sufficient reported having a hoist available, they also had lower scores on the malaise index. This means that the availability of appropriate equipment at home is crucial to reducing the strain of the body work.

Similarly, the home care assistants who spent a lot of time, energy and relational skills on convincing their clients to do something (such as eating, washing, waking up) had significantly more health issues than those working for cooperative or self-sufficient clients. The former had a high malaise index in 28.2% of cases, while for the latter this was true of 21.4% (with cooperative clients) and 17.9% (with self-sufficient clients) (Table 6).

Cohabitation in the Domestic Space

The focus group participants emphasized the difficulty of the live-in formula, for both body and mind, which they attributed to loneliness, isolation in the domestic space, the extended hours of the working day, and consequently limited free time. The quantitative questionnaire (Table 7) generated less clear results concerning the correlation between the live-in formula and care workers' health, however. The proportion of respondents with a high malaise index was not particularly large among the live-in workers, though a larger proportion of live-out workers reported experiencing little or no malaise, probably because it gives them more control over their working day and the opportunity to have a social life.

The live-in formula does not appear to affect workers' health per se, but if we look at the answers to the question "What is the most difficult aspect of your job?" (Table 8), we can see that some of the problems mentioned above as being typical of the live-in regime correlate strongly with a high malaise index.

Table 7. Psychophysical Malaise Index for Live-in Formula (Absolute Number and Percentage).

Psychophysical Malaise Index	Do You Live in with Your Client?				Total	
	Yes		No			
	N	%	*N*	%	*N*	%
Absent	123	23.7	113	34.0	236	27.7
Low	152	29.3	93	28.0	245	28.8
Intermediate	116	22.4	66	19.9	182	21.4
High	128	24.7	60	18.1	188	22.1
Total	519	100.0	332	100.0	851	100.0

Note: Missing, 16.

Table 8. Psychophysical Malaise Index for the Main Difficulties of Home Care Work (Absolute Number and Percentage).

Psychophysical Malaise Index	What Is the Most Difficult Aspect of Your Job?								Total	
	Spending a Lot of Time Alone with People Who Are Ill		Living in a Foreign Country and Learning the Language		Being Separated from My Family		Managing the Relationship with My Client's Family			
	N	%	*N*	%	*N*	%	*N*	%	*N*	%
Absent	54	20.7	39	39.0	99	27.9	27	25.7	219	26.7
Low	71	27.2	28	28.0	106	29.9	23	21.9	228	27.8
Intermediate	59	22.6	21	21.0	79	22.3	25	23.8	184	22.4
High	77	29.5	12	12.0	71	20.0	30	28.6	190	23.1
Total	261	100.0	100	100.0	355	100.0	105	100.0	821	100.0

Note: Missing, 46.

Examples are: "staying a lot of time alone with ill people" and "managing the relationship with my client's family." So there are some aspects that make the live-in regime more difficult, and potentially more harmful for workers' health, including isolation and the unavoidably long periods of time spent with employers.

In the light of these data, the focus group discussions take on a clearer meaning. Participants emphasized the importance for their well-being of sleeping away from their employer's home, partly because this was the only way to interrupt their working day but also because they needed to develop their own social relations outside the workplace.

> You're alone, you can't go out, you're not free. It's essential to sleep somewhere else two or three times a week. I wish I could go to sleep at my sister's house. The time issue for us workers is important. The years we work as home care assistants are lost, because we live far away from our families, stuck in a house. Having at least some free time is important. (Treviso focus group)

Although the quality of life improves for many home care assistants when they switch from living in to living out, they say they never switch off completely, their work follows them home. For instance, some workers said that, even when on holiday in their country of origin, they would wake up in the night imagining that somebody is calling them. Even so, preventing their isolation, providing them with a private space and enabling them to develop social relations seem to be the best ways to protect home care workers' health.

Violence in the Workplace

Finally, I consider violence in the workplace as a factor closely connected with both the care assistant's body and emotional work, as well as with their domesticity and isolation. In this section, I concentrate on how the implications of experiences of violence of various kinds correlate with home care assistants' health.

The issue of gender violence emerged especially in the Cosenza focus group, taking the specific form of sexual harassment. Participants reported that it was quite common to be exposed to their employers' advances and sexual proposals. Sometimes sexual services are even considered part of the job, and if they refuse to comply they are dismissed, often without payment, or simply not employed in the first place. That is why, according to one home care worker, employers prefer young and unmarried home care assistants.

> They want beautiful young girls, because you don't only do the duties of the home care assistant, you must have sex with them too. They ask you to have sex and, if you don't want to sleep with the old guy, or with his son, they fire you without paying you for the work you've done. When they call you to fix a job interview, they ask you: Are you tall? Are you beautiful? Are you married? If you're married they don't want you. (Cosenza focus group)

The topic of violence emerged in other focus groups too, but it was more a case of verbal abuse and physical aggression inflicted by clients with Alzheimer's disease. Participants described with such clients as particularly dangerous.

> I can't tell you what kind of woman I worked with. She wouldn't let me touch her. She hit me. She scratched me. She suffered from Alzheimer's disease. She refused everything. I didn't know what to do or how to deal with her. I was always anxious. (Treviso focus group)

Such experiences of violence leave a deep mark on workers. Sexual harassment in the workplace was reflected in rather high psychophysical malaise indexes: 38% of those reporting such experiences had a high malaise index, and another 26.4% had intermediate scores, while the malaise index was much lower for the home care assistants who had never been victims of sexual harassment (Table 9).

Table 9. Psychophysical Malaise Index for Sexual Harassment in the Workplace (Absolute Number and Percentage).

Psychophysical Malaise Index	Sexual Harassment in the Workplace				Total	
	No		Yes			
	N	%	*N*	%	*N*	%
Absent	213	29.1	19	15.7	232	27.2
Low	221	30.3	24	19.8	245	28.8
Intermediate	153	20.9	32	26.4	185	21.7
High	144	19.7	46	38.0	190	22.3
Total	731	100.0	121	100.0	852	100.0

Note: Missing, 15.

Table 10. Psychophysical Malaise Index for Physical Aggressions (Absolute Number and Percentage).

Psychophysical Malaise Index	Does the Person You Work with Throw Things at You?						Total	
	Yes, Often		Yes, Sometimes		Never			
	N	%	*N*	%	*N*	%	*N*	%
Absent	4	10.3	25	23.6	192	30.4	221	28.4
Low	7	17.9	24	22.6	178	28.2	209	26.9
Intermediate	8	20.5	31	29.2	133	21	172	22.1
High	20	51.3	26	24.5	129	20.4	175	22.5
Total	39	100	106	100	632	100	777	100

Note: Missing, 90.

The violence experienced by home care assistants is not always clearly gender-related, as in the case of sexual harassment. These workers also face other kinds of violent behavior on the part of their clients. This is sometimes involuntary (due to mental disease), as mentioned earlier, but in some cases it can stem from a complex combination of gendered, racialized, and sometimes class-hierarchical relations between employer and employee. These data analysis shows a strong correlation between experiences of violence in the workplace and workers' health. Looking after someone who is violent carries high levels of psychophysical malaise, particularly for workers assisting people who throw things at them (51.3% of whom had a high malaise index) (Table 10).

CONCLUSIONS

This chapter explored the relationship between home care work and psychophysical malaise, adding an original contribution to the literature on domiciliary care services for the elderly or disabled in an effort to improve these workers' well-being and, as a consequence, that of the people in their care as well.

While analyses on home care work usually stress its immaterial and emotional dimension, here I have highlighted the bodily implications of this work. Looking at the body from a holistic perspective enabled me to go beyond the traditional binary view of body and mind, and to focus on how any job and its effects on body and mind are always inseparable. We adopted an index of malaise that does not distinguish between the different (physical and psychological) kinds of discomfort to which home care workers are exposed, and I have linked their malaise with the most significant risks characterizing their job.

The findings may suffer from limitations concerning the data collected. For a start, a convenience survey (not a representative survey) was used, so the results are not generalizable, and they may have been negatively influenced by bias relating to sample self-selection. Second, this empirical research was not designed to investigate occupational health, so no detailed and accurate information was collected on any symptoms, causes of disease, experiences of violence, or the significance of any malaise or violent episodes. Third, with the help of an epidemiologist, we could have included some diagnostic tests to objectively assess the workers' health.

The chapter nonetheless offers some new insight for sociological studies on occupational health hazards from a gender-specific perspective. It investigates workers' health risks in an understudied and highly feminized and ethnicized occupational sector. The analysis also includes the implications of both emotional strain and body work on workers' health, and deals with the correlation between cohabitation and health problems. Finally, it examines the impact on workers' health of violence in the workplace, another strongly gendered issue that is rooted in social processes of stigmatization and racialization of migrant women employed as home care workers.

The data show a strong correlation between the physical and emotional complexity of the work relating to the clients' poor health and the workers' malaise. Home care assistants are aware of the hazards of their job, and particularly stress the importance of keeping the right distance from clients and their families to avoid becoming emotionally exhausted. The burden of their responsibilities, and the multiplicity and complexity of their tasks nonetheless engender physical problems too, which in turn add to their stress levels.

An interesting, but unexpected finding in this study is the lack of a clear link between the live-in formula and higher levels of psychophysical malaise, although the workers living out seemed to be in generally better health. What emerged as being much more strongly associated with a high malaise index is the social isolation experienced by home care workers. Their prolonged and complex relationships with their employers alone is one of the problems workers mentioned among the negative aspects of the live-in formula. I therefore argue that isolation, rather than the overlap between working and living spaces, is one of the most significant causes of home assistants' malaise. More research is needed, however, to clarify this ambiguous result.

Finally, violence in the workplace is clearly one of the most relevant perils for home care workers. Those who experience violence (in its various forms) at work suffer from higher levels of psychophysical strain. Analyzing the focus groups' output suggests, however, that violence is not a topic home care workers are accustomed to discussing. Further research is needed to clarify the different meanings of the various forms of violence, and its phenomenology in relation to the interwoven power axes of gender, race and class (Toffanin, 2015).

In conclusion, the present findings should be helpful to policy-makers interested in reducing the occupational health risks for home care workers, and consequently for the many migrant women in this line of work. First, these workers should be trained to work as home care assistants: it is a very demanding job in many ways and should not be considered merely as something that any woman can naturally do. But qualifying care workers is only a first step, and not enough to reduce the related health risks. Clients' homes should be equipped to cope with the client's medical and mobility needs, and workers should be able to access professional psychological support.

Then we can combat the social isolation of live-in home care assistants by encouraging families to employ two home care assistants, so that they can work shifts and have a private life. Horizontal shifts might enable these workers to have their own home and develop social relations in their adopted country, while vertical shifts would enable them to return home for longer periods and spend time with their relatives.

Lastly, specific policies for the prevention of violence should be adopted to reduce the risk to home care workers. Counseling centers could be set up in the places where migrant women meet, and efforts should be made to improve the awareness of workers, employers and trade unions concerning violence against women. All these measures demand more public and private investment in care activities, so to protect and improve home care workers' health we need a radical cultural shift in the social meaning attributed to home care, not as an unacknowledged and underestimated form of menial labor, but as an activity crucial to the well-being of our whole society.

DISCLOSURE STATEMENT

The author has no potential conflict of interest to disclose.

ACKNOWLEDGMENTS

I am most grateful to the study participants. Thanks also go to ACLI Colf for involving me in the research project and allowing me to use their data. I am also grateful to Gianfranco Zucca and Francesca Scrinzi for their thoughtful comments on earlier drafts of this chapter.

REFERENCES

Ahonen, E. M., Lopez-Jacob, M. J., Vazquez, M. L., Porthe, V., Gil-Gonzalez, D.,Garcia, A. M., … Benavides, F. (2010). Invisible work, unseen hazards: the health of women immigrant household service workers in Spain. *American Journal of Industrial Medicine*, *53*, 405–416.

Aiken, L. H., Clarke, S. P., & Sloane, D. M. (2002). Hospital staffing, organization, and quality of care: Cross-national findings. *International Journal of Quality in Health Care*, *14*(1), 5–13.

Alemani, C., Maioni, R., Marchetti, S., Sarti, R., Vianello, F. A., & Zucca, G. (2016). *Viaggio nel lavoro di cura. Chi sono, cosa fanno e come vivono le badanti che lavorano nelle famiglie italiane*, Ediesse, Roma.

Ambrosini, M. (2013). *Irregular migration and invisible welfare*. London: Palgrave.

Andall, J. (2000). *Gender, migration and domestic service: The politics of Black women in Italy*. Aldershot: Ashgate.

Anderson, B. (2000). *Doing the dirty work*. London: Zed Books.

Ayalon, L. (2012). Suicidal and depressive symptoms in Filipino home care workers in Israel. *Journal of Cross-Cultural Gerontology*, *27*, 51–63.

Bettio, F., Simonazzi, A., & Villa, P. (2006). Change in care regimes and female migration: The 'care drain' in the Mediterranean. *Journal of European Social Policy*, *16*(3), 271–285.

Catanzaro, R., & Colombo, A. (Eds.) (2009). *Badanti & Co.: Il lavoro domestico straniero in Italia*. Bologna: Il Mulino.

Christensen, K., & Manthorpe, J. (2016). Personalised risk: New risk encounters facing migrant care workers. *Health, Risk & Society*, *18*(3–4), 137–152.

Demir, D., & Rodwell, J. (2012). Psychosocial antecedents and consequences of workplace aggression for hospital nurses. *Journal of Nursing Scholarship*, *44*(4), 376–384.

DeSouza, E. R., & Cerqueira, E. (2009). From the kitchen to the bedroom. Frequency rates and consequences of sexual harassment among female domestic workers in Brazil. *Journal of Interpersonal Violence*, *24*(8), 1264–1284.

Duffy, M. (2007). Doing the dirty work: Gender, race, and reproductive labour in historical perspective. *Gender and Society*, *21*(3), 313–336.

Dyer, S., McDowell, L., & Batnitzky, A. (2008). Emotional labour/body work: The caring labours of migrants in the UK's National Health Service. *Geoforum*, *39*, 2030–2038.

England, P. (2005). Emerging theories of care work. *Annual Review of Sociology*, *31*, 381–399.

European Institute for Gender Equality. (2016). *Poverty, gender and intersecting inequalities in the EU*. Vilnius: EIGE.

Federici, S. (2012). *Revolution at point zero. Housework, reproduction and feminist struggle*. Oakland, CA: PM Press.

George, E., Hale, L., & Angelo, J. (2017). Valuing the health of the support worker in the aged care sector. *Ageing & Society*, *37*(5), 1006–1024.

Gimlin, D. (2007). What is 'body work'? A review of literature. *Sociology Compass*, *1*(1), 353–370.

Goffman, E. (1959). *The presentation of self in everyday life*. New York, NY: Doubleday Anchor Books.

Hochschild, A. R. (1983). *The managed heart*. Berkeley, CA: University of California Press.

Huang, S., & Yeoh, B. S. A. (2007). Emotional labour and transnational domestic work: The moving geographies of 'maid abuse' in Singapore. *Mobilities*, *2*(2), 195–217.

Inps. (2015, 08, 17). *Osservatorio sui lavoratori domestici*. Retrieved from www.inps.it/webidentity/banchedatistatistiche/menu/domestici/main.html

James, N. (1992). Care = organization + physical labour + emotional labour. *Sociology of Health & Illness*, *14*(4), 488–509.

Kang, M. (2003). The managed hand: The commercialization of bodies and emotions in Korean immigrant-owned nail salons. *Gender and Society*, *17*(6), 820–839.

Lan, P. C. (2003). Negotiating social boundaries and private zones: The micropolitics of employing migrant domestic workers. *Social Problems*, *50*(4), 525–549.

Lutz, H. (Ed.) (2008). *Migration and domestic work. A European perspective on a global theme*. Aldershot: Ashgate.

Magnavita, N., & Heponiemi, T. (2011). Workplace violence against nursing students and nurses: An Italian experience. *Journal of Nursing Scholarship*, *43*(2), 203–210.

Marchetti, S. (2014). *Black girls. Migrant domestic workers and colonial legacies*. Leiden: Brill.

Maslach, C. (2003). *Burnout: The cost of caring*. Los Altos: ISHK.

Mies, M. (1986). *Patriarchy and accumulation on a world scale: Women in the international division of labour*. London: Zed Books.

Miranda, H., Punnett, L., Gore, R. J., & ProCare Research Team. (2014). Musculoskeletal pain and reported workplace assault: A prospective study of clinical staff in nursing homes. *Human Factors*, *56*(1), 215–227.

Moore, J. (2006). Homeworking and work-life balance: Does it add to quality of life? *Revue européenne de psychologie appliquée*, *56*, 5–13.

Parreñas, R. S. (2001). *Servants of globalisation: Women, migration, and domestic work*. Stanford, CA: Stanford University Press.

Poghosyan, L., Clarke, S. P., Finlayson, M., & Aiken, L. H. (2010). Nurse burnout and quality of care: cross-national investigation in six countries. *Research in Nursing & Health*, *33*(4), 288–299.

Rakovski, C., & Price-Glynn, K. (2012). Intersectional identities and worker experiences in home health care: The National Home Health Aide Survey. In J. Jacobs Kronenfeld (Ed.), *Health and health care related to race/etnicity, immigration, SES and gender. Research in the Sociology of Health Care* (Vol. 30, pp. 261–280). Emerald.

Rechel, B., Mladovsky, P., Devillé, W., Rijks, B., Petrova-Benedict, R., & McKee, M. (2011). *Migration and health in the European Union*. London: Open University Press.

Rollins, J. (1985). *Between women: Domestics and their employers*. Philadelphia, PA: Temple University Press.

Sarli, A. (2014). The psycho-social malaise of migrant private carers in Italy: A rampant, but hidden health demand. *Acta Biomed for Health Professions*, *85*(3), 62–73.

Sarti, R. (Ed.) (2010). *Il lavoro domestic e di cura: quali diritti?* Roma: Ediesse.

Schenker, M. (2008). Work-related injuries among immigrants: A growing global health disparity. *Occupational and Environmental Medicine*, *65*(11), 717–718.

Schenker, M. B. (2010). A global perspective of migration and occupational health. *American Journal of Industrial Medicine*, *53*(4), 329–337.

Scrinzi, F. (2013). *Genre, migrations et emplois domestiques en France et en Italie construction de la non-qualification et de l'altérité ethnique*. Paris: Pétra.

Smith, C. (2003). Living at work: Management control and the dormitory labour system in China. *Asia Pacific Journal of Management*, *20*, 333–358.

Taylor, B. J., & Donnelly, R. (2006). Risks to home care workers: Professional perspectives. *Health, Risk & Society*, *8*(3), 239–256.

Toffanin, A. M. (2015). *Controcanto. Donne latinoamericane tra violenza e riconoscimento*. Milano: Guerini.

Trees Bolt, E. E., & Lashley, C. (2015). All at sea: Insights into crew work experiences on a cruise liner. *Research in Hospitality Management*, *5*(2), 199–206.

Triandafyllidou, A., & Marchetti, S. (Eds.) (2015). *Employers, agencies and immigration*. London: Routledge.

Vianello, F. A. (2009). *Migrando sole. Legami transnazionali tra Ucraina e Italia*. Milano: Franco Angeli.

Walsh, K., & Shutes, I. (2013). Care relationships, quality of care and migrant workers caring for older people. *Ageing & Society*, *33*, 393–420.

Williams, F. (2012). Converging variations in migrant care work in Europe. *Journal of European Social Policy*, *22*(4), 363–376.

Wolkowitz, C. (2002). *Bodies at work*. London: Sage.

Yeoh, B., & Huang, S. (1998). Negotiating public space: Strategies and styles of migrant female domestic workers in Singapore. *Urban Studies*, *35*, 583–602.

Zampieron, A., Galeazzo, M., Turra, S., & Buja, A. (2009). Perceived aggression towards nurses: Study in two Italian health institutions. *Journal of Clinical Nursing*, *19*, 2329–2341.

INDEX